Cystic Fibrosis

Editors

SUSAN G. MARSHALL
DRUCY BOROWITZ

PEDIATRIC CLINICS
OF NORTH AMERICA

www.pediatric.theclinics.com

Consulting Editor
BONITA F. STANTON

August 2016 • Volume 63 • Number 4

ELSEVIER

1600 John F. Kennedy Boulevard • Suite 1800 • Philadelphia, Pennsylvania, 19103-2899

http://www.theclinics.com

THE PEDIATRIC CLINICS OF NORTH AMERICA Volume 63, Number 4
August 2016 ISSN 0031-3955, ISBN-13: 978-0-323-45983-9

Editor: Kerry Holland
Developmental Editor: Casey Jackson

The Pediatric Clinics of North America (ISSN 0031-3955) is published bimonthly by Elsevier Inc., 360 Park Avenue South, New York, NY 10010-1710. Months of issue are February, April, June, August, October, and December. Periodicals postage paid at New York, NY and additional mailing offices. Subscription prices are $200.00 per year (US individuals), $556.00 per year (US institutions), $270.00 per year (Canadian individuals), $740.00 per year (Canadian institutions), $325.00 per year (international individuals), $740.00 per year (international institutions), $100.00 per year (US students and residents), and $165.00 per year (international and Canadian residents and students). To receive students/resident rare, orders must be accompanied by name of affiliated institution, date of term, and the signature of program/residency coordinator on institution letterhead. Orders will be billed at individual rate until proof of status is received. Foreign air speed delivery is included in all *Clinics* subscription prices. All prices are subject to change without notice. **POSTMASTER:** Send address changes to *The Pediatric Clinics of North America*, Elsevier Health Sciences Division, Subscription Customer Service, 3251 Riverport Lane, Maryland Heights, MO 63043. **Customer Service: 1-800-654-2452 (US and Canada). From outside of the US and Canada: 1-314-447-8871. Fax: 1-314-447-8029. For print support, E-mail: JournalsCustomerService-usa@elsevier.com. For online support, E-mail: JournalsOnlineSupport-usa@elsevier.com.**

Reprints. For copies of 100 or more, of articles in this publication, please contact the Commercial Reprints Department, Elsevier Inc., 360 Park Avenue South, New York, NY 10010-1710. Tel.: 212-633-3874; Fax: 212-633-3820; E-mail: reprints@elsevier.com.

The Pediatric Clinics of North America is also published in Spanish by McGraw-Hill Inter-americana Editores S.A., Mexico City, Mexico; in Portuguese by Riechmann and Affonso Editores, Rua Comandante Coelho 1085, CEP 21250, Rio de Janeiro, Brazil; and in Greek by Althayia SA, Athens, Greece.

The Pediatric Clinics of North America is covered in *MEDLINE/PubMed (Index Medicus), Excerpta Medica, Current Contents, Current Contents/Clinical Medicine, Science Citation Index, ASCA, ISI/BIOMED,* and *BIOSIS*.

PROGRAM OBJECTIVE

The goal of the *Pediatric Clinics of North America* is to keep practicing physicians and residents up to date with current clinical practice in pediatrics by providing timely articles reviewing the state-of-the-art in patient care.

TARGET AUDIENCE

All practicing pediatricians, physicians and healthcare professionals who provide patient care to pediatric patients.

LEARNING OBJECTIVES

Upon completion of this activity, participants will be able to:
1. Review the screening and diagnosis of cystic fibrosis.
2. Discuss nutrition, growth, and psychosocial challenges associated with cystic fibrosis.
3. Recognize new therapies and treatments for cystic fibrosis and its manifestations.

ACCREDITATION

The Elsevier Office of Continuing Medical Education (EOCME) is accredited by the Accreditation Council for Continuing Medical Education (ACCME) to provide continuing medical education for physicians.

The EOCME designates this enduring material for a maximum of 15 *AMA PRA Category 1 Credit*(s)™. Physicians should claim only the credit commensurate with the extent of their participation in the activity.

All other health care professionals requesting continuing education credit for this enduring material will be issued a certificate of participation.

DISCLOSURE OF CONFLICTS OF INTEREST

The EOCME assesses conflict of interest with its instructors, faculty, planners, and other individuals who are in a position to control the content of CME activities. All relevant conflicts of interest that are identified are thoroughly vetted by EOCME for fair balance, scientific objectivity, and patient care recommendations. EOCME is committed to providing its learners with CME activities that promote improvements or quality in healthcare and not a specific proprietary business or a commercial interest.

The planning committee, staff, authors and editors listed below have identified no financial relationships or relationships to products or devices they or their spouse/life partner have with commercial interest related to the content of this CME activity:

Scott M. Blackman, MD, PhD; Drucy Borowitz, MD; Albert Faro, MD; Aliza K. Fink, DSc; Anjali Fortna; Carla Frederick, MD; Alvin Jay Freeman, MD; Danielle M. Goetz, MD; Lucas R. Hoffman, MD, PhD; Kerry Holland; Indu Kumari; Sarah Lusman, MD; Susan G. Marshall, MD; Thida Ong, MD; Karen S. Raraigh, MGC; Clement L. Ren, MD; Margaret Rosenfeld, MD, MPH; Meghana Nitin Sathe, MD; Shipra Singh, MD, MPH; Marci K. Sontag, PhD; Bonita F. Stanton, MD; Megan Suermann; Jillian Sullivan, MD, MSCS; Vin Tangpricha, MD, PhD; Alexander Weymann, MD; Edith T. Zemanick, MD, MSCS.

The planning committee, staff, authors and editors listed below have identified financial relationships or relationships to products or devices they or their spouse/life partner have with commercial interest related to the content of this CME activity:

Ronald L. Gibson, MD, PhD is a consultant/advisor for the Cystic Fibrosis Foundation, with research support from the Cystic Fibrosis Foundation; Vertex Pharmaceuticals Incorporated; Nivalis Therapeutics; and the National Institutes of Health.
Bonnie W. Ramsey, MD is a consultant/advisor for Aridis Pharmaceuticals, Inc; Celtaxsys; KaloBios; Flatley Discover Lab; Vertex Pharmaceuticals Incorporated; Laurent Pharmaceuticals, Inc; Nivalis Therapeutics; and Synedgen, Inc.
Don B. Sanders, MD, MS is a consultant/advisor for, with research support from, the Cystic Fibrosis Foundation.
Patrick R. Sosnay, MD is a consultant/advisor for Genetech, A Member of the Roche Group, with research support from Vertex Pharmaceuticals Incorporated.

UNAPPROVED/OFF-LABEL USE DISCLOSURE

The EOCME requires CME faculty to disclose to the participants:
1. When products or procedures being discussed are off-label, unlabelled, experimental, and/or investigational (not US Food and Drug Administration [FDA] approved); and

2. Any limitations on the information presented, such as data that are preliminary or that represent ongoing research, interim analyses, and/or unsupported opinions. Faculty may discuss information about pharmaceutical agents that is outside of FDA-approved labelling. This information is intended solely for CME and is not intended to promote off-label use of these medications. If you have any questions, contact the medical affairs department of the manufacturer for the most recent prescribing information.

TO ENROLL

To enroll in the *Pediatric Clinics of North America* Continuing Medical Education program, call customer service at 1-800-654-2452 or sign up online at http://www.theclinics.com/home/cme. The CME program is available to subscribers for an additional annual fee of USD 290.

METHOD OF PARTICIPATION

In order to claim credit, participants must complete the following:
1. Complete enrolment as indicated above.
2. Read the activity.
3. Complete the CME Test and Evaluation. Participants must achieve a score of 70% on the test. All CME Tests and Evaluations must be completed online.

CME INQUIRIES/SPECIAL NEEDS

For all CME inquiries or special needs, please contact elsevierCME@elsevier.com.

Contributors

CONSULTING EDITOR

BONITA F. STANTON, MD
Founding Dean, School of Medicine, Professor of Pediatrics, Seton Hall University, South Orange, New Jersey

EDITORS

SUSAN G. MARSHALL, MD
Director of Medical Education and Attending Physician, Pulmonary Division, Professor and Vice Chair of Education, Department of Pediatrics, Seattle Children's Hospital, University of Washington School of Medicine, Seattle, Washington

DRUCY BOROWITZ, MD
Professor of Clinical Pediatrics, Jacobs School of Medicine and Biomedical Sciences, University at Buffalo, Vice President of Community Partnerships, Cystic Fibrosis Foundation, Bethesda, Maryland

AUTHORS

SCOTT M. BLACKMAN, MD, PhD
Associate Professor of Pediatrics, Division of Pediatric Endocrinology, Johns Hopkins University, Attending, Johns Hopkins Hospital, Baltimore, Maryland

ALBERT FARO, MD
Professor, Department of Pediatrics, Washington University in St. Louis, St Louis, Missouri

ALIZA K. FINK, DSc
Director of Epidemiology, Cystic Fibrosis Foundation, Bethesda, Maryland

CARLA FREDERICK, MD
Assistant Clinical Professor, Department of Medicine, WCHOB Lung and Cystic Fibrosis Center, State University of New York at Buffalo, Buffalo, New York

ALVIN JAY FREEMAN, MD
Assistant Professor Pediatrics, Division of Pediatric Gastroenterology, Hepatology and Nutrition, Children's Healthcare of Atlanta, Emory University, Atlanta, Georgia

RONALD L. GIBSON, MD, PhD
Professor, Division of Pulmonary and Sleep Medicine, Department of Pediatrics, Seattle Children's Hospital, University of Washington School of Medicine, Seattle, Maryland

DANIELLE M. GOETZ, MD
CF Center Director; Clinical Assistant Professor of Pediatrics, Pediatric Pulmonology, Jacobs School of Medicine, Women and Children's Hospital of Buffalo, State University of New York, Buffalo, New York

LUCAS R. HOFFMAN, MD, PhD
Associate Professor of Pediatrics, Adjunct Associate Professor of Microbiology, University of Washington, Seattle, Washington

SARAH LUSMAN, MD
Assistant Professor, Department of Pediatrics, Columbia University Medical Center, New York, New York

THIDA ONG, MD
Assistant Professor, Division of Pulmonary and Sleep Medicine, Department of Pediatrics, Seattle Children's Hospital, University of Washington, Seattle, Washington

BONNIE W. RAMSEY, MD
Professor; Vice Chair for Research, Department of Pediatrics, Seattle Children's Research Institute, Director, Center for Clinical and Translational Research, University of Washington, Seattle, Washington

KAREN S. RARAIGH, MGC
Genetic Counselor, McKusick-Nathans Institute of Genetic Medicine, Johns Hopkins University, Baltimore, Maryland

CLEMENT L. REN, MD
Professor of Pediatrics, Section of Pediatric Pulmonology, Allergy, and Sleep Medicine, James Whitcomb Riley Hospital for Children, Indiana University School of Medicine, Indianapolis, Indiana

MARGARET ROSENFELD, MD, MPH
Professor of Pediatrics, Division of Pulmonary Medicine, Seattle Children's Hospital, University of Washington School of Medicine, Seattle, Washington

DON B. SANDERS, MD, MS
Associate Professor, Department of Pediatrics, Riley Hospital for Children at IU Health, Indiana University, Indianapolis, Indiana

MEGHANA NITIN SATHE, MD
Assistant Professor of Pediatrics, Associate Fellowship Director, Co-Director Pediatric Cystic Fibrosis Clinic and Therapeutic Drug Center, Division of Pediatric Gastroenterology and Nutrition, Children's Health, University of Texas Southwestern, Dallas, Texas

SHIPRA SINGH, MD, MPH
Associate CF Center Director; Clinical Assistant Professor of Pulmonology, Pediatric Pulmonology, Jacobs School of Medicine, Women and Children's Hospital of Buffalo, State University of New York, Buffalo, New York

MARCI K. SONTAG, PhD
Professor, Department of Epidemiology, Colorado School of Public Health, Anshutz Medical Center, University of Colorado, Aurora, Colorado

PATRICK R. SOSNAY, MD
Assistant Professor, Division of Pulmonary and Critical Care Medicine, Department of Medicine, Johns Hopkins University, Baltimore, Maryland

JILLIAN SULLIVAN, MD, MSCS
Assistant Professor, Department of Pediatrics, University of Vermont College of Medicine, Burlington, Vermont

VIN TANGPRICHA, MD, PhD
Associate Professor of Medicine, Division of Endocrinology, Metabolism and Lipids, Department of Medicine, Emory University School of Medicine, Atlanta VA Medical Center, Atlanta, Georgia

ALEXANDER WEYMANN, MD
Assistant Professor, Department of Pediatrics, Washington University in St. Louis, St Louis, Missouri

EDITH T. ZEMANICK, MD, MSCS
Children's Hospital Colorado, Associate Professor of Pediatrics, University of Colorado School of Medicine, Aurora, Colorado

Contents

Cystic fibrosis (CF) is the most common autosomal-recessive disease in white persons. Significant advances in therapies and outcomes have occurred for people with CF over the past 30 years. Many of these improvements have come about through the concerted efforts of the CF Foundation and international CF societies; networks of CF care centers; and the worldwide community of care providers, researchers, and patients and families. There are still hurdles to overcome to continue to improve the quality of life, reduce CF complications, prolong survival, and ultimately cure CF. This article reviews the epidemiology of CF, including trends in incidence and prevalence, clinical characteristics, common complications, and survival.

The cystic fibrosis (CF) transmembrane conductance regulator (*CFTR*) gene encodes an epithelial ion channel. Although one mutation remains the most common cause of CF (F508del), there have been more than 2000 reported variations in *CFTR*. For the most part, individuals who carry only one mutation (heterozygotes) have no symptoms; individuals who inherit deleterious mutations from both parents have CF. However, growing awareness of *CFTR* mutations that do not ever or do not always cause CF, and individuals with mild or single-organ system manifestations of CFTR-related disease have made this Mendelian relationship more complex.

The diagnosis of cystic fibrosis (CF) has evolved over the past decade as newborn screening has become universal in the United States and elsewhere. The heterogeneity of phenotypes associated with CF transmembrane conductance regulator (CFTR) dysfunction and mutations in the CFTR gene has become clearer, ranging from classic pancreatic-insufficient CF to manifestations in only 1 organ system to indeterminate diagnoses identified by newborn screening. The tools available for diagnosis have also expanded. This article reviews the newest diagnostic criteria for CF, newborn screening,

pancreatic, and hepatobiliary systems occurs as well. As in the airways, defects in CFTR alter epithelial surface fluid, mucus viscosity, and pH, increasing risk of stasis through the various hollow epithelial-lined structures of the gastrointestinal tract. This exerts secondary influences that are responsible for most gastrointestinal, pancreatic, and hepatobiliary manifestations of CF. Understanding these gastrointestinal morbidities of CF is essential in understanding and treating CF as a multisystem disease process and improving overall patient care.

individuals with cystic fibrosis (CF) to target the underlying defect of disease. This review summarizes strategies used to develop CFTR modulators as therapies that improve function and availability of CFTR protein. Lessons learned from dissemination of ivacaftor across the CF population responsive to this therapy and future approaches to predict and monitor treatment response of CFTR modulators are discussed. The goal remains to expand patient-centered and personalized therapy to all patients with CF, ultimately improving life expectancy and quality of life for this disease.

PEDIATRIC CLINICS OF NORTH AMERICA

THE CLINICS ARE AVAILABLE ONLINE!
Access your subscription at:
www.theclinics.com

Foreword
Cystic Fibrosis

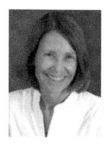

Bonita F. Stanton, MD
Consulting Editor

Our understanding of cystic fibrosis (CF) has exploded over the last several decades, with substantial advances in disease treatment and life expectancy. Given dramatic advances in newborn screening, approximately 80% of patients living in the United States with CF are diagnosed by age 2. Through the 1950s, the majority of children with CF died before age 5. A substantial increase in life expectancy was derived from the understanding of the high salt concentration in sweat associated with CF and the role of pancreatic enzymes. The emphasis on early and aggressive airway clearance and use of antibiotics resulted in further increases in life expectancy such that by the 1980s a majority of patients with CF were surviving into their late teens. With the early diagnosis and the treatment modalities described in these articles, the average lifespan now hovers close to 40 years of age, with many patients living into and past their 50s. As CF is no longer just a disease of childhood, this issue should be of interest to pediatricians, family medicine practitioners, and internists. The articles clearly and effectively describe the history of these breakthroughs and the current standard of care.

Bonita F. Stanton, MD
School of Medicine
Seton Hall University
400 South Orange Avenue
South Orange, NJ 07079, USA

E-mail address:
bonita.stanton@shu.edu

http://dx.doi.org/10.1016/j.pcl.2016.06.002
0031-3955/16/$ – see front matter © 2016 Published by Elsevier Inc.
pediatric.theclinics.com

Preface

Cystic Fibrosis

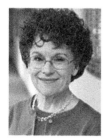 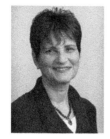

Susan G. Marshall, MD   Drucy Borowitz, MD
Editors

Living with Cystic Fibrosis (CF) is a challenge, but advances in medical care for people with CF have opened new opportunities for health. The scientific breakthroughs in recent years are a tribute to the extraordinary work of our clinical and research colleagues, to the Cystic Fibrosis Foundation, and especially, to our patients and their families, true partners in all of our endeavors. As "older" physicians, we have observed the evolution of this disease from the early days of our medical careers, when most people with CF did not plan for graduations, weddings, births, and productive professional careers, to the current era when expectations are high. The changes in CF care have been remarkable. Understanding the molecular genetics of cystic fibrosis transmembrane regulator protein (CFTR), the "CF gene" product, has been central to many of our new insights. It has helped us to see phenotype-genotype correlations, placed into context some of the long-observed but poorly understood microbiologic perturbations in CF, and has played a part in newborn screening and our current approach to the diagnosis of CF. A multisystem approach to this complex condition has led us not only to focus on the respiratory complications of the disease but also to recognize the influence of growth and nutrition, gastroenterologic, and endocrine aspects of the disorder as well. Despite advances in treatment, transplantation ultimately remains the best option for some individuals. Now that adults make up half the CF population in the United States, issues related to transition of care need to be addressed. Furthermore, we must expand our view to take into account not only the physical but also the psychosocial challenges of living with chronic illness. In the words of Sir William Osler, "the good physician treats the disease; the great physician treats the person who has the disease." By taking both a translational and a holistic approach, we are convinced that people with CF will have steadily improved medical and personal outcomes. As you read the articles included in this issue, we hope you will share our optimism for the bright future ahead for those with CF.

It has been wonderful to collaborate with our exceptional colleagues, the outstanding authors who contributed to this compendium. Their enthusiasm to bring

Pediatr Clin N Am 63 (2016) xvii–xviii
http://dx.doi.org/10.1016/j.pcl.2016.06.001
0031-3955/16/$ – see front matter © 2016 Published by Elsevier Inc.

a wealth of new basic and clinical information to you in a comprehensive and understandable format is inspiring. We have enjoyed and appreciated working with them to create this issue of *Pediatric Clinics of North America* focused on Cystic Fibrosis.

This issue is dedicated to our fathers, Rabbi Eugene B. Borowitz and Victor M. Marshall, MD, both scholars and teachers, who passed away within days of each other as we were in the final stages of editing this issue. They inspired us to seek, understand, and transmit knowledge in an enduring quest to benefit others. We hope that as you read this issue you will take away new insights, and through our part in that process of ongoing education, their legacy will live on.

Susan G. Marshall, MD
Department of Pediatrics
University of Washington School of Medicine
Pulmonary Division
Seattle Children's Hospital
1959 NE Pacific Street
Seattle, WA 98195, USA

Drucy Borowitz, MD
Jacobs School of Medicine and Biomedical Sciences
University at Buffalo
Vice President of Community Partnerships
Cystic Fibrosis Foundation
6931 Arlington Road
2nd Floor
Bethesda, MD 20814, USA

E-mail addresses:
susan.marshall@seattlechildrens.org (S.G. Marshall)
dborowitz@cff.org (D. Borowitz)

Background and Epidemiology

Don B. Sanders, MD, MS[a],*, Aliza K. Fink, DSc[b]

KEYWORDS

- Cystic fibrosis • Newborn screening • FEV$_1$ • BMI • *Pseudomonas aeruginosa*
- MRSA • Mortality

KEY POINTS

- Survival for people with CF has improved greatly and for the first time adults with CF outnumber children with CF.
- The introduction of newborn screening has changed how CF is recognized; today, most people with CF are diagnosed in the neonatal period.
- Changes in CF therapies, disease measures, and outcomes can be tracked longitudinally using large registries, such as the CF Foundation Patient Registry.
- Progressive lung disease can be detected in early life via sensitive measures, such as chest CT scans and the lung clearance index.
- CF is a multisystem disease with complications that include pancreatic insufficiency, sinusitis, CF-related diabetes, infertility, and depression and anxiety.

INTRODUCTION

Cystic fibrosis (CF) is the most common autosomal-recessive cause of early mortality in caucasians worldwide.[1] However, significant advances in therapies and outcomes for people with CF over the past 30 years have brought hope and optimism to clinicians, researchers, and most importantly, individuals and families with CF. In just the past few years, therapies that directly correct errors caused by mutations of the Cystic Fibrosis Transmembrane Conductance Regulator (*CFTR*) gene have received regulatory approval,[2,3] the current median predicted survival is approaching 40 years (and even longer in Canada and some other countries),[4,5] and the number of adults with CF outnumber the number of children with CF in the United States for the first time.[6]

Disclosure Statement: D.B. Sanders has received grant support and honoraria from the CFF (SANDER11A0) for serving as a member of the Patient Registry Committee. A. Fink has nothing to disclose.
Funding Source: NIH (KL2 TR000428; UL1 TR000427).
[a] Department of Pediatrics, Riley Hospital for Children at IU Health, Indiana University, 705 Riley Hospital Drive, Suite 4270, Indianapolis, IN 46202, USA; [b] Cystic Fibrosis Foundation, 6931 Arlington Road, Bethesda, MD 20814, USA
* Corresponding author.
E-mail address: dbsand@iu.edu

Pediatr Clin N Am 63 (2016) 567–584
http://dx.doi.org/10.1016/j.pcl.2016.04.001
0031-3955/16/$ – see front matter © 2016 Elsevier Inc. All rights reserved.

pediatric.theclinics.com

These recent successes illustrate the great strides that have occurred since "cystic fibrosis of the pancreas" was first described by Dorothy Anderson in 1938.[7] At that time, few children with CF lived beyond 5 years, and it was not until the introduction of airway clearance, pancreatic enzyme replacement therapy, nutritional supplements, and anti-*Staphylococcus* antibiotics in the 1960s to 1970s that life expectancy began to extend into adolescence.[1]

CYSTIC FIBROSIS FOUNDATION PATIENT REGISTRY

Many of the developments in CF have occurred at care centers accredited by the CF Foundation (CFF). Modeled on the first successful therapeutic program developed in the 1950s,[8] CF care centers follow CFF Care Guidelines, deliver multidisciplinary care, and have appropriate inpatient and outpatient medical, diagnostic, and laboratory facilities.[9] They are part of a network that includes pediatric, adult, and affiliate programs. As of 2014, there were 121 CF care centers geographically dispersed within the United States. All accredited care centers must contribute data to the CFF Patient Registry (CFFPR).[10] The CFFPR is an ongoing, observational study that is the primary tool for monitoring the health of individuals with CF in the United States. Starting in the 1960s, the CFFPR has evolved to expand the quantity and frequency of the information collected from individuals with CF. Data entered into the CFFPR include demographic and diagnostic information, anthropometric values, pulmonary function test (PFT) results, cultures of respiratory secretions, CF complications, comorbidities, and prescribed CF medications. Thus, the CFFPR is a valuable resource used extensively to inform clinical care, support quality improvement initiatives, and conduct research. Outside of the United States, CF registries exist in Canada, the United Kingdom, Europe, and Oceania, all of which are used to better the understanding of individuals with CF and the course of the disease.[11]

INCIDENCE

Among white persons, CF occurs in approximately 1 in 3000 to 4000 live births.[12] Approximately 1 in 25 to 30 white persons are carriers of a pathogenic mutation of the *CFTR* gene. In other races and ethnicities CF occurs less commonly, including approximately 1 in 4000 to 10,000 Latin Americans, 1 in 15,000 to 20,000 African Americans, and even less commonly in Asian Americans.[12] In the United States, approximately 1000 individuals are diagnosed with CF each year (**Fig. 1**).[6]

Before the widespread use of newborn screening (NBS), individuals with CF were diagnosed either after presenting symptomatically, or via family history. The list of presenting signs and symptoms indicates the multiorgan system nature of the disease (**Box 1**). In 2004, the Centers for Disease Control and Prevention recommended that all states consider NBS for CF.[13] Since then, the proportion of individuals diagnosed via NBS has risen to account for nearly two-thirds of all diagnoses.[6] The early diagnosis of CF after NBS is associated with improved nutritional outcomes and may improve later pulmonary function.[14–16] Similar to NBS, prenatal screening is also widely available, although it accounts for only a minority of diagnoses (4% in 2014).[6] Overall, reports are inconsistent regarding the impact prenatal screening and NBS have had on incidence rates; some reported differences may be in part caused by changes in racial and ethnic distributions over time.[17–19]

The introduction of NBS for CF has also led to the recognition of patients who have abnormal NBS results, but do not meet the diagnostic criteria for CF. The terms "CFTR metabolic syndrome" in the United States and "CF screened positive, inconclusive diagnosis" in Europe have been introduced to characterize the symptoms of these

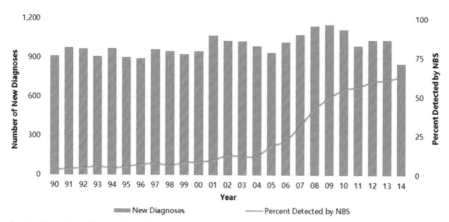

Fig. 1. Number of people with CF and new diagnoses of CF in the United States each year. NBS, newborn screening. (*From* Cystic Fibrosis Foundation Patient Registry 2014 annual data report. Bethesda (MD): Cystic Fibrosis Foundation; 2015; with permission. ©2015 Cystic Fibrosis Foundation.)

individuals (**Table 1**).[20,21] Although the frequency of the diagnosis of CFTR metabolic syndrome/CF screened positive, inconclusive diagnosis depends on the NBS algorithm used (**Box 2**),[22–25] both the CFF and European CF Society recommend that these individuals be followed at specialized CF centers. This population of patients is different than the patients who present clinically with some degree of CFTR dysfunction, such as congenital bilateral absence of the vas deferens, recurrent pancreatitis, or bronchiectasis; these patients are considered to have CFTR-related disorders (see **Table 1**).[26]

PREVALENCE AND TRENDS

The CFFPR captures most individuals with CF living in the United States, but does not include those who seek care outside of a CFF care center, who do not consent to participate in the CFFPR, or who are lost to follow-up in a given calendar year. To estimate the total number of individuals with CF living in the United States, the CFF combined CFFPR data with national data sources.[27] They estimated that there were around 33,200 individuals with CF living in the United States in 2012,[28] of whom approximately 28,700 had data entered into the CFFPR.[6]

Demographics

The prevalence of CF varies throughout the 50 United States and the District of Columbia (**Fig. 2**), ranging from 1.2 per 100,000 people in Hawaii to 24.6 per 100,000 in Vermont.[6,29] The variability across states is likely related to the proportion of the state that is white. In 2014, a total of 93.9% of the individuals in the CFFPR were white, 4.6% were African American, 3.1% were other races, and 8.2% were Hispanics. This is in contrast to the population of the United States that is 62% white, 12% African American, and 17% Hispanic.[30]

In 1966, CF was a disease primarily affecting children with only 6% of the CFFPR population older than age 18 and only 0.1% older than age 30.[31] However, over the last 30 years, there have been steady increases in the adult population of people with CF, leading to an increase in the prevalence of CF. For the first time in 2014, the adult population made up more than half of individuals in the CFFPR (**Fig. 3**).

Box 1
Signs and symptoms of CF

General

Family history of CF

Salty-tasting skin

Clubbing of fingers and toes

Productive cough

Pseudomonas aeruginosa isolated from airway secretions

Hypochloremic metabolic alkalosis

Neonatal

Meconium ileus

Prolonged neonatal jaundice

Abdominal or scrotal calcifications (secondary to meconium peritonitis)

Intestinal atresia

Infancy

Persistent infiltrate on chest radiographs

Failure to thrive

Anasarca or hypoproteinemia

Chronic diarrhea

Abdominal distention

Cholestasis

Staphylococcus aureus pneumonia

Pseudotumor cerebri (vitamin A deficiency)

Hemolytic anemia (vitamin E deficiency)

Childhood

Chronic pansinusitis

Nasal polyps

Steatorrhea

Rectal prolapse

Distal intestinal obstruction syndrome

Recurrent or chronic pancreatitis

Liver disease

Adolescence or adulthood

Allergic bronchopulmonary aspergillosis

Chronic pansinusitis or nasal polyps

Bronchiectasis

Hemoptysis

Recurrent or chronic pancreatitis

Portal hypertension

Delayed puberty

Congenital bilateral absence of the vas deferens

Adapted from O'Sullivan BP. Cystic fibrosis. Lancet 2009;373:1894; with permission.

Table 1
Potential results from diagnostic tests and clinical presentations for CF, CRMS, and CFTR-RDs

	CF	CRMS	CFTR-RDs
Identified via NBS	+	+	−
Sweat test results[a]			
Abnormal	+	−	−
Intermediate	+	+	+
Normal	−	+	−
Typical CFTR mutation analysis	2 disease-causing mutations	1–2 mutations, 1 of which is not clearly disease-causing	1–2 mutations, 1 of which is not clearly disease-causing
Symptomatic at presentation	+ or −	−	+
Diagnostic criteria	Abnormal sweat test and/or 2 disease-causing mutations	Intermediate sweat test and <2 disease-causing mutations or normal sweat test and 2 CFTR mutations, including <2 disease-causing mutations	Intermediate sweat test and 2 CFTR mutations, including <2 disease-causing mutations

Abbreviations: CFTR-RD, CFTR-related disorder; CRMS, CF transmembrane conductance regulator metabolic syndrome.

[a] Abnormal sweat chloride test ≥60 mmol/L: intermediate, 40–59 mmol/L in children >6 months of age and adults or 30–59 mmol/L in children <6 months of age; normal, <40 mmol/L in children >6 months of age and adults or <30 mmol/L in children <6 months of age.

Reprinted with permission of the American Thoracic Society. Copyright © 2016 American Thoracic Society. *From* Boyer D, Nevin M, Thomson CC, et al. ATS core curriculum 2015: Part III: pediatric pulmonary medicine. Ann Am Thorac Soc 2015;12(11):1689. The Annals of the American Thoracic Society is an official journal of the American Thoracic Society.

CF care is multifaceted and involves substantial costs for outpatient medical care, hospitalizations, and medications thereby making health insurance for individuals with CF a necessity. Federal- and state-supported insurance is used extensively within the population (**Fig. 4**). In 2014, CFFPR data showed 41% of children received Medicaid only, 8% received insurance through state special needs programs, and an additional 6% received both types. Among adults, 18% received Medicare disability benefits and an additional 21% received Medicaid. Only a small percentage of individuals report no insurance for the entire year (0.4% of children and 1.3% of adults). The impact of the costs of care are even wider-reaching because of days missed from school and work for patients and caregivers.

Box 2
Reported ratios of CFTR-related metabolic syndrome/CF screened positive, inconclusive diagnosis to CF

New York state, 0.5:1

California, 2.9:1

Canada/Italy, 0.3–0.7:1

Entire United States, 0.2:1

Data from Refs.[22–25]

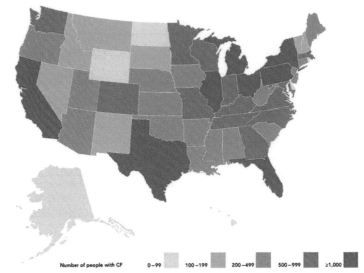

Fig. 2. Map indicating distribution of individuals with CF in the United States. (*From* Cystic Fibrosis Foundation. Patient registry 2014 annual data report. Bethesda (MD): Cystic Fibrosis Foundation; 2015; with permission. ©2015 Cystic Fibrosis Foundation.)

CLINICAL CHARACTERISTICS
Lung Disease

Lung disease is the major source of morbidity and mortality for people with CF. The most commonly tracked measure of lung disease forced expiratory volume in

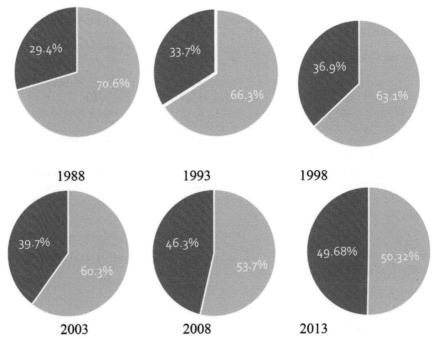

Fig. 3. Proportion of pediatric (*green*) and adult (*blue*) patients in the CFFPR every 5 years from 1988 to 2013. (*From* Cystic Fibrosis Foundation Patient Registry 2014 annual data report. Bethesda (MD): Cystic Fibrosis Foundation; 2015; with permission. ©2015 Cystic Fibrosis Foundation.)

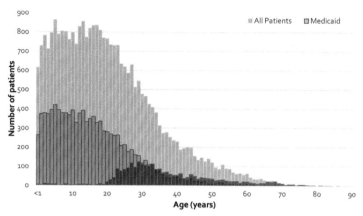

Fig. 4. Distribution of patients with CF by age in the CFFPR. The number receiving Medicare and/or Medicaid insurances is highlighted. (*From* Cystic Fibrosis Foundation Patient Registry 2014 annual data report. Bethesda (MD): Cystic Fibrosis Foundation; 2015; with permission. ©2015 Cystic Fibrosis Foundation.)

1 second (FEV_1). Expressed as percent predicted or z scores adjusted for age, gender, race, and height, FEV_1 can first be measured in children approaching school-age.[32] FEV_1% predicted has improved markedly: the average FEV_1 is nearly 100% predicted (ie, normal) among 6 year olds in the most recent birth cohort (**Fig. 5**).[6] Among 18 year olds, the proportion with FEV_1 greater than or equal to 70% predicted increased from 43% in 1994% to 72% in 2014.[6]

Children less than 6 years of age are unable to reliably perform spirometry, and FEV_1 has poor sensitivity for early CF lung disease.[33–35] There are several complementary measures that overcome these limitations, including infant PFTs, chest imaging, and lung clearance index (LCI), a research tool that identifies abnormalities in the distribution of ventilation.[36–38] The Australian Respiratory Early Surveillance Team for CF (AREST CF) and London CF Collaborative studies have followed children with CF prospectively from diagnosis after NBS with routine infant PFTs, bronchoscopies, chest computed

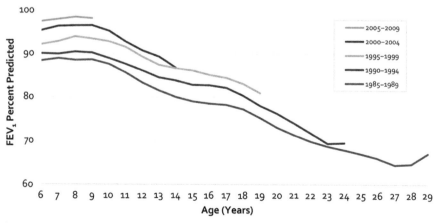

Fig. 5. Mean FEV_1% predicted by age for birth cohorts of people with CF. The population average for people without CF is 100% predicted at every age. (*From* Cystic Fibrosis Foundation Patient Registry 2014 annual data report. Bethesda (MD): Cystic Fibrosis Foundation; 2015; with permission. ©2015 Cystic Fibrosis Foundation.)

tomography (CT) scans, and LCI measurements.[39,40] These studies have shown that infant PFTs are abnormal in approximately 25% of 3 month olds and in greater than 50% of 2 year olds with CF,[40,41] although they may stabilize with conventional CF evaluations and treatment.[42] LCI is abnormal even in 3 month olds.[40] Early abnormalities in LCI may correlate with later abnormalities on chest CT scans,[43] and are more likely to be abnormal than traditional spirometry in the early school years.[44] Results of chest CT scans are inconsistent between the two studies; bronchiectasis, the most severe manifestation of CF lung disease, is often present in infants of the AREST CF cohort[45,46] but not in the 1 year olds of the London CF Collaborative cohort.[47] The use of complementary measures, although not yet used widely, has advanced the understanding of early CF lung disease.

Nutrition

People with CF can develop malnutrition and failure to thrive even in the first few weeks after birth.[48] This is caused by pancreatic insufficiency, which prevents the absorption of fats, proteins, and fat-soluble vitamins.[12] Approximately 85% of individuals with CF are prescribed pancreatic enzyme replacement therapy to treat pancreatic insufficiency. As demonstrated by Corey and colleagues,[49] improved survival is associated with better measures of nutrition among people with CF. Furthermore, nutritional status and severity of lung disease are tightly linked (**Fig. 6**) and there are data to suggest that improvements in nutritional status are associated with improved lung function.[50–52] As a result, the CFF nutrition guidelines recommend that all children maintain a body mass index (BMI) greater than or equal to 50th percentile for age on the Centers for Disease Control and Prevention growth charts and that all adult females and males achieve a BMI greater than or equal to 22 and 23 kg/m^2, respectively.[53] Substantial progress has been made toward this goal, with a median weight for length percentile of 63% among children younger than age 2, a median BMI percentile of 50% among individuals aged 2 to 19, and a median BMI of 22.3 among adults.[6] However, despite the improvements, there is still evidence of stunting with median height percentiles of 32% in children younger than age 2 and 35% among individuals aged 2 to 19.[54] At the other end of the spectrum, there is concern that the number of people with CF who are overweight or obese is increasing.[55]

Microbiology

Chronic endobronchial infections have long been recognized as playing an important role in morbidity and mortality in CF.[1] The identification of organisms considered to be proinflammatory (*Pseudomonas aeruginosa*, *Staphylococcus aureus*, *Haemophilus influenza*, *Streptococcus pneumonia*, and *Aspergillus* species) in the first 2 years of life is associated with worse spirometry in school-age children.[56] S aureus is often the first respiratory pathogen identified in respiratory secretions in young children with CF (**Fig. 7**), although there is some controversy as to whether they should receive antibiotic prophylaxis to treat an S aureus infection.[57,58]

P aeruginosa is the most common pathogen encountered in adults with CF (see **Fig. 7**) and its appearance, especially the mucoid phenotype, is associated with the course of lung disease in CF.[59–61] Over time, the prevalence of P aeruginosa has been significantly decreasing, likely attributable to improved infection control and the more recent strategy of eradicating P aeruginosa when it first appears.[62]

The presence of methicillin-resistant S aureus (MRSA) is associated with worsening lung disease and increased mortality for people with CF.[63,64] The prevalence of MRSA has increased substantially over the past 20 years, similar to the general non-CF population; however, in recent years it seems to be stabilizing (**Fig. 8**). The prevalence of *Burkholderia cepacia* complex has decreased significantly since 1995, whereas the prevalence of nontuberculous *Mycobacteria* has increased since 2010.[62]

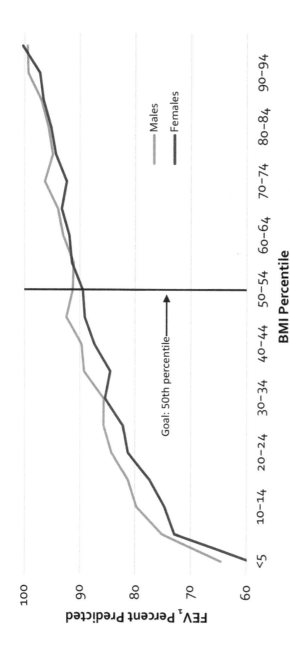

Fig. 6. Median FEV$_1$% predicted versus median body mass index (BMI) percentile for children ages 6 to 19 years of age. The CF Foundation goal is a BMI ≥50th percentile. (*From* Cystic Fibrosis Foundation Patient Registry 2014 annual data report. Bethesda (MD): Cystic Fibrosis Foundation; 2015; with permission. ©2015 Cystic Fibrosis Foundation.)

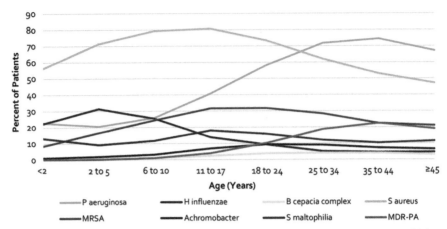

Fig. 7. Prevalence of bacteria in respiratory secretions by age in 2014. MDR-PA, multidrug resistant *Pseudomonas aeruginosa*; MRSA, methicillin-resistant *Staphylococcus aureus*. (*From* Cystic Fibrosis Foundation Patient Registry 2014 annual data report. Bethesda (MD): Cystic Fibrosis Foundation; 2015; with permission. ©2015 Cystic Fibrosis Foundation.)

Recently developed bacterial detection techniques that do not rely on routine microbial culture techniques have identified the diversity and complexity of the microbiome of the airways in CF.[65] Decreases in diversity of the microbiome and the presence of specific CF pathogens are strongly associated with more severe CF lung disease.[66,67]

CHRONIC AND ACUTE MANAGEMENT

Daily airway clearance to help remove respiratory secretions has been a cornerstone of CF care since the 1950s.[68] Dornase alfa, the first medication designed specifically to treat symptoms of CF, received regulatory approval in 1994.[69] Since then, several additional mucolytic, antibacterial, and CFTR-modulator therapies have been developed for CF (**Box 3**).[2,3,70–74] Once introduced, the uptake of medication prescriptions differs. Within a year of approval, about 80% of eligible individuals received a prescription for ivacaftor, with other medications having more gradual uptake (**Fig. 9**). The daily

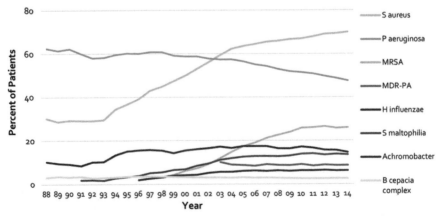

Fig. 8. Prevalence of bacteria in respiratory secretions from 1989 to 2014. (*From* Cystic Fibrosis Foundation Patient Registry 2014 annual data report. Bethesda (MD): Cystic Fibrosis Foundation; 2015; with permission. ©2015 Cystic Fibrosis Foundation.)

Box 3
Chronic therapies developed for patients with CF

Dornase alfa (approved by the Food and Drug Administration in 1994)

High-dose ibuprofen

Inhaled tobramycin (1996)

Chronic azithromycin

Hypertonic saline

Inhaled aztreonam (2007)

Ivacaftor (2012)

Lumacaftor-ivacaftor (2015)

Data from Refs.[2,3,69–74]

---

treatment complexity for patients with CF has increased substantially, which may decrease overall medication adherence.[75]

Pulmonary exacerbations are diagnosed clinically based on a combination of respiratory and systemic signs and symptoms,[76] and are typically treated with a combination of antibiotics (oral, inhaled, and/or intravenous), airway clearance techniques, and attention to nutrition.[77] Pulmonary exacerbations are linked to increased mortality, higher health care costs, and reduced quality of life.[78–80] They occur commonly, and despite overall improvements over the past 30 years, the proportion of CF individuals treated with intravenous antibiotics has not decreased (**Fig. 10**).

Pulmonary exacerbations are frequently associated with adverse outcomes, including reduced FEV_1, prolonged duration of treatment, and the need for additional treatments in the near future.[81–84] Risk factors for pulmonary exacerbations include age, severity of baseline FEV_1, gender, chronic endobronchial infections, allergic bronchopulmonary aspergillosis, CF-related diabetes, and a history of having been treated previously for a pulmonary exacerbation.[84–87]

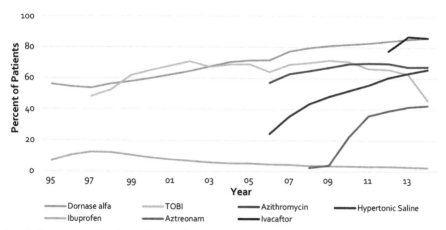

Fig. 9. Proportion of patients with CF who meet CF Foundation–recommended eligibility requirements and who are prescribed chronic CF therapies. Each line starts in the year that Food and Drug Administration approval was received or when high-level evidence was published supporting its use in CF. (*From* Cystic Fibrosis Foundation Patient Registry 2014 annual data report. Bethesda (MD): Cystic Fibrosis Foundation; 2015; with permission. ©2015 Cystic Fibrosis Foundation.)

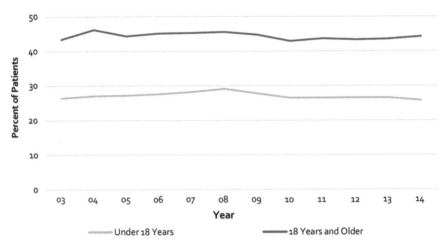

Fig. 10. Proportion of patients treated for a pulmonary exacerbation with intravenous anti-biotics. (*From* Cystic Fibrosis Foundation Patient Registry 2014 annual data report. Bethesda (MD): Cystic Fibrosis Foundation; 2015; with permission. ©2015 Cystic Fibrosis Foundation.)

For some CF individuals with advanced lung disease, bilateral lung transplants are a treatment option. In the United States during 2014, a total of 244 individuals received a lung transplant.[6] Compared with other individuals on the lung transplant wait list, patients with CF have higher wait list mortality but higher posttransplant survival; however, debate continues about selecting patients most likely to benefit from lung transplant.[88]

COMMON COMPLICATIONS OF CYSTIC FIBROSIS

Beyond poor nutrition and progressive lung disease, several other manifestations of CFTR dysfunction or absence are common in people with CF. Chronic sinusitis, reported in 30% of all patients with CF,[6] is associated with poorer quality of life[89] and often requires surgical intervention. Liver disease occurs in approximately 15% to 30% of people with CF and typically has minimal clinical consequences[90]; however, it can progress to cirrhosis and in severe cases require a liver transplant.

CF-related diabetes occurs with increasing frequency as patients age and progressive destruction of the pancreatic islet cells occurs, leading to insulin deficiency.[90] The presence of CF-related diabetes is associated with more severe lung disease, more frequent pulmonary exacerbations, and poorer nutritional status.[91]

Depression and anxiety occur commonly in individuals with CF and their caregivers and routine screening is recommended for all individuals with CF and their caregivers.[92] The presence of depression or anxiety is associated with decreases in adherence, increased risk of pulmonary exacerbations, and worsening lung disease.[92]

In general, complications of CF occur in individuals with more severe genotypes and pancreatic insufficiency. Those with milder CFTR mutations are typically pancreatic sufficient and may have no demonstrable lung disease, or at least have delayed onset of measurable abnormalities.[93] These individuals may suffer from male infertility (congenital bilateral absence of the vas deferens) or recurrent or chronic pancreatitis.[94,95]

SURVIVAL

Over time there have been steady increases in survival for individuals with CF. The main metric used to measure survival is the median predicted survival, which

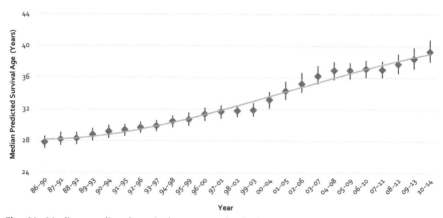

Fig. 11. Median predicted survival among individuals included in the CFFPR from 1986 to 2014. (*From* Cystic Fibrosis Foundation Patient Registry 2014 annual data report. Bethesda (MD): Cystic Fibrosis Foundation; 2015; with permission. ©2015 Cystic Fibrosis Foundation.)

represents the age that half of the current individuals are expected to survive until, assuming that mortality rates stay constant. For the years 2010 to 2014, the median predicted survival is 39.3. Over the past 20 years, the median survival has increased 10 years (**Fig. 11**). MacKenzie and colleagues[4] examined mortality rates from 2000 to 2010 and observed decreases in the mortality rate of 1.8% per year. If the rate of decrease continues, they predicted that the median predicted survival for individuals born in 2010 would be 56 years of age. Among individuals in the registry in 2009 and followed through 2014, children younger than age 15 had greater than 97% probability of surviving 5 years. The steepest drop in probability of survival was between those currently ages 15 to 20 who have a 92% probability of surviving 5 years and those age 20 to 25 who had an 84% probability of surviving 5 years.

Several risk factors for early mortality in people with CF have been identified. Although the number of individuals with CF is evenly split between males and females, the risk of death is greater among females.[96] The cause of this difference is unclear, but is likely multifactorial. Early mortality is also associated with ethnicity (Hispanic patients tend to have poorer survival), poorer nutritional status, specific respiratory infections (eg, *B cepacia* complex, MRSA), and pulmonary exacerbations.[49,64,79,80,97]

SUMMARY

The outlook for people with CF has improved substantially over the past 30 years. Many of the improvements in morbidity and mortality have come about through the concerted efforts of the US CFF and international CF societies, care center networks, and the worldwide community of care providers, researchers, and patients and families. Despite these gains, there are still hurdles to overcome to continue to improve quality of life, reduce CF complications, prolong survival, and ultimately cure CF.

REFERENCES

1. Davis PB. Cystic fibrosis since 1938. Am J Respir Crit Care Med 2006;173(5):475–82.
2. Ramsey BW, Davies J, McElvaney NG, et al. A CFTR potentiator in patients with cystic fibrosis and the G551D mutation. N Engl J Med 2011;365(18):1663–72.
3. Wainwright CE, Elborn JS, Ramsey BW, et al. Lumacaftor-ivacaftor in patients with cystic fibrosis homozygous for Phe508del CFTR. N Engl J Med 2015;373(3):220–31.

4. MacKenzie T, Gifford AH, Sabadosa KA, et al. Longevity of patients with cystic fibrosis in 2000 to 2010 and beyond: survival analysis of the Cystic Fibrosis Foundation patient registry. Ann Intern Med 2014;161(4):233–41.

5. Goss CH. Country to country variation: what can be learnt from national cystic fibrosis registries. Curr Opin Pulm Med 2015;21(6):585–90.

6. Cystic Fibrosis Foundation. Patient registry 2014 annual report. Bethesda (MD): Cystic Fibrosis Foundation; 2015.

7. Anderson DH. Cystic fibrosis of the pancreas and its relation to celiac disease: a clinical and pathologic study. Am J Dis Child 1938;56(2):344.

8. Doershuk CF, Matthews LW, Tucker AS, et al. A 5 year clinical evaluation of a therapeutic program for patients with cystic fibrosis. J Pediatr 1964;65:677–93.

9. Mogayzel PJ Jr, Dunitz J, Marrow LC, et al. Improving chronic care delivery and outcomes: the impact of the cystic fibrosis Care Center Network. BMJ Qual Saf 2014;23(Suppl 1):i3–8.

10. Schechter MS, Fink AK, Homa K, et al. The Cystic Fibrosis Foundation Patient Registry as a tool for use in quality improvement. BMJ Qual Saf 2014; 23(Suppl 1):i9–14.

11. Salvatore D, Buzzetti R, Baldo E, et al. An overview of international literature from cystic fibrosis registries. Part 4: update 2011. J Cyst Fibros 2012;11(6):480–93.

12. O'Sullivan BP, Freedman SD. Cystic fibrosis. Lancet 2009;373(9678):1891–904.

13. Grosse SD, Boyle CA, Botkin JR, et al. Newborn screening for cystic fibrosis: evaluation of benefits and risks and recommendations for state newborn screening programs. MMWR Recomm Rep 2004;53(RR-13):1–36.

14. Farrell P, Kosorok M, Rock M, et al. Early diagnosis of cystic fibrosis through neonatal screening prevents severe malnutrition and improves long-term growth. Wisconsin Cystic Fibrosis Neonatal Screening Study Group. Pediatrics 2001;107(1):1–13.

15. Farrell P, Kosorok M, Laxova A, et al. Nutritional benefits of neonatal screening for cystic fibrosis. Wisconsin Cystic Fibrosis Neonatal Screening Study Group. N Engl J Med 1997;337(14):963–9.

16. McKay KO, Waters DL, Gaskin KJ. The influence of newborn screening for cystic fibrosis on pulmonary outcomes in new South Wales. J Pediatr 2005; 147(Suppl 3):S47–50.

17. Hale JE, Parad RB, Comeau AM. Newborn screening showing decreasing incidence of cystic fibrosis. N Engl J Med 2008;358(9):973–4.

18. Castellani C, Picci L, Tamanini A, et al. Association between carrier screening and incidence of cystic fibrosis. JAMA 2009;302(23):2573–9.

19. Levy H, Farrell PM. New challenges in the diagnosis and management of cystic fibrosis. J Pediatr 2015;166(6):1337–41.

20. Cystic Fibrosis Foundation, Borowitz D, Parad RB, Sharp JK, et al. Cystic Fibrosis Foundation practice guidelines for the management of infants with cystic fibrosis transmembrane conductance regulator-related metabolic syndrome during the first two years of life and beyond. J Pediatr 2009;155(Suppl 6):S106–16.

21. Munck A, Mayell SJ, Winters V, et al. Cystic fibrosis screen positive, inconclusive diagnosis (CFSPID): a new designation and management recommendations for infants with an inconclusive diagnosis following newborn screening. J Cyst Fibros 2015;14(6):706–13.

22. Ren CL, Desai H, Platt M, et al. Clinical outcomes in infants with cystic fibrosis transmembrane conductance regulator (CFTR) related metabolic syndrome. Pediatr Pulmonol 2011;46(11):1079–84.

23. Prach L, Koepke R, Kharrazi M, et al. Novel CFTR variants identified during the first 3 years of cystic fibrosis newborn screening in California. J Mol Diagn 2013;15(5):710–22.
24. Ooi CY, Castellani C, Keenan K, et al. Inconclusive diagnosis of cystic fibrosis after newborn screening. Pediatrics 2015;135(6):e1377–85.
25. Ren CL, Fink AK, Petren K, et al. Outcomes of infants with indeterminate diagnosis detected by cystic fibrosis newborn screening. Pediatrics 2015;135(6):e1386–92.
26. Bombieri C, Claustres M, De Boeck K, et al. Recommendations for the classification of diseases as CFTR-related disorders. J Cyst Fibros 2011;10(Suppl 2):S86–102.
27. Statistics Centers for Disease Control and Prevention - National Center for Health Statistics. Vital Statistics Data. Available at: http://www.cdc.gov/nchs/data_access/Vitalstatsonline.htm. Accessed November 1, 2015.
28. Knapp EA, Fink AK, Goss CH, et al. The Cystic Fibrosis Foundation Patient Registry: Design and Methods of a National Observational Disease Registry. Ann Am Thorac Soc 2016. [Epub ahead of print].
29. US Census Bureau. Annual Estimates of the Resident Population: April 1, 2010 to July 1, 2014. 2014. Available at: www.census.gov/popest. Accessed November 1, 2015.
30. US Census Bureau. Annual estimates of the resident population by sex, race alone or in combination, and Hispanic origin for the United States, states, and counties: April 1, 2010 to July 1, 2014. Available at: www.census.gov/popest. Accessed November 1, 2015.
31. Cystic Fibrosis Foundation. Patient registry 1975 annual report. Atlanta (GA): Cystic Fibrosis Foundation; 1975.
32. Quanjer PH, Stanojevic S, Cole TJ, et al. Multi-ethnic reference values for spirometry for the 3-95-yr age range: the global lung function 2012 equations. Eur Respir J 2012;40(6):1324–43.
33. Brody A, Klein J, Molina P, et al. High-resolution computed tomography in young patients with cystic fibrosis: distribution of abnormalities and correlation with pulmonary function tests. J Pediatr 2004;145(1):32–8.
34. de Jong P, Lindblad A, Rubin L, et al. Progression of lung disease on computed tomography and pulmonary function tests in children and adults with cystic fibrosis. Thorax 2006;61(1):80–5.
35. Gustafsson P, De Jong P, Tiddens H, et al. Multiple-breath inert gas washout and spirometry versus structural lung disease in cystic fibrosis. Thorax 2008;63(2):129–34.
36. Davis SD, Rosenfeld M, Kerby GS, et al. Multicenter evaluation of infant lung function tests as cystic fibrosis clinical trial endpoints. Am J Respir Crit Care Med 2010;182(11):1387–97.
37. Lum S, Gustafsson P, Ljungberg H, et al. Early detection of cystic fibrosis lung disease: multiple-breath washout versus raised volume tests. Thorax 2007;62(4):341–7.
38. Stick S, Brennan S, Murray C, et al. Bronchiectasis in infants and preschool children diagnosed with cystic fibrosis after newborn screening. J Pediatr 2009;155(5):623–8.e1.
39. Ranganathan SC, Parsons F, Gangell C, et al. Evolution of pulmonary inflammation and nutritional status in infants and young children with cystic fibrosis. Thorax 2011;66(5):408–13.
40. Hoo AF, Thia LP, Nguyen TT, et al. Lung function is abnormal in 3-month-old infants with cystic fibrosis diagnosed by newborn screening. Thorax 2012;67(10):874–81.
41. Pillarisetti N, Williamson E, Linnane B, et al. Infection, inflammation, and lung function decline in infants with cystic fibrosis. Am J Respir Crit Care Med 2011;184(1):75–81.

42. Nguyen TT, Thia LP, Hoo AF, et al. Evolution of lung function during the first year of life in newborn screened cystic fibrosis infants. Thorax 2014;69(10):910–7.

43. Aurora P, Stanojevic S, Wade A, et al. Lung clearance index at 4 years predicts subsequent lung function in children with cystic fibrosis. Am J Respir Crit Care Med 2011;183(6):752–8.

44. Aurora P, Bush A, Gustafsson P, et al. Multiple-breath washout as a marker of lung disease in preschool children with cystic fibrosis. Am J Respir Crit Care Med 2005;171(3):249–56.

45. Sly PD, Gangell CL, Chen L, et al. Risk factors for bronchiectasis in children with cystic fibrosis. N Engl J Med 2013;368(21):1963–70.

46. Mott LS, Park J, Murray CP, et al. Progression of early structural lung disease in young children with cystic fibrosis assessed using CT. Thorax 2012;67(6):509–16.

47. Thia LP, Calder A, Stocks J, et al. Is chest CT useful in newborn screened infants with cystic fibrosis at 1 year of age? Thorax 2014;69(4):320–7.

48. O'Sullivan BP, Baker D, Leung KG, et al. Evolution of pancreatic function during the first year in infants with cystic fibrosis. J Pediatr 2013;162(4):808–12.e1.

49. Corey M, McLaughlin F, Williams M, et al. A comparison of survival, growth, and pulmonary function in patients with cystic fibrosis in Boston and Toronto. J Clin Epidemiol 1988;41(6):583–91.

50. Sanders DB, Fink A, Mayer-Hamblett N, et al. Early life growth trajectories in cystic fibrosis are associated with pulmonary function at age 6 years. J Pediatr 2015;167(5):1081–8.e1.

51. Konstan M, Butler S, Wohl M, et al. Growth and nutritional indexes in early life predict pulmonary function in cystic fibrosis. J Pediatr 2003;142(6):624–30.

52. Lai H, Shoff S, Farrell P. Wisconsin Cystic Fibrosis Neonatal Screening Group. Recovery of birth weight z score within 2 years of diagnosis is positively associated with pulmonary status at 6 years of age in children with cystic fibrosis. Pediatrics 2009;123(2):714–22.

53. Stallings VA, Stark LJ, Robinson KA, et al. Evidence-based practice recommendations for nutrition-related management of children and adults with cystic fibrosis and pancreatic insufficiency: results of a systematic review. J Am Diet Assoc 2008;108(5):832–9.

54. Comeau AM, Accurso FJ, White TB, et al. Guidelines for implementation of cystic fibrosis newborn screening programs: Cystic Fibrosis Foundation workshop report. Pediatrics 2007;119(2):e495–518.

55. Stephenson AL, Mannik LA, Walsh S, et al. Longitudinal trends in nutritional status and the relation between lung function and BMI in cystic fibrosis: a population-based cohort study. Am J Clin Nutr 2013;97(4):872–7.

56. Ramsey KA, Ranganathan S, Park J, et al. Early respiratory infection is associated with reduced spirometry in children with cystic fibrosis. Am J Respir Crit Care Med 2014;190(10):1111–6.

57. Stutman HR, Lieberman JM, Nussbaum E, et al. Antibiotic prophylaxis in infants and young children with cystic fibrosis: a randomized controlled trial. J Pediatr 2002;140(3):299–305.

58. Smyth AR. Pseudomonas eradication in cystic fibrosis: who will join the ELITE? Thorax 2010;65(4):281–2.

59. Lee TW, Brownlee KG, Conway SP, et al. Evaluation of a new definition for chronic *Pseudomonas aeruginosa* infection in cystic fibrosis patients. J Cyst Fibros 2003; 2(1):29–34.

60. Li Z, Kosorok M, Farrell P, et al. Longitudinal development of mucoid *Pseudomonas aeruginosa* infection and lung disease progression in children with cystic fibrosis. JAMA 2005;293(5):581–8.

61. Konstan M, Morgan W, Butler S, et al. Risk factors for rate of decline in forced expiratory volume in one second in children and adolescents with cystic fibrosis. J Pediatr 2007;151(2):134–9, 139.e1.

62. Salsgiver EL, Fink AK, Knapp EA, et al. Changing epidemiology of the respiratory bacteriology of patients with cystic fibrosis. Chest 2015;149(2):390–400.

63. Dasenbrook E, Merlo C, Diener-West M, et al. Persistent methicillin-resistant *Staphylococcus aureus* and rate of FEV1 decline in cystic fibrosis. Am J Respir Crit Care Med 2008;178(8):814–21.

64. Dasenbrook EC, Checkley W, Merlo CA, et al. Association between respiratory tract methicillin-resistant *Staphylococcus aureus* and survival in cystic fibrosis. JAMA 2010;303(23):2386–92.

65. Zhao J, Schloss PD, Kalikin LM, et al. Decade-long bacterial community dynamics in cystic fibrosis airways. Proc Natl Acad Sci U S A 2012;109(15):5809–14.

66. Carmody LA, Zhao J, Schloss PD, et al. Changes in cystic fibrosis airway microbiota at pulmonary exacerbation. Ann Am Thorac Soc 2013;10(3):179–87.

67. Cox MJ, Allgaier M, Taylor B, et al. Airway microbiota and pathogen abundance in age-stratified cystic fibrosis patients. PLoS One 2010;5(6):e11044.

68. Bradley JM, Moran FM, Elborn JS. Evidence for physical therapies (airway clearance and physical training) in cystic fibrosis: an overview of five Cochrane systematic reviews. Respir Med 2006;100(2):191–201.

69. Fuchs H, Borowitz D, Christiansen D, et al. Effect of aerosolized recombinant human DNase on exacerbations of respiratory symptoms and on pulmonary function in patients with cystic fibrosis. The Pulmozyme Study Group. N Engl J Med 1994;331(10):637–42.

70. Konstan MW, Byard PJ, Hoppel CL, et al. Effect of high-dose ibuprofen in patients with cystic fibrosis. N Engl J Med 1995;332(13):848–54.

71. Ramsey B, Pepe M, Quan J, et al. Intermittent administration of inhaled tobramycin in patients with cystic fibrosis. Cystic Fibrosis Inhaled Tobramycin Study Group. N Engl J Med 1999;340(1):23–30.

72. Saiman L, Marshall B, Mayer-Hamblett N, et al. Azithromycin in patients with cystic fibrosis chronically infected with *Pseudomonas aeruginosa*: a randomized controlled trial. JAMA 2003;290(13):1749–56.

73. Elkins MR, Robinson M, Rose BR, et al. A controlled trial of long-term inhaled hypertonic saline in patients with cystic fibrosis. N Engl J Med 2006;354(3):229–40.

74. McCoy KS, Quittner AL, Oermann CM, et al. Inhaled aztreonam lysine for chronic airway *Pseudomonas aeruginosa* in cystic fibrosis. Am J Respir Crit Care Med 2008;178(9):921–8.

75. Sawicki GS, Ren CL, Konstan MW, et al. Treatment complexity in cystic fibrosis: trends over time and associations with site-specific outcomes. J Cyst Fibros 2013;12(5):461–7.

76. Rosenfeld M, Emerson J, Williams-Warren J, et al. Defining a pulmonary exacerbation in cystic fibrosis. J Pediatr 2001;139(3):359–65.

77. Ferkol T, Rosenfeld M, Milla CE. Cystic fibrosis pulmonary exacerbations. J Pediatr 2006;148:259–64.

78. Britto M, Kotagal U, Hornung R, et al. Impact of recent pulmonary exacerbations on quality of life in patients with cystic fibrosis. Chest 2002;121(1):64–72.

79. Ellaffi M, Vinsonneau C, Coste J, et al. One-year outcome after severe pulmonary exacerbation in adults with cystic fibrosis. Am J Respir Crit Care Med 2005; 171(2):158–64.

80. Lieu T, Ray G, Farmer G, et al. The cost of medical care for patients with cystic fibrosis in a health maintenance organization. Pediatrics 1999;103(6):e72.

81. Sanders DB, Bittner RC, Rosenfeld M, et al. Pulmonary exacerbations are associated with subsequent FEV(1) decline in both adults and children with cystic fibrosis. Pediatr Pulmonol 2011;46(4):393–400.

82. Waters V, Stanojevic S, Atenafu EG, et al. Effect of pulmonary exacerbations on long-term lung function decline in cystic fibrosis. Eur Respir J 2012;40(1):61–6.

83. Parkins MD, Rendall JC, Elborn JS. Incidence and risk factors for pulmonary exacerbation treatment failures in patients with cystic fibrosis chronically infected with *Pseudomonas aeruginosa*. Chest 2012;141(2):485–93.

84. VanDevanter DR, Pasta DJ, Konstan MW. Treatment and demographic factors affecting time to next pulmonary exacerbation in cystic fibrosis. J Cyst Fibros 2015;14(6):763–9.

85. Corey M, Edwards L, Levison H, et al. Longitudinal analysis of pulmonary function decline in patients with cystic fibrosis. J Pediatr 1997;131(6):809–14.

86. Goss C, Burns J. Exacerbations in cystic fibrosis. 1: epidemiology and pathogenesis. Thorax 2007;62(4):360–7.

87. Sawicki GS, Ayyagari R, Zhang J, et al. A pulmonary exacerbation risk score among cystic fibrosis patients not receiving recommended care. Pediatr Pulmonol 2013;48(10):954–61.

88. Lynch JP 3rd, Sayah DM, Belperio JA, et al. Lung transplantation for cystic fibrosis: results, indications, complications, and controversies. Semin Respir Crit Care Med 2015;36(2):299–320.

89. Habib AR, Buxton JA, Singer J, et al. Association between chronic rhinosinusitis and health-related quality of life in adults with cystic fibrosis. Ann Am Thorac Soc 2015;12(8):1163–9.

90. Ledder O, Haller W, Couper RT, et al. Cystic fibrosis: an update for clinicians. Part 2: hepatobiliary and pancreatic manifestations. J Gastroenterol Hepatol 2014; 29(12):1954–62.

91. Moran A, Dunitz J, Nathan B, et al. Cystic fibrosis-related diabetes: current trends in prevalence, incidence, and mortality. Diabetes Care 2009;32(9):1626–31.

92. Quittner AL, Abbott J, Georgiopoulos AM, et al. International Committee on Mental Health in Cystic Fibrosis: Cystic Fibrosis Foundation and European Cystic Fibrosis Society consensus statements for screening and treating depression and anxiety. Thorax 2015;71(1):26–34.

93. Braun AT, Farrell PM, Ferec C, et al. Cystic fibrosis mutations and genotype-pulmonary phenotype analysis. J Cyst Fibros 2006;5(1):33–41.

94. Boyle MP. Nonclassic cystic fibrosis and CFTR-related diseases. Curr Opin Pulm Med 2003;9(6):498–503.

95. Pall H, Zielenski J, Jonas MM, et al. Primary sclerosing cholangitis in childhood is associated with abnormalities in cystic fibrosis-mediated chloride channel function. J Pediatr 2007;151(3):255–9.

96. Liou T, Adler F, Fitzsimmons S, et al. Predictive 5-year survivorship model of cystic fibrosis. Am J Epidemiol 2001;153(4):345–52.

97. Buu MC, Sanders LM, Mayo J, et al. Assessing differences in mortality rates and risk factors between Hispanic and non-Hispanic patients with cystic fibrosis in California. Chest 2015;149(2):380–9.

Molecular Genetics of Cystic Fibrosis Transmembrane Conductance Regulator: Genotype and Phenotype

Patrick R. Sosnay, MD[a],*, Karen S. Raraigh, MGC[b],
Ronald L. Gibson, MD, PhD[c]

KEYWORDS

- CFTR mutations • Genotype/phenotype correlations • Cystic fibrosis

KEY POINTS

- There are more than 2000 mutations in the cystic fibrosis (CF) transmembrane conductance regulator (*CFTR*) gene described, though not all result in CF.
- Genotyping *CFTR* can help establish a CF diagnosis (if mutations are characterized) and can be helpful to identify patients eligible for mutation-specific therapies.
- There is a wide range of phenotypes and severity among patients with CF.
- The traditional legacy manner of naming mutations used by CF clinicians and scientists is not in line with other genetic nomenclatures.

THE HISTORY OF THE DISCOVERY OF CYSTIC FIBROSIS TRANSMEMBRANE CONDUCTANCE REGULATOR AS THE GENE RESPONSIBLE FOR CYSTIC FIBROSIS

Very soon after cystic fibrosis (CF) was recognized and characterized, clinicians caring for patients with CF observed that the disease occurred in families with a Mendelian autosomal recessive inheritance pattern.[1] The study of CF was an important test case for the molecular tools used to study how DNA and genes are responsible for inherited traits. Beginning with restriction fragment length polymorphism analysis that allowed DNA segments differing by restriction enzyme sites to be sorted with

Disclosures: PRS has received consulting fees from Genetech and have received research grants from Vertex. KSR has received consulting fees from Pro-QR.
[a] Division of Pulmonary & Critical Care Medicine, Department of Medicine, Johns Hopkins University, 1830 E. Monument Street, Baltimore, MD 21205, USA; [b] McKusick-Nathans Institute of Genetic Medicine, Johns Hopkins University, 733 N. Broadway, Baltimore, MD 21205, USA; [c] Division of Pulmonary and Sleep Medicine, Department of Pediatrics, Seattle Children's Hospital, University of Washington School of Medicine, 4800 Sand Point Way, Seattle, WA 98105, USA
* Corresponding author.
E-mail address: psosnay@jhmi.edu

inheritance of a phenotype, the gene responsible for CF could be localized to the long arm of chromosome 7.[2] Coincident with these genetic advances, researchers examining the biochemical defect in the disease by studying the epithelial tissues affected by CF discovered that these tissues did not allow normal chloride transport.[3] The genetic and biochemical investigational pathways converged with the identification of the CF transmembrane conductance regulator (CFTR) gene and its most common mutation (F508del) in 1989.[4–6] Immediately after the gene was identified, it became apparent that multiple mutations in this gene could be responsible for CF[7,8] (**Box 1**).

RESOURCES TO DESCRIBE AND CHARACTERIZE VARIATION IN CYSTIC FIBROSIS TRANSMEMBRANE CONDUCTANCE REGULATOR

As understanding of CF has increased and more patients have been identified, advancing DNA technology has become a greater part of regular medical care and the number of CFTR mutations recognized has grown to more than 2000.[9] Researchers at the University of Toronto and the Hospital for Sick Children began cataloging CFTR mutations in 1989 and continue to curate a publicly available online database of all genetic variations described in CFTR (the CF Mutation Database; http://www.genet.sickkids.on.ca/cftr/app). This resource has limited clinical information and/or laboratory-based functional testing in some cases but was not established as a resource to determine whether or not a mutation causes CF. There are examples of benign CFTR variants being mistaken for causative mutations if functional investigations are not carried out or if other variants present are not recognized.[10] The ramifications of an incorrect mutation annotation are now more severe as the CFTR genotype is increasingly being used as part of the CF diagnosis and to inform treatment.

To meet the growing need for a resource that characterizes mutations, the US CF Foundation amassed a team of international CF researchers to create the Clinical and Functional Translation of CFTR (CFTR2) database.[11] CFTR2 was designed with the goal to identify and annotate the mutations that cause CF among all the mutations described in CFTR. The research group, with tremendous assistance of registries and national CF foundations, has collected genotype and phenotype data from patients

---

Box 1
Terminology

The terms *mutation* and *variant* can both be used to describe a genetic difference from that which is commonly seen in a population (sometimes referred to as wild-type). In some writing, *mutation* implies that the genetic change is deleterious and *variant* is used when the change does not result in disease; however, both terms are used in the literature, somewhat interchangeably. The Human Genome Variation Society, American College of Medical Genetics and Genomics, and the Association for Molecular Pathology recommend use of the term *variant*, recognizing the potential negative connotations of the term *mutation*. Similarly, the terms *polymorphism* or *single nucleotide polymorphism* have been used to describe sequence changes occurring at greater than 1% frequency in the population but also to describe sequence changes that do not lead to disease (regardless of frequency). Therefore, consensus has been to use the term *variant* or *sequence alteration* to describe any DNA change, with further explanation given if the variant has been deemed to have an effect on the gene, protein, or person. However, for the purpose of this article and this issue, *mutation* is used to describe DNA changes because it is more familiar to most clinicians. When known, terms such as *CF-causing mutation* or *mutation of unknown significance* may be used to appropriately define disease liability.

with CF around the world (though most hail from North America and Europe). From the list of *CFTR* mutations observed in patients with CF, 3 separate analyses were used to evaluate and annotate these mutations: clinical characteristics, functional testing, and population/penetrance analysis. Sweat chloride concentration was used as a clinical filter because it is standardized, widely performed, and reflects CF severity.[12] Functional evaluation was performed to quantify the effect of the mutation on how much protein is made, how it is processed, and whether the protein functions normally. Finally, population and penetrance analysis compared how much the mutation is seen in CF cases versus in the general population. *CFTR* mutations seen more commonly in the general population are suspicious that they are nonpenetrant (do not always result in CF) (see **Box 3** on penetrance/expressivity later). This evaluation yields 3 possible outcomes (**Box 2**): a mutation could be characterized as CF causing, as a mutation of varying clinical consequence (MVCC), or as non-CF causing.[13] The initial phase of the project studied the most common 159 *CFTR* mutations that had an allele frequency of 0.01% or greater in a group of nearly 40,000 patients, with subsequent updates resulting in 88,664 patients with CF studied and a total of 276 mutations annotated. **Table 1** summarizes available online resources to help interpret *CFTR* mutations.

Box 2

Categories of cystic fibrosis transmembrane conductance regulator mutations as defined by Clinical and Functional Translation of CFTR

The CFTR2 group is performing ongoing analysis of *CFTR* mutations to determine their likelihood to result in CF (disease liability). The following annotations are made based on the criteria detailed here:

CF-causing mutations: Mutations satisfying the 3 criteria listed next are characterized as CF-causing mutations.

- Clinical: Patients with one copy of the mutation and another copy of a known CF-causing mutation (such as F508del) have clinical features that satisfy the CF diagnostic criteria[14]; specifically, the mean sweat chloride of these patients is 60 mEq/L or greater.
- Functional: Mutations expected to result in a premature termination codon (class 1) are presumed dysfunctional and undergo no further testing. Mutations expected to result in an amino acid substitution or alter splicing efficiency are tested experimentally and deemed CF causing if they result in less than 10% of wild-type (nonmutated) CFTR protein levels or chloride conductance.
- Population/penetrance: Mutations with no evidence of reduced or nonpenetrance (that is, evidence supports that they will always cause CF when in *trans* with another CF-causing mutation) were used. Because there is no way to confirm full penetrance (without knowing everyone in the world's genotype and whether or not they have CF), the double negative of the following is intentional: CF-causing mutations have *no* evidence of *non*penetrance.

Mutation of varying clinical consequence (MVCC): Mutations not meeting clinical or functional criteria listed earlier but that have no evidence of nonpenetrance are characterized as MVCCs. These mutations may not always result in CF.

Non–CF-causing mutations: Mutations not meeting clinical and/or functional criteria listed earlier and that *do* have evidence of nonpenetrance are characterized as non-CF causing. Mutations are deemed to be nonpenetrant based on a study of fathers of CF offspring and evaluations of population frequencies of mutations. Rare individuals who have one non–CF-causing mutation in *trans* with a CF-causing mutation have presented with CFTR-related disorders or mild CF symptoms. For this reason, non–CF-causing mutations are not labeled as neutral or benign. However, these individuals are not expected to have life-limiting CF and represent only a small portion of those carrying non–CF-causing mutation in *trans* with a CF-causing mutation.

Table 1
Online resources to help characterize cystic fibrosis transmembrane conductance regulator mutations

Resource	Web Address	Information
CF Mutation Database	http://www.genet.sickkids.on.ca/app	Original site that described all variation in *CFTR* gene; useful to determine if a mutation has ever been seen before, describing a mutation using legacy and new nomenclature, and searching by location; contains some clinical and functional information, submitted by the clinic or laboratory that described the mutation
CFTR2	http://cftr2.org/index.php	Database of *CFTR* mutations seen in patients with CF; mutations annotated to describe their disease liability; useful to determine if a mutation is CF causing, of varying clinical consequence, or non-CF causing
The following Web sites are not CF specific but may be helpful as they describe variation across the genome.		
1000 genomes	http://browser.1000genomes.org/index.html	Data from the HapMAP project; variants in exon as well as intron
UCSC	https://genome.ucsc.edu/	Source that allows examination of variation in the entire genome
ExAC	http://exac.broadinstitute.org/	Summary information from several bioinformatics resources; mostly exonic data

Abbreviations: ExAC, Exome Aggregation Consortium; UCSC, University of California, Santa Cruz.

NOMENCLATURE AND TERMINOLOGY

Nomenclature recommendations for mutations within *CFTR* have changed over time, creating a challenge for clinicians, patients, and researchers. The same mutation within *CFTR* may have different names that are, or were at one time, accurate.

The *CFTR* DNA sequence (like nearly all genes) contains both exons (sections of DNA that code for the protein) and introns (sections between exons that do not code for protein). As DNA is transcribed into mRNA, the introns are removed in a process called splicing. The *CFTR* gene was originally thought to have 24 exons, which were numbered as such.[5] Subsequent findings indicated that there were actually 27, resulting in the addition of exons 6b, 14b, and 17b (exons 6, 14, and 17 renamed to 6a, 14a, and 17a, respectively).[15] Codon (protein) numbering has always begun with the first ATG (methionine) being codon 1, but the original nucleotide numbering of the *CFTR* gene began 132 bases 5′ from the A of the ATG initiation codon, such that this A existed at nucleotide position 133.

Following the development of the Human Genome Variation Society (HGVS), an attempt to standardize genetic nomenclature across all genes was undertaken.[16] This attempt resulted in the renumbering of *CFTR* nucleotides such that coding DNA position +1 now begins at the A of the initiation codon and differs from the colloquial numbering system by 132 bases. The amino acid numbering remains unchanged. Thus, the common mutation F508del ([delta]F508) was previously numbered to nucleotide position 1653 but now corresponds to c.1521. The 27 exons were also renumbered 1 to 27, eliminating the *a* and *b* versions. The *CFTR* mutation names before these changes are referred to as the legacy system.

The HGVS recommendations state that mutations should be described first at the DNA level and may also be described at the protein level. But because the CF community initially characterized most mutations using legacy nomenclature, most *CFTR* mutations have at least 3 names that may be recognizable and used in medical records. The legacy mutation G542X is now referred to as c.1624G>T (HGVS cDNA nomenclature) or p.Gly542Ter (HGVS protein nomenclature). Similarly, legacy mutation 2184insA is now known as c.2052delA or p.Lys684AsnfsX38. The difference in nucleotide numbering is due to the change in starting point described earlier.

When referring to a specific mutation in a patient's medical record, it is recommended to list HGVS and legacy names, if known. This practice decreases the chance for misinterpretation by those reviewing the medical records and gives greater assurance that a patient's mutations will be correctly recorded. It is also recommended to either include a copy of the genetic testing report in a patient's record or, if original records cannot be included, copy the nomenclature from the report verbatim, as incorrect transcription of a mutation name can result in confusion. Nomenclature for several common *CFTR* mutations is described in **Table 2**. Online resources, such as the CF Mutation Database and CFTR2, can be used to translate nomenclature.

CYSTIC FIBROSIS TRANSMEMBRANE CONDUCTANCE REGULATOR GENETIC TESTS

Genetic testing for *CFTR* has expanded tremendously. When considering which test to order, there are now a multitude of options, all with different capabilities and detection rates. These options are summarized in **Table 3**.

CFTR panels, which use a variety of technologies to test for a limited (23–150) number of known mutations, are the most common and least expensive. The percentage of true positives (detection rate) varies both by size of panel and by ethnicity of patient. Common CF mutations are more likely to be found in those of European and/or Ashkenazi Jewish ancestry and less likely to be found in those of Asian or African ancestry.[17,18]

Traditional full-gene *CFTR* sequencing will detect any sequence change in the exon or intron/exon border but will not detect large deletions or duplications. Sequencing is more expensive and has a longer turnaround time but is more comprehensive and is thought to detect 98% to 99% of sequence changes.

Table 2
Example nomenclature for select cystic fibrosis transmembrane conductance regulator mutations

Legacy Name	HGVS cDNA	HGVS Protein	Other Known or Accepted Names
[delta]F508	c.1521_1523delCTT	p.Phe508del	F508del, 1653delCTT, ΔF508
G551D	c.1652G>A	p.Gly551Asp	—
3849 + 10kbC>T	c.3717 + 12191C>T	No protein name	—
N1303K	c.3909C>G	c.Asn1303Lys	—
621 + 1G>T	c.489 + 1G>T	No protein name	—
3659delC	c.3528delC	p.Lys1177SerfsX15	—
2183AA>G	c.2051_2052delAAinsG	p.Lys684SerfsX38	2183delAA>G
1716G/A	c.1584G>A	p.(Glu528 =)	E528E

Table 3
Molecular testing options for cystic fibrosis transmembrane conductance regulator

CFTR Test	Capability and Limitations	Cost[a] ($)	Best Use
Mutation panel	Will detect specific mutations only; will not detect mutations not on panel; varied detection rate by panel size and patient ethnicity	300–600	For carrier screening or in patients with clear CF diagnosis who are Ashkenazi Jewish or of European ancestry
Traditional sequencing	Will detect all sequence variations in the exons and exon/intron junctions; will not detect large deletions or duplications	1500–2300	Patients with clear CF diagnosis who are not white; patients who have had incomplete results after panel testing
Deletion/ duplication testing	Will detect large deletions and duplication within *CFTR*; will not detect sequence changes	600–900	Patients who have had CFTR sequencing and <2 causative mutations have been identified
Next-generation sequencing	Will detect all sequence variations in exons and exon/intron junctions	>2500	Patients with clear CF diagnosis who are not white; screening algorithms where a staged approach is needed
Targeted mutation testing	Custom designed to detect only one or 2 specific mutations previously identified in a family	300–600	To confirm presence/absence of mutations in close relatives of patient (such as for carrier screening); may be useful in parental or sibling follow-up testing

[a] Costs are estimated based on US dollars, January 2016.

Some mutations are the result of large sections of the gene being duplicated or deleted (such as CFTRdele2,3 [deletion of exons 2 and 3]). A specialized test is usually necessary to detect these, although common deletions/duplications may be part of panels. Deletion and duplications are sometimes referred to as copy number variants. Testing is normally done by multiplex ligation probe amplification or array comparative genomic hybridization and is an entirely different method from sequencing. Typically these tests may need to be performed if sequencing has not identified 2 CF-causing mutations.

Next-generation sequencing (NGS) is a faster way to test large segments of DNA. Although the initial platforms are extremely expensive, the cost per test is cheaper than traditional sequencing. This technology is being used by more laboratories and will continue to grow as genetic analysis is used in more medical situations. NGS allows flexibility by customizing the bioinformatics analysis programs that interpret the raw sequencing results. As an example, this approach is being used for newborn screening.[19] Confirmed CF-causing mutations are reported out first, similar to a mutation panel. If 2 CF-causing mutations are not detected, subsequent results of MVCCs or uncharacterized variants are unblinded without the need to redraw blood or even reanalyze the specimen. In addition to saving unnecessary testing, this tiered approach also helps clinicians avoid the burden of interpreting variants of unknown significance, unless or until this is deemed clinically necessary for a patient in whom 2 obvious CF-causing mutations were not initially found.

GENETIC TESTING INTERPRETATION

A genetic counselor may be helpful in ordering and/or interpreting CF testing results and can work with the primary care physician and/or a CF provider. In some cases, CF genetic testing results may not be straightforward and will require follow-up or further explanation. Examples of this may include

- If more than two mutations are found, parental testing may be recommended to determine which mutations are in cis (on the same *CFTR* allele).
- Carrier screening and family planning may be done in coordination between the obstetrician, primary care doctor, and CF specialty clinic.
- For a positive family history of CF, appropriate review of previous familial genetic testing records is needed to choose the most appropriate testing strategy.

Despite improvements in genetic testing, there will remain a small number of patients with suspected CF who have fewer than 2 causative mutations identified after comprehensive studies. In these cases, the care team will need to consider one of the following: either the diagnosis of CF is incorrect; or CF is the correct diagnosis but current genetic testing technology is unable to find 2 causative mutations. Further physiologic testing, such as repeat sweat chloride measurement, nasal potential difference, or intestinal current measurement, may be helpful to determine if there is in vivo evidence of CFTR dysfunction. Alternative diagnoses may provide an explanation for a patient's symptoms, as conditions such as primary ciliary dyskinesia and pseudohypoaldosteronism, among others, are known to mimic some symptoms of CF. Diagnostic and/or genetic testing beyond *CFTR* should be based on the clinical manifestations that are most abnormal. For example, *SPINK1* and *PRSS1* may be considered for patients with pancreatitis. However, further diagnostic studies should be dictated by the severity of symptoms and clinical manifestations; some patients with only a few mild symptoms and a lack of compelling evidence of CFTR dysfunction may represent normal variation with no specific underlying condition. For instances in which all clinical history does indicate an underlying condition and diagnostic testing points to *CFTR* as the causative gene, further options for clinical genetic testing are limited. However, ongoing research studies may allow for additional investigation:

- Although sequencing and deletion/duplication testing are thought to detect greater than 99% of *CFTR* mutations, a significant portion of genetic material remains untouched after clinical testing. Intronic sequences are large and typically only interrogated in areas around the intron/exon junction and in regions with known intronic mutations. Deep sequencing of all introns and/or the promoter region may identify causative mutations not previously detected, though mutations identified using this method may remain categorized as mutations of unknown significance until or unless functional studies demonstrate an effect on CFTR. Deep sequencing is currently done on a research basis, though a limited number of laboratories are starting to offer this clinically; the spread of NGS technology may result in deep sequencing becoming more ubiquitous.
- Other studies may be performed on cells from patients with less than 2 causative *CFTR* mutations to determine whether or not CFTR is present in the correct quantity and conformation and whether or not it conducts chloride. Studies done on nasal scraping or brushing samples can interrogate *CFTR* on a transcriptional level (RNA). Even when a sequence change cannot be identified, determining whether or not *CFTR* transcript is affected can shed light on the

effect of the unidentified genetic change. These studies are currently done on a research basis.

Ultimately, CF is a clinical diagnosis. An experienced clinician with a strong suspicion should not delay treatment in the absence of a genetic diagnosis. Likewise, when genetic evidence of CF does not correlate with the clinical scenario (for example, when a homozygous mutation is found in asymptomatic carrier screening), the clinical information takes precedent. It is important to note that for the many CFTR mutations that are not annotated or are known to have varying clinical consequences, clinical criteria must be used to determine if an individual has CF. (See Rosenfeld M, Sontag M, Ren CL: Cystic Fibrosis Diagnosis and Newborn Screening, in this issue.) (**Box 3**).

GENOTYPE AND PHENOTYPE RELATIONSHIPS IN CYSTIC FIBROSIS

Heterogeneity in CF disease severity was noted decades before the discovery of CFTR.[20] Before knowledge of a specific genetic defect, patients with CF were noted to have a wide spectrum of survival as well as nutritional and pulmonary outcomes.[20,21] Patients with CF and normal fat absorption had milder clinical symptoms, lower mean sweat chloride values, and higher lung function compared with those with steatorrhea.[21] It was speculated that variation in disease severity was the result of genetic and environmental factors.[22]

Over the past 25 years since CFTR was identified, the more commonly seen mutations have been delineated as high risk or low risk.[23,24] Patients with 2 CFTR mutations with minimal CFTR function (high risk) are generally pancreatic insufficient with more severe lung disease, and those with at least one CFTR mutation with residual CFTR function (low risk) are generally pancreatic sufficient with improved pulmonary outcomes and survival.[23]

Fundamentally, all mutations must disrupt CFTR protein quantity or function in order to cause CF. The best-established paradigm to categorize the molecular

---

Box 3
Defining penetrance and expressivity

Within CF and other genetic conditions, it is also important to differentiate between the terms penetrance and expressivity when discussing a CF phenotype. Penetrance refers to the proportion of people with a given genetic mutation who will exhibit symptoms of a condition. In CF, this refers to the proportion of people with a specific genotype or mutation who will meet the diagnostic criteria for CF. Mutations or genotypes that always lead to CF are said to be 100% penetrant. The common mutation F508del is thought to be 100% penetrant, when combined with another 100% penetrant mutation, meaning that every person with the genotype F508del/F508del is expected to have CF. Other mutations, such as the more variable D1152H, are less than 100% penetrant because not all people with this mutation, even in combination with something like F508del, will have CF.

The term expressivity refers to the phenotypic signs and symptoms expressed by different people with the same condition. For example, 2 people who both have CF may have different features of the condition: one may have pancreatic insufficiency and CF-related diabetes, whereas the other may have pancreatic insufficiency and CF-related liver disease but no diabetes. This situation is called variable expressivity. Although penetrance refers to whether or not someone will have a condition, expressivity refers to how that condition will manifest.

There are many factors that influence a mutation's penetrance and expressivity. Haplotype background (variation within CFTR), modifier genes, and environment all play a role in whether or not a mutation will cause CF and how the disease will manifest.

consequences has grouped mutations in *CFTR* into functional classes based on the mechanism by which the CFTR protein is disrupted.[25–27] These classes are described in **Table 4** and shown in **Fig. 1**. This scheme provides a framework to categorize mutations in *CFTR*, but there are some drawbacks. For example, several mutations have characteristics of more than one functional class (eg, F508del and R117H).[28] Class for missense mutations resulting in an amino acid substitution cannot be predicted from sequence alone, requiring that the mutation be functionally evaluated in a laboratory. Clinical circumstances in which a patient's disease severity does match the predicted severity of their genotype have been clues to detect mutations that may disrupt CFTR function in unexpected or novel ways, such as leading to alternative splicing of the mRNA.[29,30]

Better molecular understanding of *CFTR* mutations is a necessary step to inform the emerging arsenal of CFTR modulators that it is hoped will permit personalized medicine for patients with CF.[31] The categories of CFTR modulators being investigated include (1) stop codon read-through agents, (2) potentiators that increase CFTR channel function at the cell surface (eg, ivacaftor), and (3) correctors that improve trafficking of mutant CFTR to the cell surface (eg, lumacaftor). (See a detailed description in Ong T, Ramsey BW: New Therapeutic Approaches to Modulate and Correct CFTR, in this issue.)[31] The response of a given mutation to a CFTR-specific therapy will be an important complement to the traditional mutation classes. It will be helpful to know not only that a given mutation is class II but also whether or not it responds to a specific CFTR potentiator and corrector. Functional testing to evaluate and class mutations will need to also test for these "theratypes."[27,31] It is essential that care providers know each patient's *CFTR* mutations for optimal patient education and care.

SPECTRUM OF DISORDERS WITH MUTATIONS IN CYSTIC FIBROSIS TRANSMEMBRANE CONDUCTANCE REGULATOR

Most of the emphasis on *CFTR* mutations has been on individuals with CF. However, there are related phenotypes in which CFTR dysfunction may be playing a role but that do not meet the diagnostic criteria of CF. There are 2 entities that describe individuals with an inconclusive diagnosis of CF based on sweat chloride testing and *CFTR* mutational analyses. (See Rosenfeld M, Sontag M, Ren CL: Cystic Fibrosis Diagnosis and Newborn Screening, in this issue.)

First, the entities CFTR-related metabolic syndrome (CRMS, United States) and Cystic Fibrosis Screen-Positive-Inconclusive Diagnosis (CFSPID, Europe) both

Table 4
Cystic fibrosis transmembrane conductance regulator mutation classes

Mutation Class	CFTR Defect	Examples	Risk Category
I	Defective biosynthesis; little to no protein made	G542X, 1717-1G->A	High risk (associated with pancreatic insufficiency)
II	Defective protein processing and trafficking to the cell surface	F508del, N1303K	
III	Abnormal gating	G551D, S549N	
IV	Defective chloride conductance	D1152H, R334W	Low risk (associated with pancreatic sufficiency)
V	Reduced protein quantity	3849+10kbC->T, 5T	
VI	Reduced stability at cell surface	4236delTC	Risk not classified

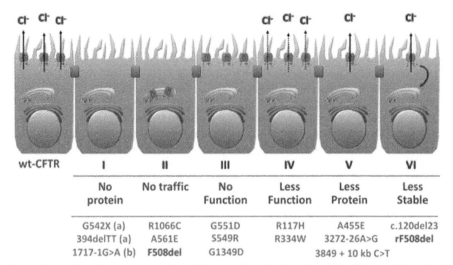

wt-CFTR	I	II	III	IV	V	VI
	No protein	No traffic	No Function	Less Function	Less Protein	Less Stable
	G542X (a)	R1066C	G551D	R117H	A455E	c.120del23
	394delTT (a)	A561E	S549R	R334W	3272-26A>G	rF508del
	1717-1G>A (b)	F508del	G1349D		3849 + 10 kb C>T	

Fig. 1. Mutations classes grouped by CFTR protein. Cl⁻, chloride; WT, wild type. (*From* Bell SC, De Boeck K, Amaral MD. New pharmacological approaches for cystic fibrosis: promises, progress, pitfalls. Pharmacol Ther 2015;145:19–34; with permission.)

describe infants with a positive newborn screen but indeterminate diagnostic testing.[37,38] The specific results of *CFTR* mutation analysis and sweat chloride values associated with these conditions, but both include generally asymptomatic infants recommended for ongoing monitoring in a CF center as a small proportion may develop clinical features of CF. Second, CFTR-related disorder (CFTR-RD) describes symptomatic individuals with single-organ system clinical features associated with CFTR dysfunction but who do not fulfill diagnostic criteria for CF.[39] The most common clinical conditions in the spectrum of CFTR-RD are (1) bronchiectasis, (2) acute recurrent or chronic pancreatitis, (3) congenital bilateral absence of the vas deferens (CBAVD), and (4) chronic sinusitis.[39–41] There are no specific *CFTR* mutations associated with either CRMS/CFSPID or CFTR-RD, but such individuals typically have at least one mild *CFTR* mutation. Evaluation of an individual with these conditions may require a *CFTR* mutational analysis that includes mutations with residual CFTR function or that are associated with partial penetrance.

Approximately 3% of cases of male infertility are explained by CBAVD, with an estimated prevalence of 1:1000 males. The vas deferens seems to be the tissue most sensitive to reduced CFTR function. Although not all individuals with CBAVD have *CFTR* mutations, a higher-than-expected proportion of those with CBAVD have either one (CF carriers) or 2 identified mutations.[42] The two most common compound heterozygotes are F508del in *trans* with 5T or with R117H. *CFTR* mutation analysis, including the poly-thymidine and TG tracts, is recommended for a complete evaluation for male infertility (**Box 4**).[39,40]

Approximately 30% of patients who have idiopathic chronic pancreatitis have one or 2 *CFTR* mutations (with no preexisting CF diagnosis). As with CBAVD, most patients have at least one mutation associated with residual function. The risk of pancreatitis is increased 40-fold if patients have 2 mild CFTR mutations and is increased much more if individuals have 1 mild CFTR mutation and coinheritance of a common mutation in either *SPINK1* or *PRSS1*.[39,43]

There is also increased incidence of *CFTR* mutations in patients with non-CF bronchiectasis.[44] There are widely varying estimates for the prevalence of such patients

---

Box 4
R117H and intron 9 modifiers

The CFTR mutation R117H is relatively common and a recognized cause of CF but is heavily influenced by another element in the same *CFTR* gene. Following its discovery shortly after *CFTR* was identified, R117H was noted to have reduced penetrance for CF.[32,33] This reduction in penetrance was found to depend on variation within the ninth intron (IVS8 in legacy numbering), which affects the amount of correctly spliced exon 10. The variation responsible is a series of thymidine nucleotides present in all individuals, typically in the form of 5, 7, or 9 thymidine repeats. Decreasing length of the poly-thymidine (poly-T) tract correlates with the decreasing amount of full-length *CFTR* (containing all exons) and higher risk of a CF phenotype.

- R117H with 5T: acts as a CF-causing mutation; expected to cause CF when combined with another CF-causing mutation on the other allele (such as F508del)

- R117H with 7T: acts as a MVCC; may result in CF when combined with a CF-causing mutation on the other allele but more commonly results in a CFTR-related disorder or no phenotype[34]

- R117H with 9T: a very rare combination that is thought to result in no disease

In the absence of R117H, the 5T variation of the poly-T tract may still affect CFTR. This effect depends on another intragenic modifier with intron 9: the TG dinucleotide repeat tract, which further influences the effect of 5T on exon 10 splicing.[35,36] Each *CFTR* gene has a TG tract of varying length, usually with 11, 12, or 13 TG repeats. Increasing TG tract length correlates with the decreased amount of full-length *CFTR*, thereby leading to higher likelihood of a CF phenotype.

- 5T with TG13: may cause CF when combined with a CF-causing mutation on the other allele

- 5T with TG12: may cause CF when combined with a CF-causing mutation on the other allele

- 5T with TG11: unlikely to result in CF

---

having at least one *CFTR* mutation (range 10%–50%) or 2 *CFTR* mutations (range 5%–20%).[39] Most associated *CFTR* mutations in patients with non-CF bronchiectasis have residual CFTR function, and there is a high incidence of the 5T allele.

BEYOND CYSTIC FIBROSIS TRANSMEMBRANE CONDUCTANCE REGULATOR: GENETIC MODIFIERS OF CYSTIC FIBROSIS

The wide range in lung function, nutritional status, and survival among patients with CF with the most common *CFTR* genotype, F508del homozygous, provides evidence that the *CFTR* genotype is not the only determinant of the CF phenotype.[22,28] The genotype-phenotype relationships in CF are tissue specific and impacted by other factors. These factors include stochastic (random) variables, environmental factors, as well as genetic factors apart from *CFTR* genotype. Common or rare variants in other genes can significantly affect clinical outcomes in CF.[45–47] Genetic modifiers have been identified for nutritional outcomes (eg, body mass index, locus on Chr1p36.1), meconium ileus (eg, *SLC6A14*), cirrhotic liver disease (Z-allele of *SERPINA*), CF-related diabetes (eg, *TCF7L2, SLC26A9*), severity of airway obstruction (eg, *TGFbeta-1, APIP*), and infection with *Pseudomonas aeruginosa* (eg, *MBL2, SLC6A14, DCTN4, CAV2, TMC6*).[28,47–49] Thus, future personalized medicine may include knowledge of a patient's *CFTR* mutations and key genetic modifiers. In the future, patients with confirmed high-risk genetic modifiers for specific traits may have more frequent monitoring and more intensive therapeutic interventions. More importantly, the knowledge gained from genetic modifiers may provide new therapeutic targets to improve outcomes for patients with CF.

REFERENCES

1. Andersen DH, Hodges RG. Celiac syndrome; genetics of cystic fibrosis of the pancreas, with a consideration of etiology. Am J Dis Child 1946;72:62–80.
2. Botstein D, White RL, Skolnick M, et al. Construction of a genetic linkage map in man using restriction fragment length polymorphisms. Am J Hum Genet 1980;32: 314–31.
3. Quinton PM. Chloride impermeability in cystic fibrosis. Nature 1983;301:421–2.
4. Kerem B, Rollins BM, Tarran R. Identification of the cystic fibrosis gene: genetic analysis. Science 1989;245:1073–80.
5. Riordan JR, Rommens JM, Kerem B, et al. Identification of the cystic fibrosis gene: cloning and characterization of complementary DNA. Science 1989;245: 1066–73.
6. Rommens JM, Iannuzzi MC, Kerem B, et al. Identification of the cystic fibrosis gene: chromosome walking and jumping. Science 1989;245:1059–65.
7. Cutting GR, Antonarakis SE, Buetow KH, et al. Analysis of DNA polymorphism haplotypes linked to the cystic fibrosis locus in North American black and Caucasian families supports the existence of multiple mutations of the cystic fibrosis gene. Am J Hum Genet 1989;44:307–18.
8. Cutting GR, Kasch LM, Rosenstein BJ, et al. A cluster of cystic fibrosis mutations in the first nucleotide-binding fold of the cystic fibrosis conductance regulator protein. Nature 1990;346:366–9.
9. Cystic Fibrosis Mutation Database. Available at: http://www.genet.sickkids.on.ca/app. Accessed January 7, 2016.
10. Rohlfs EM, Zhou Z, Sugarman EA, et al. The I148T CFTR allele occurs on multiple haplotypes: a complex allele is associated with cystic fibrosis. Genet Med 2002; 4:319–23.
11. CFTR2@Johns Hopkins - Home Page. Available at: http://cftr2.org/. Accessed January 7, 2016.
12. McKone EF, Velentgas P, Swenson AJ, et al. Association of sweat chloride concentration at time of diagnosis and CFTR genotype with mortality and cystic fibrosis phenotype. J Cyst Fibros 2015;14:580–6.
13. Sosnay PR, Siklosi KR, Van Goor F, et al. Defining the disease liability of variants in the cystic fibrosis transmembrane conductance regulator gene. Nat Genet 2013;45:1160–7.
14. Farrell PM, Rosenstein BJ, White TB, et al. Guidelines for diagnosis of cystic fibrosis in newborns through older adults: Cystic Fibrosis Foundation consensus report. J Pediatr 2008;153:S4–14.
15. Tsui L-C, Romeo G, Greger R, et al. The identification of the CF (cystic fibrosis) gene: recent progress and new research strategies. Springer Science & Business Media; 2013. Available at: http://www.ncbi.nlm.nih.gov/pmc/articles/PMC1682659/?page=1.
16. Beaudet AL, Tsui LC. A suggested nomenclature for designating mutations. Hum Mutat 1993;2:245–8.
17. Bobadilla JL, Macek M, Fine JP, et al. Cystic fibrosis: a worldwide analysis of CFTR mutations–correlation with incidence data and application to screening. Hum Mutat 2002;19:575–606.
18. Schrijver I, Pique L, Graham S, et al. The spectrum of CFTR variants in nonwhite cystic fibrosis patients: implications for molecular diagnostic testing. J Mol Diagn 2016;18:39–50.

19. Baker MW, Atkins AE, Cordovado SK, et al. Improving newborn screening for cystic fibrosis using next-generation sequencing technology: a technical feasibility study. Genet Med 2015;18(3):231–8.
20. Gurwitz D, Corey M, Francis PW, et al. Perspectives in cystic fibrosis. Pediatr Clin North Am 1979;26:603–15.
21. Gaskin K, Gurwitz D, Durie P, et al. Improved respiratory prognosis in patients with cystic fibrosis with normal fat absorption. J Pediatr 1982;100:857–62.
22. Kerem E, Corey M, Kerem BS, et al. The relation between genotype and phenotype in cystic fibrosis–analysis of the most common mutation (delta F508). N Engl J Med 1990;323:1517–22.
23. McKone EF, Goss CH, Aitken ML. CFTR genotype as a predictor of prognosis in cystic fibrosis. Chest 2006;130:1441–7.
24. Green DM, McDougal KE, Blackman SM, et al. Mutations that permit residual CFTR function delay acquisition of multiple respiratory pathogens in CF patients. Respir Res 2010;11:140.
25. Welsh MJ, Smith AE. Molecular mechanisms of CFTR chloride channel dysfunction in cystic fibrosis. Cell 1993;73:1251–4.
26. Bombieri C, Seia M, Castellani C. Genotypes and phenotypes in cystic fibrosis and cystic fibrosis transmembrane regulator-related disorders. Semin Respir Crit Care Med 2015;36:180–93.
27. Bell SC, De Boeck K, Amaral MD. New pharmacological approaches for cystic fibrosis: promises, progress, pitfalls. Pharmacol Ther 2015;145:19–34.
28. Cutting GR. Cystic fibrosis genetics: from molecular understanding to clinical application. Nat Rev Genet 2015;16:45–56.
29. Molinski SV, Gonska T, Huan LJ, et al. Genetic, cell biological, and clinical interrogation of the CFTR mutation c.3700 A>G (p.Ile1234Val) informs strategies for future medical intervention. Genet Med 2014;16:625–32.
30. Hinzpeter A, Aissat A, Sondo E, et al. Alternative splicing at a NAGNAG acceptor site as a novel phenotype modifier. PLoS Genet 2010;6. Available at: http://www.ncbi.nlm.nih.gov/pubmed/20949073.
31. Elborn JS. Personalised medicine for cystic fibrosis: treating the basic defect. Eur Respir Rev 2013;22:3–5.
32. Kiesewetter S, Macek M Jr, Davis C, et al. A mutation in CFTR produces different phenotypes depending on chromosomal background. Nat Genet 1993;5:274–8.
33. Chu CS, Trapnell BC, Curristin S, et al. Genetic basis of variable exon 9 skipping in cystic fibrosis transmembrane conductance regulator mRNA. Nat Genet 1993;3:151–6.
34. Thauvin-Robinet C, Munck A, Huet F, et al. The very low penetrance of cystic fibrosis for the R117H mutation: a reappraisal for genetic counselling and newborn screening. J Med Genet 2009;46:752–8.
35. Cuppens H, Lin W, Jaspers M, et al. Polyvariant mutant cystic fibrosis transmembrane conductance regulator genes. The polymorphic (Tg)m locus explains the partial penetrance of the T5 polymorphism as a disease mutation. J Clin Invest 1998;101:487–96.
36. Sun W, Anderson B, Redman J, et al. CFTR 5T variant has a low penetrance in females that is partially attributable to its haplotype. Genet Med 2006;8:339–45.
37. Cystic Fibrosis Foundation, Borowitz D, Parad RB, et al. Cystic Fibrosis Foundation practice guidelines for the management of infants with cystic fibrosis transmembrane conductance regulator-related metabolic syndrome during the first two years of life and beyond. J Pediatr 2009;155:S106–16.

38. Munck A, Mayell SJ, Winters V, et al. Cystic Fibrosis Screen Positive, Inconclusive Diagnosis (CFSPID): a new designation and management recommendations for infants with an inconclusive diagnosis following newborn screening. J Cyst Fibros 2015;14:706–13.

39. Bombieri C, Claustres M, De Boeck K, et al. Recommendations for the classification of diseases as CFTR-related disorders. J Cyst Fibros 2011;10(Suppl 2): S86–102.

40. Moskowitz S, Chmiel JF, Sternen DL, et al. Clinical practice and genetic counseling for cystic fibrosis and CFTR-related disorders. Genet Med 2008;10: 851–68.

41. Wang X, Moylan B, Leopold DA, et al. Mutation in the gene responsible for cystic fibrosis and predisposition to chronic rhinosinusitis in the general population. JAMA 2000;284:1814–9.

42. Wilschanski M, Dupuis A, Ellis L, et al. Mutations in the cystic fibrosis transmembrane regulator gene and in vivo transepithelial potentials. Am J Respir Crit Care Med 2006;174:787–94.

43. Masson E, Chen J-M. A conservative assessment of the major genetic causes of idiopathic chronic pancreatitis: data from a comprehensive analysis of PRSS1, SPINK1, CTRC and CFTR genes in 253 young French patients. PLoS One 2013;8:e73522.

44. Gonska T, Choi P, Stephenson A, et al. Role of cystic fibrosis transmembrane conductance regulator in patients with chronic sinopulmonary disease. Chest 2012;142:996–1004.

45. Drumm ML, Konstan MW, Schluchter MD, et al. Genetic modifiers of lung disease in cystic fibrosis. N Engl J Med 2005;353:1443–53.

46. Blackman SM, Commander CW, Watson C, et al. Genetic modifiers of cystic fibrosis-related diabetes. Diabetes 2013;62:3627–35.

47. Corvol H, Blackman SM, Boëlle PY, et al. Genome-wide association meta-analysis identifies five modifier loci of lung disease severity in cystic fibrosis. Nat Commun 2015;6:8382.

48. Emond MJ, Louie T, Emerson J, et al. Exome sequencing of phenotypic extremes identifies CAV2 and TMC6 as interacting modifiers of chronic pseudomonas aeruginosa infection in cystic fibrosis. PLoS Genet 2015;11:e1005273.

49. Bartlett JR, Friedman KJ, Ling SC, et al. Genetic modifiers of liver disease in cystic fibrosis. JAMA 2009;302:1076–83.

Cystic Fibrosis Diagnosis and Newborn Screening

Margaret Rosenfeld, MD, MPH[a],*, Marci K. Sontag, PhD[b], Clement L. Ren, MD[c]

KEYWORDS

- Cystic fibrosis • Diagnosis • Newborn screening • Sweat chloride • Mutation

KEY POINTS

- Most new diagnoses of cystic fibrosis (CF) are now identified by newborn screening, which provides the opportunity to improve outcomes by initiating monitoring and treatments in the presymptomatic period.
- The sweat chloride measurement is still the cornerstone of CF diagnosis. It should be performed according to national guidelines. Sweat conductivity and osmolality are not acceptable substitutes.
- In the United States, newborn screening algorithms vary by state, although all involve measurement of immunoreactive trypsinogen in the dried blood spot and most involve genetic testing with a panel of CF transmembrane conductance regulator (CFTR) mutations.
- CF newborn screening inevitably identifies infants with indeterminate diagnoses (referred to interchangeably as CF-related metabolic syndrome in the United States and CF screen–positive, inconclusive diagnosis in Europe). Although most of these infants do not develop signs or symptoms of CF, they should be monitored regularly at least in the first few years of life, because some will develop evidence of CFTR dysfunction.

INTRODUCTION

The landscape of the diagnosis of cystic fibrosis (CF) has changed dramatically over the past decade, as universal screening for CF has become a reality in all 50 states in the United States since 2010. Most countries with a high prevalence of CF around the world have also implemented universal CF newborn screening. Now, instead of being diagnosed based on symptoms, typically after having endured a long, difficult, and expensive diagnostic odyssey, most individuals are diagnosed after a positive

Disclosures: The authors have no relationships with commercial entities to disclose.
[a] Division of Pulmonary Medicine, Seattle Children's Hospital, University of Washington School of Medicine, 4800 Sand Point Way Northeast, Seattle, WA 98105, USA; [b] Department of Epidemiology, Colorado School of Public Health, Anshutz Medical Center, University of Colorado, 13001 East 17th, Aurora, CO 80045, USA; [c] Section of Pediatric Pulmonology, Allergy, and Sleep Medicine, James Whitcomb Riley Hospital for Children, Indiana University School of Medicine, 705 Riley Hospital Drive, ROC 4270, Indianapolis, IN 46202, USA
* Corresponding author.
E-mail address: margaret.rosenfeld@seattlechildrens.org

Pediatr Clin N Am 63 (2016) 599–615
http://dx.doi.org/10.1016/j.pcl.2016.04.004
0031-3955/16/$ – see front matter © 2016 Elsevier Inc. All rights reserved.

pediatric.theclinics.com

newborn screen. In 2013, 62% of new diagnoses in the United States were detected by newborn screening.[1] Early diagnosis affords the opportunity to improve long-term outcomes through close monitoring and appropriate interventions beginning before severe nutritional deficits or irreversible airway damage have occurred. As CF transmembrane conductance regulator (CFTR) modulator therapies that treat the basic defect in CF become available across a broad range of ages and CFTR genotypes, initiation of these therapies in infancy holds the promise of being disease modifying.

However, even in the current era of universal newborn screening, some individuals are diagnosed symptomatically, either because they were born before implementation of newborn screening or in regions in which newborn screening was not offered, or because of a false-negative newborn screen. Thus, clinicians must always maintain an index of suspicion for CF in individuals with 1 or more signs or symptoms of CF, regardless of age or newborn screening results.

Since identification of the *CFTR* gene on the long arm of chromosome 7 in 1989, it has become increasingly clear that CFTR dysfunction encompasses a wide range of phenotypes, from classic pancreatic-insufficient CF, to single-organ-system manifestations often diagnosed in adulthood, to indeterminate diagnoses in infants identified by newborn screening. Thus, although the diagnosis of CF is straightforward in most cases, with a sweat chloride level greater than or equal to 60 mmol/L and/or 2 CF-causing mutations identified, establishing the diagnosis in the minority of patients in whom these diagnostic conditions are not met can be challenging and time consuming. Newer diagnostic modalities, such as nasal potential difference and intestinal current measurements, can also be used to assess CFTR dysfunction and aid in diagnosis, but are currently only conducted at specialized centers.

ESTABLISHING THE DIAGNOSIS OF CYSTIC FIBROSIS
General Principles

The US CF Foundation has convened 3 panels of experts to establish and then refine the diagnostic criteria for CF (**Box 1**), first in 1996,[2] then in 2007,[3] and most recently in 2015. As of the writing of this article, the most recent guidelines are still in draft form. In addition, a European consensus conference established a similar diagnostic algorithm.[4] Although understanding of the heterogeneity of disease presentation and of the complexity of *CFTR* mutations has greatly increased, many of the basic tenets of establishing the diagnosis have remained virtually unchanged. The sweat chloride test remains the cornerstone of diagnosis, because it directly measures CFTR function. Proper performance of the sweat chloride test, which is crucial for the accurate diagnosis of CF, requires skill and experience. The sweat chloride test should be

---

Box 1
Diagnostic criteria for CF

Positive newborn screen

Or signs/symptoms suggestive of CF

Or positive family history in a parent or sibling

And:

Either a sweat chloride level greater than or equal to 60 mmol/L

Or identification of 2 CF-causing mutations in *trans*

Or nasal potential difference measurement consistent with CF

conducted in accordance with established guidelines.[5] It involves transdermal administration of pilocarpine by iontophoresis to stimulate sweat gland secretion, followed by sweat collection into a Macroduct coil, gauze, or filter paper, and analysis of chloride concentration. A sweat chloride level greater than or equal to 60 mmol/L is consistent with a diagnosis of CF.[3] In this era of precision medicine, it is recommended that *CFTR* mutation analysis also be performed as part of the diagnostic evaluation. Identification of 2 CF-causing mutations in *trans* is consistent with the diagnosis of CF.[3] Although ~ 1800 mutations have been identified in the *CFTR* gene, to date the minority have been established to be disease causing. The CFTR2 Web site (http://www.cftr2. org/) has the most up-to-date information on *CFTR* mutations and their phenotypic consequences (see Sosnay PR, Raraigh KS, Gibson RL: Molecular Genetics of CFTR: Genotype and Phenotype, in this issue).

Diagnosing Cystic Fibrosis in Newborn-screened Infants

It is critical to acknowledge that newborn screening is only a screening test and does not establish the diagnosis of CF. Even infants with 2 CF-causing mutations identified on the dried blood spot need a sweat chloride test to establish the diagnosis, although they may carry a presumptive diagnosis of CF so that initiation of therapies such as pancreatic enzymes is not delayed. Infants with a positive CF newborn screen should be rapidly referred for sweat chloride testing in order to avoid delays in treatment. Sweat chloride testing can be performed in infants more than 2 kg and 10 days of age, and ideally should be performed in the neonatal period (ie, before 30 days of age).

- A sweat chloride value greater than or equal to 60 mmol/L in an infant with a positive newborn screen is consistent with a diagnosis of CF. Genetic testing should also be performed to confirm the diagnosis and potentially aid in treatment and discussions of prognosis.
- A value less than 30 mmol/L makes CF unlikely, although on rare occasions infants with 2 CF-causing mutations can have a normal sweat chloride value.
- A value of 30 to 59 mmol/L suggests possible CF and further testing is required, generally to include extended CFTR mutation analysis.
  - If 2 CF-causing mutations are identified, the diagnosis of CF can be established.
  - If 0 or 1 CF-causing mutations are identified, the infant is diagnosed with CFTR-related metabolic syndrome (CRMS)/CF screen–positive, inconclusive diagnosis (CFSPID), which is discussed later.
- All infants with a diagnosis of CF or an indeterminate diagnosis should be referred to a specialized CF center for ongoing monitoring and care. Guidelines for the care of infants with CF have been published.[6]
- Meconium ileus may produce a false-negative CF newborn screen, but is highly likely to be associated with CF. Therefore, all infants presenting with meconium ileus, regardless of newborn screening result, should carry the presumptive diagnosis of CF until further testing can be accomplished.

Diagnosing Cystic Fibrosis in Symptomatic Individuals

Any child or adult presenting with signs of symptoms of CF (**Box 2**) or a positive family history should undergo diagnostic testing, regardless of newborn screening results. In general, the sweat chloride test is the initial procedure.

- A sweat chloride level greater than or equal to 60 mmol/L is consistent with a diagnosis of CF. A second, confirmatory sweat chloride test is recommended unless 2 CF-causing mutations are identified by genetic testing.

Box 2
Signs and symptoms suggestive of CFTR dysfunction in children and adolescents

Nutritional and gastrointestinal:
- Nutritional/metabolic: failure to thrive, hypoproteinemia, hypochloremic dehydration, chronic metabolic alkalosis
- Intestinal: meconium ileus, rectal prolapse, distal intestinal obstructive syndrome, steatorrhea
- Pancreatic: exocrine pancreatic insufficiency, recurrent pancreatitis
- Hepatic: protracted neonatal jaundice, biliary cirrhosis

Sinopulmonary:
- Chronic wet or productive cough
- Bronchiectasis on chest imaging
- Respiratory infection with *Pseudomonas aeruginosa* or other atypical gram-negative organisms
- Nasal polyposis in children
- Digital clubbing
- Allergic bronchopulmonary aspergillosis

Obstructive azoospermia in boys

- A sweat chloride level less than or equal to 39 mmol/L in individuals more than 6 months of age makes CF unlikely. If clinical suspicion remains high, genetic testing can be performed. Identification of 2 CF-causing mutations if there are symptoms or a positive family history is consistent with the diagnosis of CF.
- If the sweat chloride level is in the intermediate range (40–59 mmol/L if aged >6 months and 30–59 mmol/L if aged <6 months), extended genetic testing should be performed, potentially including gene sequencing and evaluation for deletions/duplications.
  - If 2 CF-causing mutations are identified, the diagnosis of CF is established.
  - Individuals with no or 1 CF-causing mutation and clinical signs or symptoms of CFTR dysfunction may be diagnosed with CFTR-related disorder (CFTR-RD). Sweat chloride testing should be repeated. If the sweat chloride level remains in the intermediate range, a referral should be made to a specialized CF center for further evaluation, which may include expanded genetic testing, lung function testing, chest imaging, respiratory culture, fecal elastase to evaluate exocrine pancreatic function, genital evaluation in boys and specialized tests of CFTR function such as nasal potential difference and intestinal current measurements.

CYSTIC FIBROSIS NEWBORN SCREENING
Rationale for Screening for Cystic Fibrosis: the Impact of Early Diagnosis on Cystic Fibrosis Outcomes

The natural history of CF makes it distinct among disorders that are currently on the Recommended Uniform Screening Panel (RUSP) maintained by the US Secretary of Health and Human Services.[7] Most of the disorders on the RUSP are responsive to treatment in the first weeks of life, resulting in a dramatic change in the natural history of the disorder, avoiding significant morbidity and even mortality. Although it is well known that pancreatic disease leading to malabsorption and malnutrition is present at birth,[8–13] and lung disease starts early in infancy in CF,[14–18] a definitive treatment has not been available that would stop disease progression in CF. Nonetheless, epidemiologic and clinical evidence accumulated throughout the 1980s and 1990s such that the Centers for Disease Control and Prevention (CDC) issued a statement in 2004 that newborn screening for CF is justified based on the benefits of early intervention and nutritional management.[19] The strongest evidence of the benefit of early identification through newborn screening that supported the decision by the CDC was in the treatment of early malabsorption and improved growth.[20,21] Additional reports provided evidence of screened infants experiencing decreased pulmonary complications,[22] opportunities to address early vitamin E deficiency associated with lower cognitive function,[23] and a potential survival advantage associated with an earlier diagnosis,[24,25] although the CDC decision to recommend CF newborn screening was driven by improved nutritional outcomes. The long-term pulmonary benefits of CF newborn screening remain more controversial.[26]

As newborn screening for CF has become universally adopted in the United States and internationally, studies on the early course of disease and evidence in support of early identification and treatment have become more prevalent.[27,28] Epidemiologic and clinical studies continue to provide critical information about early growth restriction in CF while providing additional evidence of the early onset of lung disease, showing the need for early therapies before onset of irreversible stunting and lung damage (**Table 1**). Despite catch-up growth in weight following newborn screening,[20] linear growth impairment occurs during the first year, even among newborn-screened infants, suggesting that earlier and more aggressive nutritional therapy may be necessary to achieve normal growth.[29] Further, it is clear that lung disease is present in the first months of life, and, despite guidelines for early care[6] and more aggressive approaches to treat CF lung disease,[30–32] the ability to change the early course of lung disease in CF has been limited. Recent studies have shown that CFTR modulators that are targeted toward specific *CFTR* mutations can improve CFTR function, with resulting improvements in weight and lung function in adults and older children with CF.[33,34] These revolutionary new drug therapies may be able to prevent the onset of lung disease and other complications of CF if started early in life; however, safety and efficacy studies in younger children must be completed, and the clinical community is proceeding with appropriate caution.[35]

General Principles of Newborn Screening

Newborn screening is based on the early tenets of Wilson and Jungner[36] that there must be (1) an acceptable treatment or intervention, (2) a cost-effective screening method, and (3) appropriate confirmatory testing. More recently, revised guidelines have been published to help guide decision makers about the inclusion of new disorders on the newborn screening panel in the era of rapid expansion of newborn

Table 1
Ongoing surveillance programs show the importance of early identification to avoid permanent growth deficits and irreversible lung damage

System	Key Findings
Pulmonary	Respiratory infection in infancy is associated with poor pulmonary function later in childhood[79]
	Lung function is abnormal early in infancy,[80] and early abnormalities are associated with poor lung function at 1 y[81]
	Structural lung disease is present in infants and progresses through childhood[82]
Growth and nutrition	Length, but not weight, in infants is stunted at 1 y, despite early interventions[29]

screening panels caused by multiplex testing and genomic screening.[37–39] In the United States, the public health system within each state is responsible for implementing newborn screening at the state level. Adoption and implementation of screening for disorders within each state can vary widely because of local resources and legislative and regulatory constraints.[40] Each state also determines the specific processes for follow-up on abnormal results.

History of Newborn Screening for Cystic Fibrosis

Crossley and colleagues[41] from Auckland, New Zealand, established the foundation for CF newborn screening in the 1970s by measuring immunoreactive trypsinogen (IRT) on a dried blood spot specimen using a radioimmunoassay.[42] Screening for CF was adopted internationally through adaptation of this technique, beginning in East Anglia, United Kingdom, and New South Wales, Australia.[17,43] In 1982, Colorado became the first US state to initiate CF newborn screening,[44] followed shortly thereafter by Wisconsin. The Wisconsin Cystic Fibrosis Neonatal Screening Project was a randomized trial of newborn screening for CF, showing both its feasibility and the long-term efficacy of newborn screening for nutritional outcomes.[20]

Initially, uptake of CF newborn screening was slow internationally as well as within the United States; however, systematic evaluation of the evidence to support the benefit of newborn screening led initially to recommendations for more focused studies,[45] and eventually to the CDC's statement that newborn screening for CF was justified.[19] Rapid uptake of CF newborn screening followed this recommendation, moving from only 8 states at the time of the recommendation in 2004 to all 50 states by 2010. Similarly, international adoption of CF newborn screening has been widespread, and most Australian, European, and North American newborn screening programs have adopted CF newborn screening.

Cystic Fibrosis Newborn Screening Algorithms

Screening for CF in the United States is implemented at a state level through 4 algorithms. The algorithms and their relative strengths and weaknesses are presented in **Fig. 1**.[46,47] All the algorithms use an increased IRT level from the dried blood spot specimen as the first stage. IRT level is increased in infants with CF presumably because of pancreatic duct dysfunction in both pancreatic-sufficient and pancreatic-insufficient infants. However, increased IRT levels can also be seen in preterm infants, associated with perinatal stress, low Apgar scores, and African American origin.[48] Thus, all states use a multistage algorithm to minimize false-positives. IRT cutoffs are typically set such that 1% to 5% of samples tested are positive at the first stage and move on for further testing; the selection of the cutoff for the IRT concentration is crucial for balancing the sensitivity and positive predictive value of the screen. All CF newborn screening algorithms in the United States have a second stage of testing, and some have 3 stages, all of which are designed to improve the positive predictive value of the screen. Most frequently, the second stage incorporates molecular testing for *CFTR* mutations on the first specimen (IRT/DNA).[49,50] In some states, IRT concentrations are analyzed on a second specimen collected between 1 and 2 weeks of life (IRT/IRT),[44] whereas other programs combine the two strategies, following 2 increased IRT results with *CFTR* mutation analysis performed on the second specimen (IRT/IRT/DNA).[51] The most recent developments in CF algorithms incorporate an extended gene analysis following an increased IRT level and identification of 1 *CFTR* mutation, allowing a more specific screening result (2 mutations).[52,53]

The careful selection of the mutations on the *CFTR* screening panel is critical in order to ensure adequate coverage for the racial and ethnic composition of the

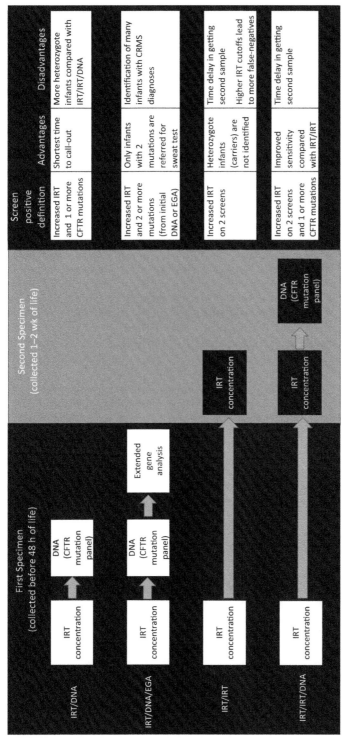

Fig. 1. CF newborn screening algorithms. EGA, extended gene analysis.

population being screened. An individual with 2 rare mutations may be missed on newborn screening because of limitations of the *CFTR* panel. This possibility is especially problematic in nonwhite populations, because they are more likely to have *CFTR* mutations not included in typical panels. To combat this challenge, an ultrahigh IRT algorithm has been proposed.[49] Infants with no mutations identified on the screening panel following an extremely increased IRT test are considered to be screen positive and are recalled for sweat chloride testing. The ultrahigh IRT algorithm results in more sweat tests and the diagnostic yield may be low; however, in some regions with ethnically diverse populations, the proportion of missed infants among the Hispanic population would have been very high without an ultrahigh IRT algorithm.[54]

Quality Improvement in Cystic Fibrosis Newborn Screening

The benefits of CF newborn screening can only be achieved if there are effective systems and processes in place to ensure prompt and accurate diagnosis. As CF newborn screening has become universal in the United States, areas for quality improvement have been identified. Data from the 2013 CF Foundation National Patient Registry evaluating age at diagnosis by state showed that the median age at diagnosis after a positive newborn screen was 19 days, but with a wide range, from a low of 4 days to a high of 45 days.[55] Ascertainment of the age at diagnosis is complicated by the Registry not having a clear definition of this metric. Some CF centers define the day of the positive newborn screen as the day of diagnosis, whereas others use the day of the confirmatory sweat test, which often takes place several weeks after the infant has been clinically diagnosed with CF. Prenatally diagnosed infants are also included in this metric, leading to a negative age at diagnosis. In addition to prompt diagnostic testing after a positive newborn screen, prompt evaluation at a CF center is also essential for reaping the benefits of early detection. The goal of CF newborn screening is for the diagnosis to be made and treatment started by 1 month of age. However, 2013 registry date showed that in 39 states the median age at which infants were seen at a CF center was greater than 30 days, and in 21 states was greater than 42 days.[55]

These data show that there is a need to improve CF newborn screening processes through quality improvement initiatives. In recognition of this need, the US CF Foundation has organized a CF Newborn Screening Quality Improvement Consortium that will use registry data to identify best practices and foster collaboration between CF centers to improve the newborn screening process. These efforts will help to deliver the optimal benefits from CF newborn screening.

PRENATAL SCREENING AND TESTING FOR CYSTIC FIBROSIS

The American College of Obstetricians and Gynecologists, the American College of Medical Genetics and Genomics (ACMG), and a European consensus statement[56] recommend that CF carrier screening be offered to prospective parents to inform them of their risk of having a child with CF, because most children with CF have no family history of the disease. CF carrier frequency is highest in non-Hispanic white people and Ashkenazi Jews (~1:30 for both), followed by Hispanic Americans (1:46), and is lowest in African Americans (1:65) and Asian Americans (1:90).[57] The mutation panel currently recommended by the ACMG includes 23 mutations.[58] It is important to understand that the limited mutation detection rate in certain racial and ethnic groups, as well as the high US rate of racial admixture, means that a couple can have an infant with CF even after negative prenatal carrier screening. If both parents are identified as carriers, the risk of CF in the offspring is 1 in 4. If desired, prenatal diagnostic testing of fetal cells for CF can be accomplished by chorionic villus sampling at 10 to 12 weeks or amniocentesis at 16 to 18 weeks. Fetal DNA testing from a maternal blood sample may be a noninvasive option in the future, but is not currently available.

For individuals with a family history of CF, general carrier screening may not be the appropriate preconception evaluation. If the affected individual has known *CFTR* mutations, those mutations should be tested in the individual's relative. If not, and the other member of the couple is a CF carrier, more extensive molecular testing, including sequencing, deletion, and/or duplication analysis, may be warranted. Consultation with a genetic counselor is recommended.

INDETERMINATE DIAGNOSES
Indeterminate Diagnosis in Infants Identified by Newborn Screening

In almost all cases, the diagnosis of CF can be easily made in patients who present with a positive CF newborn screen through a combination of sweat chloride concentration and/or genetic analysis. However, in some cases, sweat testing and genetic testing yield indeterminate results. In the United States, infants with a positive newborn screen but indeterminate diagnostic testing and no symptoms are classified as having CRMS.[59] CRMS was developed to allow entry of these infants into the US health care system while avoiding the term CF in the diagnosis. In Europe, the analogous term is CFSPID.[60,61] An international consensus conference was held in 2015 to address issues of CF diagnosis and CRMS/CFSPID. Conference participants reached consensus that the terms CRMS and CFSPID can be used interchangeably. The term CRMS/CFSPID can be applied to infants with a positive newborn screen and either (1) a sweat chloride level less than 30 mmol/L and 2 CFTR mutations, 1 of which has unclear phenotypic consequences; or (2) a sweat chloride level between 30 and 59 mmol/L and fewer than 2 CF-causing CFTR mutations (**Box 3**). Because infants with CRMS/CFSPID are identified through newborn screening, it is a condition that can only be identified through newborn screening.

Although almost all infants with CRMS/CFSPID remain asymptomatic, a small proportion ultimately develop CF. Thus, these infants should be followed on a regular basis by clinicians trained in the care of children with CF, such as those at a CF Foundation–accredited care center. The frequency and duration of this follow-up remain controversial.[59]

Parad and Comeau[62] were among the first investigators to report diagnostic dilemmas; infants who today would be classified as having CRMS. Other brief case reports described infants with CRMS, but did not report their clinical features or outcomes.[63–65] Until recently, little was known about the prevalence or outcomes of CRMS/CFSPID. Even now, the long-term outcomes remain unknown, because these

---

Box 3
Definition of indeterminate diagnosis following identification by newborn screening

The terms CRMS and CFSPID can be applied interchangeably in an asymptomatic infant with:

- A positive newborn screen

And either:
  o A sweat chloride level less than 30 mmol/L and 2 CFTR mutations, 1 of which has unclear phenotypic consequences, or
  o A sweat chloride level of 30 to 59 mmol/L and fewer than 2 CF-causing CFTR mutations

children have not yet been followed into adulthood. In a small, single-center, retrospective study of 12 infants with CRMS, 25% of infants had an oropharyngeal culture that was positive for *Pseudomonas aeruginosa*, a proportion higher than that expected in the non-CF population.[66] In 1 infant, the sweat chloride concentration increased from a mean of 46 mmol/L in the neonatal period to 73 mmol/L at 1 year of age. This infant also had an oropharyngeal culture positive for *P aeruginosa*, and his diagnosis was changed from CRMS to CF.

More recently, CRMS/CFSPID has been studied in several large cohort studies from multiple sites around the world (**Table 2**).[67–70] Differences in study populations and design make it difficult to compare across studies, but several general findings are apparent. The ratio of CF to CRMS cases ranged from 1.8:1 to 5.3:1. In California, where extended gene analysis identifies numerous mutations with unclear phenotypic consequences, CRMS is identified more frequently than CF, with a CF/CRMS ratio of 0.8:1. In general, infants with CRMS are pancreatic sufficient, and their nutritional indices are normal. However, the prevalence of *Pseudomonas*-positive oropharyngeal

Table 2
Summary of recent studies of indeterminate diagnoses following CF newborn screening, CRMS/CFSPID

	Ren et al,[69] 2015	Ooi et al,[68] 2015	Groves et al,[67] 2015	Levy et al,[70] 2015
Study Design	Prospective Cohort	Prospective Case control	Retrospective Case control	Prospective Cross sectional
Location	United States	Multinational	Australia	United States
Duration of Follow-up (y)	1	3	14[a]	20[a]
N with CF	1540	3101	225[f]	300
N with CRMS	309	82	29[c]	57
CF/CRMS Ratio	5:1	1.8:1	7.8:1	5.2:1
Of CRMS, N (%) converting to CF	NA	9[b] (10.9)	14[d] (38)	NA
Of CRMS, N (%) with sweat Cl Level ↑ to ≥60 mmol/L	NA	3 (33)	4 (14)	NA
Of CRMS, % with *Pseudomonas* Isolated from Respiratory Culture	10.7	14.6	78.6[e]	39
Of CRMS, % with *Stenotrophomonas* Isolated from Respiratory Culture	9.4	4.9	NA	NA
Of CRMS, N (%) Developing Exocrine Pancreatic Insufficiency	14 (4.5)	0	4 (13.8)	0
Of CRMS, N with CF Genotype F508del/R117H	26.1%	19.5%	4 (28.5%)[e]	36 (63%)

Abbreviation: NA, not available.
[a] Twenty-eight percent lost to follow-up.
[b] Diagnosed as CF through reclassification of a *CFTR* mutations as CF-causing or increasing sweat chloride level to greater than or equal to 60 mmol/L.
[c] CRMS definition was different from CRMS/CFSPID.
[d] Diagnosed through clinical signs and symptoms of respiratory disease (N = 8) or exocrine pancreatic insufficiency (N = 6).
[e] Denominator is 14.
[f] Estimated (not reported in the citation).

cultures ranged from 10.7% to 78.4%, and some studies have also reported respiratory cultures yielding other CF-related pathogens, such as *Stenotrophomonas maltophilia*. In one study, 11% of infants with CRMS were reclassified as having CF after additional study of their *CFTR* mutations revealed that both were CF causing.[68] In a 14-year retrospective study, 48% of infants with CRMS were subsequently diagnosed as having CF, but the clinical features on which this decision was made were not specific for CF (eg, recurrent cough).[67]

Sweat chloride concentration in the newborn period does not seem to be a predictor of which infants with CRMS will later develop clinical features of CF disease. The rate of *Pseudomonas*-positive oropharyngeal cultures was similar in infants with sweat chloride levels less than 30 mmol/L compared with infants with a sweat chloride level of 30 to 59 mmol/L.[69] An abnormal nasal potential difference measurement, which measures CFTR function in the respiratory tract, can potentially distinguish infants with CRMS who will go on to develop features of CF lung disease from those who will not.[71] However, this test is not widely available in the clinical setting. The genotype F508del/R117H/7T is also commonly found in infants with CRMS, occurring in 23% to 63% of patients in recent studies. This finding is consistent with the classification of R117H without the 5T polymorphism in *cis* as a mutation with varying clinical consequences.[72–75]

Because of its diverse ethnic and racial population, the state of California chose to incorporate gene sequencing in its newborn screening algorithm.[76] The California definition of a *CFTR* mutation is very broad, and includes poly-T and TG repeats, as well mutations with varying clinical consequences. As a result, their program detects 1.5 times as many CRMS cases as CF cases.[52] However, most of these infants seem to have benign outcomes.[77]

In summary, CRMS/CFSPID is the term used to identify infants with an abnormal CF newborn screen but inconclusive diagnostic testing. Although almost all infants with CRMS/CFSPID remain well, a small proportion develop clinical features concerning for CF or even transition into a CF phenotype. Recent studies have provided clinicians with more information regarding the prevalence and outcomes of CRMS. However, many questions remain unanswered, such as the long-term risk for development of CF and the optimal monitoring and management of these infants.

Cystic Fibrosis Transmembrane Conductance Regulator–related Disorder

Inconclusive diagnostic testing can also arise in the evaluation of older patients who present with 1 or more clinical features associated with CFTR dysfunction but who do not meet the diagnostic criteria for CF. The term CFTR-RD is used to describe this group of patients.[78] CFTR-RD is defined as a clinical entity associated with CFTR dysfunction that does not meet diagnostic criteria for CF. In contrast with infants with CRMS, patients with CFTR-RD are symptomatic (**Box 4**); the term should not be applied to newborn-screened infants. However, in both CRMS and CFTR-RD,

---

Box 4
Conditions associated with CFTR-RD

- Bronchiectasis
- Chronic sinusitis
- Recurrent/chronic pancreatitis
- Azoospermia/congenital absence of the vas deferens

diagnostic testing for CF is inconclusive. Nasal potential difference measurements in patients with CFTR-RD tend to be in an intermediate range between patients with and without CF. Similarly, patients with CFTR-RD tend to have CFTR mutations that result in diminished CFTR function, but not so reduced as to result in a full CF phenotype. For an additional description, (see Sosnay PR, Raraigh KS, Gibson RL: Molecular Genetics of CFTR: Genotype and Phenotype, in this issue).

SUMMARY

The diagnosis of CF has undergone extensive changes in the United States and around the world over the past decade because of the widespread adoption of CF newborn screening programs. In the United States, CF newborn screening has been in place in all 50 states since 2010, and most new cases are now diagnosed following a positive newborn screen. Diagnosis in the newborn period provides the opportunity for early intervention before nutritional and pulmonary deficits become irreversible. To date, the long-term nutritional benefits of CF newborn screening have been more clearly established than the long-term pulmonary benefits. However, as more effective early intervention strategies are developed, particularly in the current era of CFTR modulator therapies targeting the basic defect in CF, there is great promise that early diagnosis will dramatically improve long-term outcomes.

The diagnosis of CF is fairly straightforward in most patients. Nonetheless, rapid advances in CFTR genetics and the uptake of CF newborn screening have elucidated the varying clinical manifestations of CFTR dysfunction, complicating the diagnosis of CF. In terms of newborn screening, it is extremely challenging to balance the benefits of early detection and treatment of a life-limiting illness with the risks of inconclusive diagnoses in infants who are likely to remain healthy, but in whom there is a small risk of progression to CF.

CF newborn screening and diagnosis algorithms are likely to change greatly in the next decade based on advances in tandem mass spectrometry and extended genetic analysis, as well as better understanding of genotype-phenotype correlations. It will be critical to keep the risks and benefits of detection of the wide range of CFTR dysfunctions in mind as these standards and algorithms are developed.

REFERENCES

1. Cystic Fibrosis Foundation. 2013 annual data report to the center directors. Bethesda (MD): Cystic Fibrosis Foundation; 2014.
2. Rosenstein BJ, Cutting GR. The diagnosis of cystic fibrosis: a consensus statement. Cystic Fibrosis Foundation Consensus Panel. J Pediatr 1998;132(4): 589–95.
3. Farrell PM, Rosenstein BJ, White TB, et al. Guidelines for diagnosis of cystic fibrosis in newborns through older adults: cystic fibrosis foundation consensus report. J Pediatr 2008;153(2):S4–14.
4. De Boeck K, Wilschanski M, Castellani C, et al. Cystic fibrosis: terminology and diagnostic algorithms. Thorax 2006;61(7):627–35.
5. Legrys VA, Applequist R, Briscoe DR, et al. Sweat testing: sample collection and quantitative chloride analysis; approved guideline. 3rd edition. Wayne (PA): Clinical and Laboratory Standards Institute; 2009.
6. Borowitz D, Robinson KA, Rosenfeld M, et al. Cystic fibrosis foundation evidence-based guidelines for management of infants with cystic fibrosis. J Pediatr 2009; 155(6 Suppl):S73–93.

7. Advisory committee on heritable disorders in newborns and children recommended uniform screening panel 2013. Available at: http://www.hrsa.gov/advisorycommittees/mchbadvisory/heritabledisorders/recommendedpanel/. Accessed January 13, 2016.

8. Reardon MC, Hammond KB, Accurso FJ, et al. Nutritional deficits exist before 2 months of age in some infants with cystic fibrosis identified by screening test. J Pediatr 1984;105(2):271–4.

9. Bronstein MN, Sokol RJ, Abman SH, et al. Pancreatic insufficiency, growth, and nutrition in infants identified by newborn screening as having cystic fibrosis. J Pediatr 1992;120(4 Pt 1):533–40.

10. Sokol RJ, Reardon MC, Accurso FJ, et al. Fat-soluble-vitamin status during the first year of life in infants with cystic fibrosis identified by screening of newborns. Am J Clin Nutr 1989;50(5):1064–71.

11. Gaskin K, Waters D, Allen J, et al. Nutritional status of infants with cystic fibrosis. Am J Clin Nutr 1992;56(5):955–7.

12. Gaskin K, Waters D, Dorney S, et al. Assessment of pancreatic function in screened infants with cystic fibrosis. Pediatr Pulmonol Suppl 1991;7:69–71.

13. Waters DL, Dorney SF, Gaskin KJ, et al. Pancreatic function in infants identified as having cystic fibrosis in a neonatal screening program. N Engl J Med 1990;322(5):303–8.

14. Khan TZ, Wagener JS, Bost T, et al. Early pulmonary inflammation in infants with cystic fibrosis. Am J Respir Crit Care Med 1995;151(4):1075–82.

15. Armstrong DS, Grimwood K, Carlin JB, et al. Lower airway inflammation in infants and young children with cystic fibrosis. Am J Respir Crit Care Med 1997;156(4 Pt 1):1197–204.

16. Abman SH, Ogle JW, Harbeck RJ, et al. Early bacteriologic, immunologic, and clinical courses of young infants with cystic fibrosis identified by neonatal screening. J Pediatr 1991;119(2):211–7.

17. Wilcken B, Brown AR, Urwin R, et al. Cystic fibrosis screening by dried blood spot trypsin assay: results in 75,000 newborn infants. J Pediatr 1983;102(3):383–7.

18. Farrell PM, Li Z, Kosorok MR, et al. Bronchopulmonary disease in children with cystic fibrosis after early or delayed diagnosis. Am J Respir Crit Care Med 2003;168(9):1100–8.

19. Grosse SD, Boyle CA, Botkin JR, et al. Newborn screening for cystic fibrosis: evaluation of benefits and risks and recommendations for state newborn screening programs. MMWR Recomm Rep 2004;53(RR–13):1–36.

20. Farrell PM, Kosorok MR, Rock MJ, et al. Early diagnosis of cystic fibrosis through neonatal screening prevents severe malnutrition and improves long-term growth. Wisconsin Cystic Fibrosis Neonatal Screening Study Group. Pediatrics 2001;107(1):1–13.

21. Waters DL, Wilcken B, Irwing L, et al. Clinical outcomes of newborn screening for cystic fibrosis. Arch Dis Child Fetal Neonatal Ed 1999;80(1):F1–7.

22. Accurso FJ, Sontag MK, Wagener JS. Complications associated with symptomatic diagnosis in infants with cystic fibrosis. J Pediatr 2005;147(3 Suppl):S37–41.

23. Koscik RL, Farrell PM, Kosorok MR, et al. Cognitive function of children with cystic fibrosis: deleterious effect of early malnutrition. Pediatrics 2004;113(6):1549–58.

24. Lai HJ, Cheng Y, Farrell PM. The survival advantage of patients with cystic fibrosis diagnosed through neonatal screening: evidence from the United States Cystic Fibrosis Foundation registry data. J Pediatr 2005;147(3 Suppl):S57–63.

25. Grosse SD, Rosenfeld M, Devine OJ, et al. Potential impact of newborn screening for cystic fibrosis on child survival: a systematic review and analysis. J Pediatr 2006;149(3):362–6.

26. Southern KW, Merelle MM, Dankert-Roelse JE, et al. Newborn screening for cystic fibrosis. Cochrane Database Syst Rev 2009;(1):CD001402.
27. Gonska T, Ratjen F. Newborn screening for cystic fibrosis. Expert Rev Respir Med 2015;9(5):619–31.
28. Wagener JS, Zemanick ET, Sontag MK. Newborn screening for cystic fibrosis. Curr Opin Pediatr 2012;24(3):329–35.
29. Leung DB, Heltshe S, Kloster M, et al. CF infant growth and pulmonary status in the first year of life: the bonus study. Pediatr Pulmonol Suppl 2015;50(S41).
30. Saiman L, Marshall BC, Mayer-Hamblett N, et al. Azithromycin in patients with cystic fibrosis chronically infected with *Pseudomonas aeruginosa*: a randomized controlled trial. JAMA 2003;290(13):1749–56.
31. Mayer-Hamblett N, Rosenfeld M, Treggiari MM, et al. Standard care versus protocol based therapy for new onset *Pseudomonas aeruginosa* in cystic fibrosis. Pediatr Pulmonol 2013;48(10):943–53.
32. Fuchs HJ, Borowitz DS, Christiansen DH, et al. Effect of aerosolized recombinant human DNase on exacerbations of respiratory symptoms and on pulmonary function in patients with cystic fibrosis. The Pulmozyme Study Group. N Engl J Med 1994;331(10):637–42.
33. Accurso FJ, Rowe SM, Clancy JP, et al. Effect of VX-770 in persons with cystic fibrosis and the G551D-CFTR mutation. N Engl J Med 2010;363(21):1991–2003.
34. Wainwright CE, Elborn JS, Ramsey BW. Lumacaftor-ivacaftor in patients with cystic fibrosis homozygous for Phe508del CFTR. N Engl J Med 2015;373(18):1783–4.
35. Davies JC. The future of CFTR modulating therapies for cystic fibrosis. Curr Opin Pulm Med 2015;21(6):579–84.
36. Wilson JMG, Jungner G. Principles and practice of screening for disease. Geneva (Switzerland): World Health Organization; 1968.
37. Kemper AR, Green NS, Calonge N, et al. Decision-making process for conditions nominated to the recommended uniform screening panel: statement of the US Department of Health and Human Services Secretary's Advisory Committee on Heritable Disorders in Newborns and Children. Genet Med 2014;16(2):183–7.
38. Petros M. Revisiting the Wilson-Jungner criteria: how can supplemental criteria guide public health in the era of genetic screening? Genet Med 2012;14(1): 129–34.
39. Ross LF, Saal HM, David KL, et al. Technical report: ethical and policy issues in genetic testing and screening of children. Genet Med 2013;15(3):234–45.
40. NewSTEPs: newborn screening technical assistance and evaluation program. Silver Spring (Maryland): Association of Public Health Laboratories; 2014. cited 1901 1/5/15 AD. Available at: www.newsteps.org. Accessed January 16, 2016.
41. Crossley JR, Elliott RB, Smith PA. Dried-blood spot screening for cystic fibrosis in the newborn. Lancet 1979;1(8114):472–4.
42. Crossley JR, Smith PA, Edgar BW, et al. Neonatal screening for cystic fibrosis, using immunoreactive trypsin assay in dried blood spots. Clin Chim Acta 1981; 113(2):111–21.
43. Heeley AF, Heeley ME, King DN, et al. Screening for cystic fibrosis by died blood spot trypsin assay. Arch Dis Child 1982;57(1):18–21.
44. Hammond KB, Abman SH, Sokol RJ, et al. Efficacy of statewide neonatal screening for cystic fibrosis by assay of trypsinogen concentrations. N Engl J Med 1991;325(11):769–74.
45. Newborn screening for cystic fibrosis: a paradigm for public health genetics policy development. Proceedings of a 1997 workshop. MMWR Recomm Rep 1997; 46(RR–16):1–24.

46. Newborn screening for cystic fibrosis; approved guideline, NBS05-A. Wayne (PA): Clinical Laboratory Standards Institute (CLSI); 2011.
47. Comeau AM, Accurso FJ, White TB, et al. Guidelines for implementation of cystic fibrosis newborn screening programs: Cystic Fibrosis Foundation workshop report. Pediatrics 2007;119(2):e495–518.
48. Rock MJ, Mischler EH, Farrell PM, et al. Immunoreactive trypsinogen screening for cystic fibrosis: characterization of infants with a false-positive screening test. Pediatr Pulmonol 1989;6(1):42–8.
49. Comeau AM, Parad RB, Dorkin HL, et al. Population-based newborn screening for genetic disorders when multiple mutation DNA testing is incorporated: a cystic fibrosis newborn screening model demonstrating increased sensitivity but more carrier detections. Pediatrics 2004;113(6):1573–81.
50. Farrell PM, Aronson RA, Hoffman G, et al. Newborn screening for cystic fibrosis in Wisconsin: first application of population-based molecular genetics testing. Wis Med J 1994;93(8):415–21.
51. Sontag MK, Wright D, Beebe J, et al. A new cystic fibrosis newborn screening algorithm: IRT/IRT/DNA. J Pediatr 2009;155(5):618–22.
52. Kharrazi M, Yang J, Bishop T, et al. Newborn screening for cystic fibrosis in California. Pediatrics 2015;136(6):1062–72.
53. Brennan ML, Schrijver I. Cystic fibrosis: a review of associated phenotypes, use of molecular diagnostic approaches, genetic characteristics, progress, and dilemmas. J Mol Diagn 2016;18(1):3–14.
54. Kay DM, Langfelder-Schwind E, DeCelie-Germana J, et al. Utility of a very high IRT/No mutation referral category in cystic fibrosis newborn screening. Pediatr Pulmonol 2015;50(8):771–80.
55. McColley SA, Michelson P, Petren K, et al. A state level registry report for assessment of cystic fibrosis newborn screening programs. Pediatr Pulmonol 2014; 49(S38):S383.
56. Castellani C, Macek M Jr, Cassiman JJ, et al. Benchmarks for cystic fibrosis carrier screening: a European consensus document. J Cyst Fibros 2010;9(3): 165–78.
57. Lebo RV, Grody WW. Testing and reporting ACMG cystic fibrosis mutation panel results. Genet Test 2007;11(1):11–31.
58. Watson MS, Cutting GR, Desnick RJ, et al. Cystic fibrosis population carrier screening: 2004 revision of American College of Medical Genetics mutation panel. Genet Med 2004;6(5):387–91.
59. Borowitz D, Parad RB, Sharp JK, et al. Cystic Fibrosis Foundation practice guidelines for the management of infants with cystic fibrosis transmembrane conductance regulator-related metabolic syndrome during the first two years of life and beyond. J Pediatr 2009;155(6 Suppl):S106–16.
60. Munck A, Mayell SJ, Winters V, et al. Cystic fibrosis screen positive, inconclusive diagnosis (CFSPID): a new designation and management recommendations for infants with an inconclusive diagnosis following newborn screening. J Cyst Fibros 2015;14(6):706–13.
61. Mayell SJ, Munck A, Craig JV, et al. A European consensus for the evaluation and management of infants with an equivocal diagnosis following newborn screening for cystic fibrosis. J Cyst Fibros 2009;8(1):71–8.
62. Parad RB, Comeau AM. Diagnostic dilemmas resulting from the immunoreactive trypsinogen/DNA cystic fibrosis newborn screening algorithm. J Pediatr 2005; 147(3 Suppl):S78–82.

63. Massie J, Clements B, Australian Paediatric Respiratory Group. Diagnosis of cystic fibrosis after newborn screening: the Australasian experience–twenty years and five million babies later: a consensus statement from the Australasian Paediatric Respiratory Group. Pediatr Pulmonol 2005;39(5):440–6.

64. Narzi L, Ferraguti G, Stamato A, et al. Does cystic fibrosis neonatal screening detect atypical CF forms? Extended genetic characterization and 4-year clinical follow-up. Clin Genet 2007;72(1):39–46.

65. Roussey M, Le Bihannic A, Scotet V, et al. Neonatal screening of cystic fibrosis: diagnostic problems with CFTR mild mutations. J Inherit Metab Dis 2007;30(4):613.

66. Ren CL, Desai H, Platt M, et al. Clinical outcomes in infants with cystic fibrosis transmembrane conductance regulator (CFTR) related metabolic syndrome. Pediatr Pulmonol 2011;46(11):1079–84.

67. Groves T, Robinson P, Wiley V, et al. Long-term outcomes of children with intermediate sweat chloride values in infancy. J Pediatr 2015;166(6):1469–74.e1–3.

68. Ooi CY, Castellani C, Keenan K, et al. Inconclusive diagnosis of cystic fibrosis after newborn screening. Pediatrics 2015;135(6):e1377–85.

69. Ren CL, Fink AK, Petren K, et al. Outcomes of infants with indeterminate diagnosis detected by cystic fibrosis newborn screening. Pediatrics 2015;135(6): e1386–92.

70. Levy H, Nugent M, Schneck K, et al. Refining the continuum of CFTR-associated disorders in the era of newborn screening. Clin Genet 2015. http://dx.doi.org/10.1111/cge.12711.

71. Sermet-Gaudelus I, Girodon E, Roussel D, et al. Measurement of nasal potential difference in young children with an equivocal sweat test following newborn screening for cystic fibrosis. Thorax 2010;65(6):539–44.

72. O'Sullivan BP, Zwerdling RG, Dorkin HL, et al. Early pulmonary manifestation of cystic fibrosis in children with the DeltaF508/R117H-7T genotype. Pediatrics 2006;118(3):1260–5.

73. Ren CL. Pulmonary manifestations in deltaF508/R117H. Pediatrics 2007;119(3): 647 [author reply: 8].

74. Sosnay PR, Siklosi KR, Van Goor F, et al. Defining the disease liability of variants in the cystic fibrosis transmembrane conductance regulator gene. Nat Genet 2013;45(10):1160–7.

75. Thauvin-Robinet C, Munck A, Huet F, et al. The very low penetrance of cystic fibrosis for the R117H mutation: a reappraisal for genetic counselling and newborn screening. J Med Genet 2009;46(11):752–8.

76. Prach L, Koepke R, Kharrazi M, et al. Novel CFTR variants identified during the first 3 years of cystic fibrosis newborn screening in California. J Mol Diagn 2013;15(5):710–22.

77. Salinas DB, Sosnay PR, Azen C, et al. Benign outcome among positive cystic fibrosis newborn screen children with non-CF-causing variants. J Cyst Fibros 2015;14(6):714–9.

78. Bombieri C, Claustres M, De Boeck K, et al. Recommendations for the classification of diseases as CFTR-related disorders. J Cyst Fibros 2011;10(Suppl 2): S86–102.

79. Ramsey KA, Ranganathan S, Park J, et al. Early respiratory infection is associated with reduced spirometry in children with cystic fibrosis. Am J Respir Crit Care Med 2014;190(10):1111–6.

80. Hoo AF, Thia LP, Nguyen TT, et al. Lung function is abnormal in 3-month-old infants with cystic fibrosis diagnosed by newborn screening. Thorax 2012; 67(10):874–81.
81. Nguyen TT, Thia LP, Hoo AF, et al. Evolution of lung function during the first year of life in newborn screened cystic fibrosis infants. Thorax 2014;69(10):910–7.
82. Mott LS, Park J, Murray CP, et al. Progression of early structural lung disease in young children with cystic fibrosis assessed using CT. Thorax 2012;67(6):509–16.

Cystic Fibrosis
Microbiology and Host Response

 CrossMark

Edith T. Zemanick, MD, MSCS[a], Lucas R. Hoffman, MD, PhD[b],*

KEYWORDS

- Cystic fibrosis • Inflammation • Infection • Microbiology • Neutrophil • Biomarker

KEY POINTS

- Cystic fibrosis (CF) lung disease involves a cycle of mucus obstruction, inflammation, and infection in the airways, and each of these elements affects the others as disease progresses.
- Observations from the earliest studies of CF disease in the 1930s and 1940s showed these elements, but the understanding and treatment of each has evolved over time.
- CF respiratory microbiology has also evolved as new treatments have been introduced, as people have lived longer with this disease, and as detection methods have become more sophisticated.
- The CF airway also shows altered host-defense, and imbalances in the airway environment are important for pathophysiology and may indicate both new treatment directions and useful disease biomarkers.
- Because most information regarding the relationships between infection, inflammation, and disease severity come from observational studies, their causal relationships are not always clear.

INTRODUCTION

The earliest published descriptions of cystic fibrosis (CF) lung disease described the following triad of pathophysiologic elements that still form the basis of most current models:

- Airway obstruction
- Infection
- Inflammation

In her landmark 1938 publication describing the pathologic and clinical features of children who died of this disorder, Dorothy Andersen[1] identified the common features

Disclosure: The authors have nothing to disclose.
[a] Children's Hospital Colorado, University of Colorado School of Medicine, 13123 East 16th Avenue, B-395, Aurora, CO 80045, USA; [b] Departments of Pediatrics and Microbiology, Seattle Children's Hospital and University of Washington, 4800 Sand Point Way Northeast, MS OC.7.720, Seattle, WA 98105, USA
* Corresponding author.
E-mail address: lhoffm@uw.edu

Pediatr Clin N Am 63 (2016) 617–636
http://dx.doi.org/10.1016/j.pcl.2016.04.003
0031-3955/16/$ – see front matter © 2016 Elsevier Inc. All rights reserved.

of "bronchitis, bronchiectasis, pulmonary abscesses arising in the bronchi," which were plugged with "tenacious, greenish gray mucopurulent material," and that "*Staphylococcus aureus* was the usual bacteriologic agent."[1,2] From these findings, she and others began treating children with CF with antibiotics targeting *S aureus*, specifically sulfonamides and penicillin.[2] This approach was followed by several important developments. First, the children generally improved clinically. Second, cultures showed that they were increasingly infected with penicillin-resistant *S aureus*, as well as pathogens not seen before antibiotics, including *Pseudomonas aeruginosa*.[3]

These early observations are instructive on many levels. The primary defect that causes CF, mutational dysfunction of the CF transmembrane conductance regulator (CFTR), leads to a cycle in the airways of defective mucus clearance, obstruction, infection, and inflammation. Improvements in nutrition, mucus clearance, and treatment of inflammation and infection have led to dramatic improvements in CF respiratory morbidity and mortality[4]; however, current treatments have not been able to halt disease progression. As patients live increasingly longer, their respiratory microbiology evolves,[4] perhaps driven by elements of care intended to mitigate their lung disease (such as antibiotics and attending clinics at CF care centers). Put differently, the treatments that have so greatly helped people with CF are often followed by microbiological changes, which in turn may alter their clinical course. The causal relationships between specific pathogens, clinical changes, and constantly evolving therapies are difficult to sort out.

Andersen and di Sant'Agnese[2] made special mention of the apparent link between infection and inflammation. Although these are omnipresent features of CF lung disease, the causal relationships between them are controversial. Observations from a variety of studies of patients[5] and, most recently, animals engineered with CFTR mutations[6] have led some investigators to postulate that infection is required for CF airway inflammation, whereas others have suggested that inflammation can precede infection.[7] Although these disputes continue, great progress has been made in defining the mediators and mechanisms driving the intense inflammation within CF airways, identifying not only new candidate therapeutic targets but also promising biomarkers of early disease.

This article reviews the current understanding of the roles of infection and inflammation in CF lung disease pathogenesis. Although these two features of the CF airway are mechanistically linked by data from observational studies and, as a result, in current pathophysiologic models, for simplicity this article considers them separately. Although this article touches on therapeutic approaches to both infection and inflammation, clinicians are currently experiencing a period of particularly rapid evolution in CF treatment strategies and protocols. Therefore, where appropriate, this article refers readers to recent, in-depth reviews of CF therapeutic strategies[8,9] for more information. Similarly, there have been several excellent reviews of CF respiratory microbiology and inflammation in general that readers may find useful.[10–16]

CYSTIC FIBROSIS MICROBIOLOGY
The Evolving Role of Methodology

Dorothy Andersen and her contemporaries identified several important characteristics of CF lung disease. For example, she and others who later built on her work[17–20] noted that the microbes infecting CF lungs were nearly always confined to airway luminal mucus, rather than invading tissue. The role of *S aureus* was highlighted; however, other bacteria were quickly recognized as important CF pathogens. Blending observations from culture and microscopy, two of the most sophisticated methods available at the time, provided higher sensitivity and yielded a richer depiction of infection pathogenesis than either method alone. As both treatments and laboratory methods have evolved, so has the understanding of the pathogenesis of CF respiratory infections and the spectrum of likely pathogens. Before discussing the most common pathogens, it is instructive to consider how improvements in treatment, innovations in clinical microbiology, and increases in patient longevity combine to create constant evolution in CF microbiology.

CF clinical microbiology generally relies on conventional laboratory cultivation of respiratory samples (eg, sputum, bronchoalveolar lavage fluid (BALF), oropharyngeal swabs, or sinus samples) to identify and study causative organisms. Using these techniques, bacteria and fungi can be identified, enumerated, isolated, and characterized; their growth characteristics and in vitro antibiotic susceptibilities are defined. These methods are invaluable for diagnosing infections in individual patients, directing antibiotic treatment, and generating epidemiologic information that informs our models of CF infection pathogenesis. Despite the enormous utility and power of these conventional methods, recent work with advanced laboratory techniques has added to the ever-growing list of CF-associated microbes. To show how newer methods might complement culture, this article briefly reviews how current CF respiratory cultures are performed, and how information is generated and used to direct treatment.

Current methods rely on synthetic laboratory growth media that, together with incubation conditions (generally aerobic and at body temperature for CF microbiology), have been chosen to select for the microbes customarily associated with lung disease pathogenesis. In addition, current protocols[21] usually involve selecting a small number of isolates of those traditional pathogens from those cultures to test susceptibilities and to inform treatment.

However, conventional culture methods can introduce bias or have other shortcomings. For example, it is now known that CF airway mucus has anaerobic niches that alter microbial metabolism[18] and that are not accurately modeled by these laboratory methods. In line with this finding, both advanced culture-based and culture-independent (sequencing) techniques have identified diverse microbes, including anaerobes and other otherwise undetected bacteria together with traditionally cultured pathogens, in respiratory samples from many patients with CF.[22] Microscopic and biochemical investigations[18,23] suggest that microbes infecting CF airways may commonly exist in biofilms, which are gel-encased communities of cells that are resistant to killing compared with the liquid-suspended, dispersed microbial cells usually studied in the laboratory. In-depth studies of traditional CF pathogens (such as *P aeruginosa* and *S aureus*)[24] have also revealed that they evolve and diversify over time, meaning that 1 or a few isolates do not accurately reflect the behaviors of an entire, chronically infecting population of those bacteria. In addition, studies of the microbes in different specimen types (such as swabs, sputum, and lavages) collected concurrently from individual patients with CF indicate that each may sample different anatomic sites, raising the question of which sample is best for informing treatment or prognosis.

These new findings highlight the constantly evolving and controversial nature of CF microbiology, which has largely been, and continues to be, informed by the results of standard cultures. Accordingly, the focus here is on what is known from conventional CF microbiology, with a later discussion about how recent developments may change clinical practice.

Traditional Cystic Fibrosis Respiratory Pathogens: Epidemiology

The 2 graphs in **Fig. 1** show that CF airway infections have 3 key features:

- They are diverse.
- They are frequently polymicrobial.
- They are constantly evolving.

Fig. 1A shows the US prevalence in 2013 by patient age of the bacteria cultured most commonly from respiratory cultures (as recorded in the Cystic Fibrosis

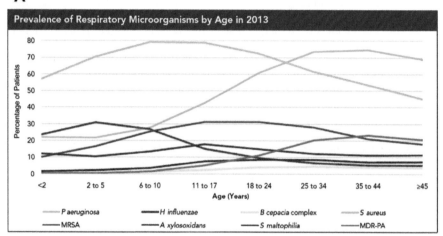

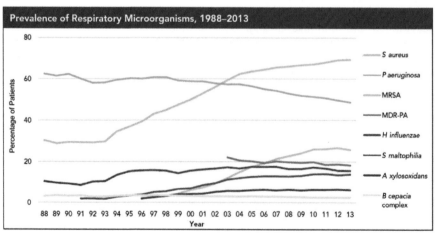

Fig. 1. Epidemiology of traditional CF pathogens in 2013, from the US CF Foundation Patient Registry. (*A*) Percentage of patients reported to be culture-positive for the indicated bacteria in 2013, by age group. (*B*) Overall prevalence of these bacteria in patients with CF per year. Patients with CF under care at CF Foundation–accredited care centers in the United States who consented to have their data entered. SOURCE OF DATA: Cystic fibrosis patients under care at CF Foundation-accredited care centers in the United States, who consented to have their data entered. Figures kindly provided by the CF Foundation.

Foundation Patient Registry[4]). This graph shows that *S aureus* was particularly common among young children, whereas *P aeruginosa* was most common in adults. The *S aureus* subtype methicillin-resistant *S aureus* (MRSA) had peak CF age prevalence in the midteens to early 20s. *P aeruginosa* resistant to multiple antibiotics (multidrug-resistant *P aeruginosa* [MDR-PA]) was uncommon but followed the same age distribution as *P aeruginosa* in general. A brief consideration of these data reveals that, for each age group, many patients must have had more than 1 of these bacteria during the year.

Fig. 1B provides a slightly different perspective of the 2013 data. For example, consider how the prevalences of *S aureus* and *P aeruginosa* have changed in the United States since 1988. *S aureus* prevalence has dramatically increased, whereas that of *P aeruginosa* has decreased. Therefore, even considering just these 6 commonly cultured bacterial species, the diverse, polymicrobial, and constantly evolving nature of CF lung infections can be appreciated. Further, some pathogens that can be cultured (such as nontuberculous mycobacteria [NTM]) are not included on these graphs. This article briefly discuss each of these species later, paying particular attention to *S aureus* and *P aeruginosa*, given their high prevalence and clinical associations. For brevity, key points are provided for less common CF respiratory microbes. Clinically relevant variants of common pathogens (such as MRSA and MDR-PA) are also discussed, as well as emerging pathogens such as NTM, with attention to their epidemiology, associations with disease, and treatment.

Staphylococcus aureus

Epidemiology and clinical associations

As described earlier, this gram-positive organism was the bacterium first identified as an important CF respiratory pathogen. The earliest CF antibiotic treatments targeted *S aureus*, and early proponents of these treatments described the substantial clinical improvements that resulted. However, the role of *S aureus* in driving CF lung disease, and the appropriate clinical response to its detection, are matters of ongoing debate. A review of published observations regarding the association between *S aureus* and lung disease clarifies the basis for this controversy.

In addition to the high prevalence of *S aureus* among children, pediatric CF studies have provided further cause for concern: *S aureus* has been associated with higher airway inflammation,[25,26] lower lung function,[27,28] and even higher subsequent mortality when detected together with *P aeruginosa*.[29] Further, these associations were for all *S aureus*; as described later, specific subtypes of *S aureus* (such as MRSA and small-colony variants of *S aureus* [SCVs]) may be associated with even worse outcomes than other *S aureus*.

However, when considering all *S aureus* in adults with CF, the picture becomes less clear. Studies of adults found *S aureus* to be associated with a lower risk of mortality,[30] better lung function,[31] and a lower risk of exacerbations.[32] Therefore, *S aureus* pathogenesis may either be context dependent (that is, perhaps it is more pathogenic either in children or in the absence of *P aeruginosa*, or it adapts over time to become less pathogenic). Alternatively, pathogenesis may be higher for specific subtypes of *S aureus* (such as MRSA or SCVs), or *S aureus* may not be universally pathogenic but rather serves as a marker of early (as with children) or mild (as with adults) disease.

Answering these questions is particularly pressing because of the recent increase in *S aureus* prevalence shown in **Fig. 1**B. Recent studies showed similar trends in parts of Europe and Australia[33] by the mid-2000s. However, *S aureus* prevalence has remained comparatively low in the United Kingdom,[33] perhaps related to differences in antibiotic use (discussed later). Importantly, both longevity and lung function have continued to improve in the general CF population,[4] including in the age groups with the highest S aureus prevalences. These combined observations make it difficult to predict the best approach to infection with S aureus.

Subtypes

As suggested earlier, 2 subtypes of S aureus are of particular significance for CF lung disease and treatment: MRSA and SCVs.

MRSA (or oxacillin-resistant S aureus [ORSA]) is usually identified either by its resistance to these β-lactams or by carriage of the mecA gene, which encodes this resistance. MRSA prevalence in CF has increased in the past 2 decades (see **Fig. 1**B) in parallel with all S aureus and methicillin-susceptible S aureus (MSSA). MRSA acquisition in CF is strongly associated with exposure to hospitals and to antibiotics,[34–36] as it is in the general population, which also experienced a parallel increase in MRSA prevalence in the United States. The increase seen in the US CF population has not occurred as dramatically elsewhere,[33] suggesting that environmental, treatment, or other factors unique to specific locations are responsible for this epidemiologic change.

The relationship between MRSA and CF lung disease outcomes is complex. Although several studies have shown an association between MRSA infection and lower lung function in patients with CF,[34,35,37] some studies indicated that patients with MRSA had faster lung function decline before MRSA detection, suggesting that MRSA may be a marker for severe disease rather than the cause.[35] However, other studies found MRSA to be an independent risk factor for failure to recover lung function during treatment of respiratory exacerbations[38] and for increased mortality.[39]

S aureus SCVs are slow-growing, antibiotic-resistant variants that are difficult to detect with conventional cultures. Small studies of both European[40–42] and US CF[43] populations have identified SCVs among 8% to 30% of patients using special laboratory methods. These studies have also found SCVs to be associated with lower lung function, faster lung function decline, and higher rates of preceding treatment with antibiotics known to select for SCVs, including aminoglycosides and sulfonamides, in addition to higher rates of coinfection with P aeruginosa, which may also select for SCVs.[44]

The similarities between MRSA and S aureus SCVs, particularly their relationships with clinical outcomes, antibiotic treatment, and resistance, are instructive. Each of these bacterial types is associated with:

- Preceding antibiotic treatment
- Subsequent antibiotic resistance
- Higher lung disease severity

However, these findings are largely from observational studies, and whether MRSA and SCVs cause worse outcomes, whether they reflect patients with worse preexisting disease and resulting higher antibiotic treatment burdens, or both, remains to be seen. Additional observational and interventional studies may resolve these questions of causality. Until then, the best therapeutic approaches to each subtype remain to be defined.

Treatment

Determining the best approach to S aureus infection in CF is a controversial subject. Some countries provide continuous antistaphylococcal prophylaxis during childhood; this practice has been associated in some trials with earlier detection of P aeruginosa, which, given its association with worse lung disease, led many countries to not adopt this approach.[45] Differences in study outcomes may have resulted from different antibiotic choices. Some centers provide antistaphylococcal antibiotics designed to eradicate *S aureus* on first detection,[46] and strategies and attitudes differ for MRSA versus MSSA; evidence supports the microbiological efficacy of this strategy, but clinical benefits for eradication of either MRSA and MSSA remain to be determined.[46,47] By comparison, for patients with *S aureus* and no other detected pathogens who have an exacerbation, there is consensus that antistaphylococcal antibiotics should be used. The drugs used most often in this case have been reviewed.[8]

Pseudomonas aeruginosa

Epidemiology and clinical associations

With the advent of effective antistaphylococcal therapy, the gram-negative bacterium *P aeruginosa* emerged as a common and important pathogen in CF lung disease (reviewed in Ref.[12]). *P aeruginosa* infection has been associated with[48]:

- Worse lung function outcomes
- Greater respiratory tract inflammation
- A greater risk of respiratory exacerbations
- Higher risk of mortality

Although chronic *P aeruginosa* infection usually cannot be eradicated, current evidence indicates that initial *P aeruginosa* detection presents an opportunity for eradication with antibiotics. There is also good evidence that suppressing *P aeruginosa* can improve measures of lung disease. For CF exacerbations among people with *P aeruginosa*, antipseudomonal antibiotics have been shown to improve outcomes.[49] However, whether early eradication provides similar clinical benefits is still under investigation.[50]

As shown in **Fig. 1**A, *P aeruginosa* prevalence tends to be higher in adults than in children; its overall prevalence has decreased slightly in the past few decades (see **Fig. 1**B), perhaps related to new eradication approaches on initial detection. Longitudinal analyses indicate that *P aeruginosa* tends to exclude other microbes that were previously detected in the respiratory tract, and that it is frequently the predominant, and often the only, bacterium identified in CF lungs during end-stage disease.[51] These aggregate findings have earned *P aeruginosa* the reputation as the most important CF respiratory pathogen.

P aeruginosa has a very large genome, encoding numerous potential toxins controlled by a complex array of regulatory elements. During chronic CF infections, *P aeruginosa* undergoes diverse adaptive changes, including inactivation of many of these so-called virulence factors and their regulators.[52] One of the most common phenotypic changes observed for *P aeruginosa* is the exuberant production of alginate, resulting in a mucoid colony appearance in vitro.[53] Mucoidy has been associated with both persistence and duration of infection; however, it was not associated with failure of early eradication in recent studies. Those studies also identified mucoid isolates on initial detection of *P aeruginosa*.[52] Because mucoidy has traditionally been thought to represent adaptation to the airway, these results may indicate that current detection methods are not perfectly sensitive for earliest infection.

Epidemiologic evidence has identified genetically related isolates of *P aeruginosa* (referred to as epidemic strains) among CF populations in several countries (reviewed in Ref.[54]). In some cases, these isolates were associated with worse outcomes than nonepidemic *P aeruginosa*, including higher risks of death and need for lung transplant. Similarly, *P aeruginosa* resistant to multiple antibiotics has been found to be associated with worse lung disease by several measures, but, as with MRSA and *S aureus* SCVs, whether these resistant *P aeruginosa* identify patients with higher antibiotic exposures, or whether they are more pathogenic than other *P aeruginosa*, remains to be determined.[55]

Treatment

Prophylaxis for *P aeruginosa* is not recommended. However, treatment with antibiotics on initial detection, with the goal of eradication, has proved to be microbiologically effective and to decrease the risk of subsequent exacerbations. Inhaled antibiotics, such as tobramycin and more recently aztreonam, form the basis of the current guidelines[56] for eradication, with no benefit found by adding an oral drug of another class (ciprofloxacin). Similarly, inhaled antibiotics are recommended as chronic maintenance medications for patients with CF with persistent *P aeruginosa*. For exacerbation treatment in patients chronically infected with *P aeruginosa*, limited evidence indicates that treatment with 2 classes of antipseudomonal antibiotics leads to longer periods of clinical stability than does a single class. Treatments for *P aeruginosa* in CF have been the subject of recent reviews and guidelines.[9,56]

Burkholderia cepacia Complex

Epidemiology and clinical associations

The *Burkholderia cepacia* complex (BCC) group of gram-negative bacteria comprises at least 18 distinct species (a related species, *Burkholderia gladioli*, is often discussed with BCC because it can cause similar infections). Of these, 2 species are among the most common and most associated with CF lung infections and disease:

- *Burkholderia cenocepacia*
- *Burkholderia multivorans*

By comparison, other BCC species are less common and their clinical associations less well defined (as is the case for *B gladioli*).[57] As shown in **Fig. 1**, *Burkholderia* species have infected between 3% and 4% of patients with CF in the United States for many years,[4,14] primarily affecting adolescents and adults. *B multivorans* prevalence was highest, followed by *B cenocepacia* and *B gladioli*.

Burkholderia CF infections are notorious for several characteristics:

They are associated with more severe lung disease These associations are more pronounced for some *Burkholderia* species than others; some small studies have shown *B cenocepacia* to be associated with more rapid lung function decline than *B multivorans*, and a recent Canadian study found the strongest association with subsequent mortality to be with *B cenocepacia*, followed by *B multivorans*.[57]

They can be transmissible between persons with cystic fibrosis Epidemic strains of *B cenocepacia* have been shown to infect patients with CF after interpatient contact at camps and clinics[58] and have even been shown to replace *B multivorans* after transmission. This transmissibility was one important driving force behind the institution of stringent infection control measures, which evidence suggests have been highly infective for controlling spread of these strains.

Clinical outcomes of Burkholderia cepacia complex infections are unpredictable Associated outcomes often range from clinical quiescence to rapidly progressive, necrotizing pneumonia and fatal septic disease (so-called "*cepacia* syndrome").

Treatment

At present, the practice of antibiotic treatment for eradication on detection is controversial, and the utility of this practice is not yet clear.[59,60] *Burkholderia* species are also notorious for their antibiotic resistance, both intrinsic and acquired, and therapy is usually limited to specific antibiotics as needed. Systematic reviews have recently been published.[61]

Considerations for the following microbes in CF infections are presented briefly.

Stenotrophomonas maltophilia

- Gram-negative[13,14]
- Increased US CF prevalence in recent years
- Particularly common among adolescents and young adults
- Conflicting data regarding clinical associations
- Both intrinsically and adaptively resistant to many antibiotics
- Inadequate evidence for the clinical impact of therapy; a Cochrane Review of current approaches recently became available

Haemophilus influenzae

- Gram-negative[14]
- Often the first organism detected in CF respiratory cultures; prevalent in children, less common in adults
- Association with CF clinical outcomes is controversial, but associated with adverse outcomes in other chronic respiratory diseases: non-CF bronchiectasis and chronic obstructive pulmonary disease
- Difficult to culture, requiring specific conditions for detection
- Since the introduction in the United States of the *H influenzae* type B vaccine, most isolates are nontypeable and unencapsulated
- Can produce β-lactamase; therefore, treatments usually include a β-lactamase inhibitor (eg, amoxicillin-clavulanate)

Achromobacter xylosoxidans

- Gram-negative bacterium similar to *P aeruginosa*[10,13]
- Increased recent US prevalence, but remains low (<10% of patients with CF; see **Fig. 1**)
- Associated with worse radiographic and spirometric measures of lung disease
- Similar to *P aeruginosa* and BCC, *Achromobacter xylosoxidans* can be the dominant, and sometimes only, bacterium isolated from patients with CF at end stage
- Notorious for resistance to many antibiotics, limiting treatment options

Nontuberculous mycobacteria

- Estimated CF prevalence 6% to 30%[11,13,14]
- Two groups of mycobacteria, accounting for 6 species, are currently considered important CF pathogens:
  - *Mycobacterium avium* complex (MAC)
  - *Mycobacterium abscessus* complex
- NTM treatment approaches usually involve 2 phases:
  - Multiple intravenous (IV) antibiotics for weeks to months
  - Multiple inhaled and oral antibiotics for months to years
  - Side effects and toxicities are common and can be troublesome

- Guidelines for NTM infection diagnosis and treatment from a joint committee based in both the United States and Europe were recently published.[62]

Fungi and Viruses

- Numerous fungi are frequently isolated from patients with CF, including:[11,14]
  - Yeasts (particularly *Candida* spp)
  - Filamentous fungi (including *Aspergillus* spp)
- Whether detection of fungi requires treatment is a matter of current debate.
- Allergic bronchopulmonary aspergillosis (ABPA): patients with CF and other chronic airway diseases can develop an immunoglobulin E–mediated allergic airway disease known as ABPA, the treatment of which primarily involves steroids, although the addition of an antifungal (such as itraconazole) may allow lower doses of steroids
- Human respiratory viruses are not thought to chronically infect the CF airway, but they have been shown to be both important and common triggers of CF respiratory exacerbations

The Cystic Fibrosis Airway Microbiome and Future Directions

The application of DNA-based microbiological techniques to CF respiratory samples has afforded a different view of their microbiota. To date, dozens of such studies using a variety of methods have been performed. This collective work provides evidence for dynamic, diverse, and highly resilient CF respiratory microbial communities (reviewed in Ref.[22]). In general, these respiratory microbiota tend to be more diverse, with more microbial species and not dominated by any individual microbe, in patients with CF who are younger, have better lung function, and/or have had fewer courses of antibiotics. In contrast, this diversity tends to be lower in patients who are older, who have more severe lung disease, and who have been treated with more antibiotics. The microbiota in lungs from patients with end-stage CF disease tend to be dominated by 1 or very few species, most often *P aeruginosa*, BCC, or *A xylosoxidans*. However, these associations between age, disease severity, microbial diversity, and antibiotic burden make it difficult to sort out cause and effect; it is not clear yet whether the decrease in diversity drives disease severity, or whether patients with worse preexisting disease receive more antibiotics that "prune" the microbiota to select for the most adaptable and resistant microbes. It is hoped that ongoing and future studies will better define the causal relationships between infection dynamics, therapy, and disease progression.

Cystic Fibrosis Microbiology: Summary

There have been remarkable changes and developments since the first descriptions of CF lung infections in the 1930s and 1940s. Antibiotics have played a central role in improving lung disease outcomes and overall longevity. However, findings over the past 70 years from both culture-based, classical microbiological methods, and those from newer culture-independent techniques, repeatedly show the resilient and dynamic nature of chronic CF lung infections. These findings warrant ongoing vigilance and innovation, and they highlight the many questions that have arisen in this rapidly moving field. In the years to come, there are certain to be new revelations regarding the mechanisms of infection and the microbial determinants of both CF lung disease and response to treatment, which will lead to new recommendations for therapy and infection control. However, the many controversies discussed earlier regarding the relationships between airway microbes and clinical outcomes underscore the importance of host response in driving CF lung disease. These inflammatory mechanisms are discussed later.

HOST RESPONSE IN CYSTIC FIBROSIS LUNG DISEASE

As emphasized earlier, chronic airway infections are a major driver of progressive airways destruction in CF. Much of the damage seen with chronic infection is mediated by a vigorous and abnormal host response to airway infections, resulting in a vicious cycle that leads to irreversible bronchiectasis and lung function decline[8,63] (**Fig. 2A**). Over the past several decades, numerous studies have documented a heightened, primarily neutrophilic inflammatory response in CF airways. Much of the inflammatory response is driven by the presence of bacterial pathogens, but the reaction is exaggerated even when accounting for the presence of infection.[64,65] Debate continues over how much of the inflammatory response is related to underlying CFTR dysfunction and whether airway inflammation precedes the onset of infection.

In this section, we consider the evidence for the role of CFTR dysfunction in altered host-defense how imbalances in the airway environment contribute to disease pathophysiology and may lead to new therapies; and how specific measures of inflammation, particularly neutrophil elastase (NE), may be useful biomarkers of disease. In addition, current and future approaches to antiinflammatory therapies are considered, and challenges in moving these therapies from the bench to bedside are highlighted.

Cystic Fibrosis Transmembrane Conductance Regulator, Impairments in Host Defense and Inflammation

The role of CFTR in altered host defense has been examined extensively using in vitro cell culture systems, in vivo animal models, and human subject studies. Two recent review articles explore this issue in depth.[15,16] Briefly, several lines of evidence now link CFTR dysfunction to altered host defense through primary and secondary

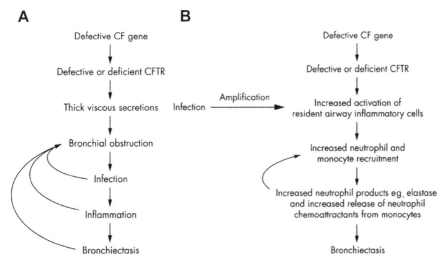

Fig. 2. Pathophysiology of lung disease in CF. (*A*) Traditional view of the development of lung disease in CF. Inflammation is triggered by chronic bacterial infection. (*B*) Potential alternative mechanism for airway inflammation in CF. Underlying CFTR dysfunction contributes to altered host response. (*From* Rao S, Grigg J. New insights into pulmonary inflammation in cystic fibrosis Arch Dis Child 2006;91(9):787; with permission.)

mechanisms (**Fig. 2**B). Airway surface liquid dehydration and acidification results from lack of CFTR function in the epithelial cells lining the airways. Loss of the airway surface liquid layer results in abnormal mucociliary clearance, which is a first layer of defense against microbes. Acidification, caused by lack of bicarbonate secretion by CFTR, likely alters periciliary mucins, resulting in a dense and overly adherent mucus layer lining the cilia.[66,67] Neutrophils and macrophages also express CFTR, and lack of functional CFTR channels likely reduce bacterial killing and clearance by these cells.[15]

In many ways, CF airways disease can be best understood as imbalances initiated by CFTR dysfunction and perpetuated by chronic infection, a necessary but overly exuberant inflammatory response, and airway structural injury that progressively worsens mucociliary clearance. Bacterial burden is typically high in CF airways; however, the neutrophilic inflammatory response is increased for a given bacterial load in patients with CF compared with patients who do not have CF.[64,65] The neutrophilic response is worsened by defects in neutrophil apoptosis and impaired clearance of debris. Defects in mucociliary clearance and macrophage dysfunction lead to accumulation of neutrophils and their products.[15,68] Proteases, primarily NE, are released by neutrophils and overwhelm the normally counteracting antiproteases (eg, alpha-1-antitrypsin, a serine protease inhibitor, and secretory leukocyte protease inhibitor), leading to airways damage.[69,70] Antioxidants in the CF airways are also overwhelmed by oxidative stress from persistent infection and inflammatory responses. CFTR dysfunction may also lead to worsening oxidative imbalance through impairment of Nrf2, a transcription factor crucial in maintaining oxidative reducing capacity. In addition, lipid mediators that regulate antiinflammatory responses to insults are likely abnormal in CF, further limiting the ability of the host to mitigate an overly vigorous inflammatory reaction. Therefore, therapies designed to restore airway equilibrium may help reduce airway injury.

Host Response and Inflammation as Biomarkers of Disease

In addition to contributing to the pathophysiology of CF airway disease, mediators of host response may serve as important biomarkers of disease progression. NE is the most well-documented inflammatory biomarker to date. NE is more abundant in induced sputum in children with CF compared with control children[71]; in school-aged children with CF, increased NE level in induced sputum has been associated with subsequent lung function decline.[72] Increased NE level in BALF is associated with bronchiectasis in infants and preschool-aged children[73] and with lung function measurements in infants with CF.[27] Sputum measures of airway inflammation have also been shown to decrease after treatment of a pulmonary exacerbation with IV antibiotics.[74] In a study of IV antibiotics, higher sputum NE level on day 14 of therapy for a pulmonary exacerbation was associated with increased risk of subsequent exacerbation.[75]

Circulating inflammatory proteins have also been examined as potential biomarkers of disease in CF. In a multicenter study measuring a panel of plasma proteins at onset of a pulmonary exacerbation and following treatment with IV antibiotics, significant reductions in the levels of 10 of 15 proteins were observed.[76] Baseline measurements of IL-8, NE-protease complexes and alpha-1 antitrypsin, when combined with changes in protein markers and lung function, predicted a better treatment response, suggesting that a panel of circulating markers may be useful clinically and for future therapeutic trials. A clinical trial in CF showed reduction in systemic inflammation following 6 months of treatment with chronic azithromycin,[77] although treatment with several agents that were expected to decrease inflammation, including ibuprofen and ivacaftor in patients with the G551D mutation, did not show this anticipated effect.[78,79]

Host Response to Pseudomonas aeruginosa

Several studies have examined the host response to *P aeruginosa* in an effort to understand the clinical associations with this pathogen.[80–82] The interaction between *P aeruginosa* and the CF host is complex and beyond the scope of this article. However, it is likely that CFTR dysfunction predisposes the host to infection with *P aeruginosa*; subsequent adaptation by the bacteria then allows chronic infection and reduced opportunity for eradication. It is also likely that *P aeruginosa* interacts with other bacterial pathogens, including *S aureus* and BCC, in a way that further alters the inflammatory response.[25,83]

Antiinflammatory Therapies in Cystic Fibrosis

As described earlier, an overly exuberant inflammatory response in CF leads to airways damage and worsening bronchiectasis. However, the CF immune response also plays a critical role in containing microbes within the airways and preventing invasive disease. Although therapies that blunt the inflammatory response theoretically may limit airway damage, they could potentially lead to worsening infections. Several antiinflammatory therapies have been studied with variable results, likely because of difficulties in maintaining this balance.

Ibuprofen

In cell and animal models, ibuprofen has been shown to inhibit neutrophil migration and aggregation, including in CF animal models.[84] The effect of chronic high-dose ibuprofen in people with CF was evaluated in a 2-center, randomized, double-blind, placebo-controlled trial.[85] Patients in the treatment group had a slower rate of lung function decline overall, although in a subgroup analysis by age the difference was significant only in patients younger than 13 years. There was no reduction in hospitalization rate seen with treatment. Several follow-up studies confirmed these findings, and showed reasonable safety data, although gastrointestinal bleeding was more common in patients on chronic therapy.[86] A recent Cochrane Review concluded that high-dose ibuprofen could slow the progression of lung disease in CF, particularly in children with mild disease.[87] Despite these findings, clinical use of ibuprofen is uncommon, particularly compared with other CF therapies.[88] Reasons are likely related to persistent clinician concerns about adverse effects (eg, kidney impairment, gastric bleeding), and the need for careful pharmacokinetic monitoring to achieve and maintain therapeutic dosing. Based on pulmonary clinical guidelines published in 2013, the CF Foundation recommends chronic use of ibuprofen in children aged 6 to 17 years with forced expiratory volume in 1 second (FEV_1) greater than 60% (grade B, moderate net benefit), but does not recommend treatment in adults with CF.[89]

Chronic azithromycin

Azithromycin is a macrolide antibiotic with immunomodulatory effects, which are likely the basis for its effectiveness in CF and other chronic inflammatory conditions.[90] Chronic azithromycin has been studied in 2 CF populations: patients with and without chronic *P aeruginosa* infection.[91,92] Patients with chronic *P aeruginosa* infection treated with thrice weekly azithromycin for 6 months had improved FEV_1, decreased risk of pulmonary exacerbation, and improved weight gain compared with placebo.[91] In a second study, patients without *P aeruginosa* treated with azithromycin had a 50% reduction in pulmonary exacerbations and a modest improvement in weight.[92] However, lung function did not improve compared with placebo. CF clinical guidelines recommend azithromycin for people with CF aged 6 years and older with chronic *P aeruginosa* (grade B, moderate net benefit), and consideration of treatment of those without *P aeruginosa* (grade C, moderate net benefit).[89] However, the durability of effect with azithromycin remains unclear, and there are concerns about emergence of bacterial resistance[93,94]; thus, treatment should be reassessed every 6 to 12 months. In addition, patients with NTM should not receive azithromycin unless it is prescribed in combination with other antimycobacterial medications as part of multidrug NTM therapy.

Corticosteroids and leukotriene receptor antagonists

Systemic and inhaled corticosteroids have been studied in patients with CF. Although systemic corticosteroids have been shown to improve lung function, the adverse effects, including poor somatic growth, outweigh any benefit.[95] Inhaled corticosteroids have also not been shown to be effective in CF.[96] Thus, the CF Foundation recommends against the use of chronic systemic or inhaled corticosteroids.[89] Montelukast, a leukotriene receptor antagonist, showed modest effects on lung function and inflammatory markers in a small pediatric study (n = 28); however, more robust data are lacking.[97] A phase 2 clinical trial of a leukotriene B_4 receptor antagonist, BIIL 284 BS, was terminated after an interim analysis revealed increased pulmonary-related, serious adverse events and incidence of pulmonary exacerbations in patients on treatment, highlighting the potential risks of suppressing the immune response in patients with chronic infections.[98]

Clinical trials

Several drugs are being developed for cystic fibrosis. Alpha-1 proteinase inhibitor (alpha-1 HC) is an aerosolized protease inhibitor with antiinflammatory properties. A phase 2 randomized, double-blind, placebo-controlled study of alpha-1 HC given for 3 weeks to adults with CF showed safety and tolerability at 2 dose levels.[99] CTX-4430 is a LTB_4 receptor antagonist that is currently in phase 2 testing; risk of pulmonary adverse events and exacerbations will be closely monitored, particularly given the previous results with BIIL 284 BS (trial number NCT02443688, clinicaltrials.gov). Ajulemic acid (JBT-101) is an oral synthetic cannabinoid agonist that binds to the CB2 receptor expressed on activated immune cells and fibroblasts, and is thought to help resolve inflammation and limit fibrosis.[100] A 12-week, phase 2 study in adults with CF is currently recruiting (trial number NCT02465450, clinicaltrials.gov).

SUMMARY

Airway obstruction, infection, and inflammation lead to much of the morbidity and mortality associated with CF. *P aeruginosa*, *S aureus*, and BCC are the bacteria most frequently associated with CF lung disease; improved and aggressive antimicrobial treatment of these pathogens has contributed greatly to improvements in life expectancy. However, airway microbial communities are complex and likely influenced by environment, host characteristics, disease progression, and antibiotic treatment. Host response to microbes in the CF airways is robust, likely in part because of underlying CFTR protein dysfunction. The overly exuberant host inflammatory response and decreased host ability to clear microbes and inflammatory debris from the airways leads to further damage. Therapies targeting airway infections and host inflammatory response are effective in reducing disease activity, but do not fully stop progression. However, several antiinflammatory and antimicrobial therapies are being developed. In addition, CFTR modulator therapy, newly available for ~50% of people with CF, and with the hope of expanded treatments for all with CF, will undoubtedly influence both airway microbiology and inflammatory responses.

REFERENCES

1. Andersen D. Cystic fibrosis of the pancreas and its relation to celiac disease: a clinical and pathological study. Am J Child 1938;56:344–99.
2. Di sant'agnese PE, Andersen DH. Celiac syndrome; chemotherapy in infections of the respiratory tract associated with cystic fibrosis of the pancreas; observations with penicillin and drugs of the sulfonamide group, with special reference to penicillin aerosol. Am J Dis Child 1946;72:17–61.
3. Lyczak JB, Cannon CL, Pier GB. Lung infections associated with cystic fibrosis. Clin Microbiol Rev 2002;15:194–222.
4. Cystic Fibrosis Foundation. Cystic Fibrosis Foundation patient registry 2013 annual data report to the center directors. 2014.
5. Armstrong DS, Hook SM, Jamsen KM, et al. Lower airway inflammation in infants with cystic fibrosis detected by newborn screening. Pediatr Pulmonol 2005;40: 500–10.
6. Stoltz DA, Meyerholz DK, Pezzulo AA, et al. Cystic fibrosis pigs develop lung disease and exhibit defective bacterial eradication at birth. Sci Transl Med 2010;2:29ra31.
7. Khan TZ, Wagener JS, Bost T, et al. Early pulmonary inflammation in infants with cystic fibrosis. Am J Respir Crit Care Med 1995;151:1075–82.
8. Gibson RL, Burns JL, Ramsey BW. Pathophysiology and management of pulmonary infections in cystic fibrosis. Am J Respir Crit Care Med 2003;168:918–51.
9. Waters V, Smyth A. Cystic fibrosis microbiology: advances in antimicrobial therapy. J Cyst Fibros 2015;14:551–60.
10. Chmiel JF, Aksamit TR, Chotirmall SH, et al. Antibiotic management of lung infections in cystic fibrosis. I. The microbiome, methicillin-resistant *Staphylococcus aureus*, gram-negative bacteria, and multiple infections. Ann Am Thorac Soc 2014;11:1120–9.
11. Chmiel JF, Aksamit TR, Chotirmall SH, et al. Antibiotic management of lung infections in cystic fibrosis. II. Nontuberculous mycobacteria, anaerobic bacteria, and fungi. Ann Am Thorac Soc 2014;11:1298–306.
12. Gilligan PH. Microbiology of airway disease in patients with cystic fibrosis. Clin Microbiol Rev 1991;4:35–51.
13. Parkins MD, Floto RA. Emerging bacterial pathogens and changing concepts of bacterial pathogenesis in cystic fibrosis. J Cyst Fibros 2015;14:293–304.
14. Lipuma JJ. The changing microbial epidemiology in cystic fibrosis. Clin Microbiol Rev 2010;23:299–323.
15. Nichols DP, Chmiel JF. Inflammation and its genesis in cystic fibrosis. Pediatr Pulmonol 2015;50(Suppl 40):S39–56.
16. Cantin AM, Hartl D, Konstan MW, et al. Inflammation in cystic fibrosis lung disease: pathogenesis and therapy. J Cyst Fibros 2015;14:419–30.
17. Ulrich M, Herbert S, Berger J, et al. Localization of *Staphylococcus aureus* in infected airways of patients with cystic fibrosis and in a cell culture model of *S. aureus* adherence. Am J Respir Cell Mol Biol 1998;19:83–91.
18. Worlitzsch D, Tarran R, Ulrich M, et al. Effects of reduced mucus oxygen concentration in airway *Pseudomonas* infections of cystic fibrosis patients. J Clin Invest 2002;109:317–25.
19. Baltimore RS, Christie CD, Smith GJ. Immunohistopathologic localization of *Pseudomonas aeruginosa* in lungs from patients with cystic fibrosis. Implications for the pathogenesis of progressive lung deterioration. Am Rev Respir Dis 1989;140:1650–61.

20. Schwab U, Abdullah LH, Perlmutt OS, et al. Localization of *Burkholderia cepacia* complex bacteria in cystic fibrosis lungs and interactions with *Pseudomonas aeruginosa* in hypoxic mucus. Infect Immun 2014;82:4729–45.

21. Saiman L, Siegel JD, LiPuma JJ, et al. Infection prevention and control guideline for cystic fibrosis: 2013 update. Infect Control Hosp Epidemiol 2014;35(Suppl 1):S1–67.

22. Caverly LJ, Zhao J, LiPuma JJ. Cystic fibrosis lung microbiome: Opportunities to reconsider management of airway infection. Pediatr Pulmonol 2015;50:S31–8.

23. Singh PK, Schaefer AL, Parsek MR, et al. Quorum-sensing signals indicate that cystic fibrosis lungs are infected with bacterial biofilms. Nature 2000;407:762–4.

24. Hauser AR, Jain M, Bar-Meir M, et al. Clinical significance of microbial infection and adaptation in cystic fibrosis. Clin Microbiol Rev 2011;24:29–70.

25. Sagel SD, Gibson RL, Emerson J, et al. Impact of *Pseudomonas* and *Staphylococcus* infection on inflammation and clinical status in young children with cystic fibrosis. J Pediatr 2009;154:183–8.

26. Gangell C, Gard S, Douglas T, et al. Inflammatory responses to individual microorganisms in the lungs of children with cystic fibrosis. Clin Infect Dis 2011;53: 425–32.

27. Pillarisetti N, Williamson E, Linnane B, et al. Infection, inflammation, and lung function decline in infants with cystic fibrosis. Am J Respir Crit Care Med 2011;184:75–81.

28. Cogen J, Emerson J, Sanders DB, et al. Risk factors for lung function decline in a large cohort of young cystic fibrosis patients. Pediatr Pulmonol 2015;50: 763–70.

29. Hudson VL, Wielinski CL, Regelmann WE. Prognostic implications of initial oropharyngeal bacterial flora in patients with cystic fibrosis diagnosed before the age of two years. J Pediatr 1993;122:854–60.

30. Liou TG, Adler FR, Fitzsimmons SC, et al. Predictive 5-year survivorship model of cystic fibrosis. Am J Epidemiol 2001;153:345–52.

31. Mayer-Hamblett N, Aitken ML, Accurso FJ, et al. Association between pulmonary function and sputum biomarkers in cystic fibrosis. Am J Respir Crit Care Med 2007;175:822–8.

32. Ahlgren HG, Benedetti A, Landry JS, et al. Clinical outcomes associated with *Staphylococcus aureus* and *Pseudomonas aeruginosa* airway infections in adult cystic fibrosis patients. BMC Pulm Med 2015;15:67.

33. Goss CH, Muhlebach MS. Review: *Staphylococcus aureus* and MRSA in cystic fibrosis. J Cyst Fibros 2011;10:298–306.

34. Ren CL, Morgan WJ, Konstan MW, et al. Presence of methicillin resistant *Staphylococcus aureus* in respiratory cultures from cystic fibrosis patients is associated with lower lung function. Pediatr Pulmonol 2007;42:513–8.

35. Sawicki GS, Rasouliyan L, Pasta DJ, et al. The impact of incident methicillin resistant *Staphylococcus aureus* detection on pulmonary function in cystic fibrosis. Pediatr Pulmonol 2008;43:1117–23.

36. Muhlebach MS, Heltshe SL, Popowitch EB, et al. Multicenter observational study on factors and outcomes associated with different MRSA types in children with cystic fibrosis. Ann Am Thorac Soc 2015. http://dx.doi.org/10.1513/AnnalsATS. 201412-596OC.

37. Dasenbrook EC, Merlo CA, Diener-West M, et al. Persistent methicillin-resistant *Staphylococcus aureus* and rate of FEV_1 decline in cystic fibrosis. Am J Respir Crit Care Med 2008;178:814–21.

38. Sanders DB, Bittner RC, Rosenfeld M, et al. Failure to recover to baseline pulmonary function after cystic fibrosis pulmonary exacerbation. Am J Respir Crit Care Med 2010;182:627–32.

39. Dasenbrook EC, Checkley W, Merlo CA, et al. Association between respiratory tract methicillin-resistant *Staphylococcus aureus* and survival in cystic fibrosis. JAMA 2010;303:2386–92.

40. Besier S, Smaczny C, von Mallinckrodt C, et al. Prevalence and clinical significance of *Staphylococcus aureus* small-colony variants in cystic fibrosis lung disease. J Clin Microbiol 2007;45:168–72.

41. Kahl B, Herrmann M, Everding AS, et al. Persistent infection with small colony variant strains of *Staphylococcus aureus* in patients with cystic fibrosis. J Infect Dis 1998;177:1023–9.

42. Schneider M, Mühlemann K, Droz S, et al. Clinical characteristics associated with isolation of small-colony variants of *Staphylococcus aureus* and *Pseudomonas aeruginosa* from respiratory secretions of patients with cystic fibrosis. J Clin Microbiol 2008;46:1832–4.

43. Wolter D, Emerson JC, McNamara S, et al. Prevalence and clinical significance of *Staphylococcus aureus* small-colony variants in children with CF: A cohort study. Pediatr Pulmonol 2012;S35:276.

44. Hoffman LR, Déziel E, D'Argenio DA, et al. Selection for *Staphylococcus aureus* small-colony variants due to growth in the presence of *Pseudomonas aeruginosa*. Proc Natl Acad Sci U S A 2006;103:19890–5.

45. Smyth AR, Walters S. Prophylactic anti-staphylococcal antibiotics for cystic fibrosis. Cochrane Database Syst Rev 2014;(11):CD001912.

46. Dalbøge CS, Pressler T, Høiby N, et al. A cohort study of the Copenhagen CF Centre eradication strategy against *Staphylococcus aureus* in patients with CF. J Cyst Fibros 2013;12:42–8.

47. Lo DKH, Hurley MN, Muhlebach MS, et al. Interventions for the eradication of methicillin-resistant *Staphylococcus aureus* (MRSA) in people with cystic fibrosis. Cochrane Database Syst Rev 2015;(2):CD009650.

48. Langton Hewer SC, Smyth AR. Antibiotic strategies for eradicating Pseudomonas aeruginosa in people with cystic fibrosis. Cochrane Database Syst Rev 2014;11:CD004197.

49. Regelmann WE, Elliott GR, Warwick WJ, et al. Reduction of sputum *Pseudomonas aeruginosa* density by antibiotics improves lung function in cystic fibrosis more than do bronchodilators and chest physiotherapy alone. Am Rev Respir Dis 1990;141:914–21.

50. Mayer-Hamblett N, Kloster M, Rosenfeld M, et al. Impact of sustained eradication of new *Pseudomonas aeruginosa* infection on long-term outcomes in cystic fibrosis. Clin Infect Dis 2015;61:707–15.

51. Zhao J, Schloss PD, Kalikin LM, et al. Decade-long bacterial community dynamics in cystic fibrosis airways. Proc Natl Acad Sci U S A 2012;109:5809–14.

52. Mayer-Hamblett N, Rosenfeld M, Gibson RL, et al. *Pseudomonas aeruginosa* in vitro phenotypes distinguish cystic fibrosis infection stages and outcomes. Am J Respir Crit Care Med 2014;190:289–97.

53. Li Z, Kosorok MR, Farrell PM, et al. Longitudinal development of mucoid *Pseudomonas aeruginosa* infection and lung disease progression in children with cystic fibrosis. JAMA 2005;293:581–8.

54. Oliver A, Mulet X, López-Causapé C, et al. The increasing threat of *Pseudomonas aeruginosa* high-risk clones. Drug Resist Updat 2015;21–22:41–59.

55. Merlo CA, Boyle MP, Diener-West M, et al. Incidence and risk factors for multiple antibiotic-resistant *Pseudomonas aeruginosa* in cystic fibrosis. Chest 2007;132: 562–8.
56. Mogayzel PJ, Naureckas ET, Robinson KA, et al. Cystic Fibrosis Foundation pulmonary guideline. Pharmacologic approaches to prevention and eradication of initial *Pseudomonas aeruginosa* infection. Ann Am Thorac Soc 2014;11: 1640–50.
57. Zlosnik JEA, Zhou G, Brant R, et al. *Burkholderia* species infections in patients with cystic fibrosis in British Columbia, Canada. 30 years' experience. Ann Am Thorac Soc 2015;12:70–8.
58. Lipuma JJ. Update on the *Burkholderia cepacia* complex. Curr Opin Pulm Med 2005;11:528–33.
59. Horsley A, Webb K, Bright-Thomas R, et al. Can early *Burkholderia cepacia* complex infection in cystic fibrosis be eradicated with antibiotic therapy? Front Cell Infect Microbiol 2011;1:18.
60. Regan KH, Bhatt J. Eradication therapy for Burkholderia cepacia complex in people with cystic fibrosis. Cochrane Database Syst Rev 2014;10:CD009876.
61. Avgeri SG, Matthaiou DK, Dimopoulos G, et al. Therapeutic options for *Burkholderia cepacia* infections beyond co-trimoxazole: a systematic review of the clinical evidence. Int J Antimicrob Agents 2009;33:394–404.
62. Floto RA, Olivier KN, Saiman L, et al. US Cystic Fibrosis Foundation and European Cystic Fibrosis Society consensus recommendations for the management of non-tuberculous mycobacteria in individuals with cystic fibrosis. Thorax 2016; 71(Suppl 1):i1–22.
63. Ratjen F, Döring G. Cystic fibrosis. Lancet 2003;361(9358):681–9.
64. Muhlebach MS, Stewart PW, Leigh MW, et al. Quantitation of inflammatory responses to bacteria in young cystic fibrosis and control patients. Am J Respir Crit Care Med 1999;160:186–91.
65. Noah TL, Black HR, Cheng PW, et al. Nasal and bronchoalveolar lavage fluid cytokines in early cystic fibrosis. J Infect Dis 1997;175:638–47.
66. Boucher RC. Airway surface dehydration in cystic fibrosis: pathogenesis and therapy. Annu Rev Med 2007;58:157–70.
67. Pezzulo AA, Tang XX, Hoegger MJ, et al. Reduced airway surface pH impairs bacterial killing in the porcine cystic fibrosis lung. Nature 2012;487:109–13.
68. Alexis NE, Muhlebach MS, Peden DB, et al. Attenuation of host defense function of lung phagocytes in young cystic fibrosis patients. J Cyst Fibros 2006;5: 17–25.
69. Birrer P, McElvaney NG, Rüdeberg A, et al. Protease-antiprotease imbalance in the lungs of children with cystic fibrosis. Am J Respir Crit Care Med 1994;150: 207–13.
70. Weldon S, McNally P, McElvaney NG, et al. Decreased levels of secretory leucoprotease inhibitor in the Pseudomonas-infected cystic fibrosis lung are due to neutrophil elastase degradation. J Immunol 2009;183:8148–56.
71. Sagel SD, Kapsner R, Osberg I, et al. Airway inflammation in children with cystic fibrosis and healthy children assessed by sputum induction. Am J Respir Crit Care Med 2001;164:1425–31.
72. Sagel SD, Wagner BD, Anthony MM, et al. Sputum biomarkers of inflammation and lung function decline in children with cystic fibrosis. Am J Respir Crit Care Med 2012;186:857–65.
73. Sly PD, Gangell CL, Chen L, et al. Risk factors for bronchiectasis in children with cystic fibrosis. N Engl J Med 2013;368:1963–70.

74. Ordonez CL, Henig NR, Mayer-Hamblett N, et al. Inflammatory and microbiologic markers in induced sputum after intravenous antibiotics in cystic fibrosis. Am J Respir Crit Care Med 2003;168:1471–5.

75. Waters VJ, Stanojevic S, Sonneveld N, et al. Factors associated with response to treatment of pulmonary exacerbations in cystic fibrosis patients. J Cyst Fibros 2015;14:755–62.

76. Sagel SD, Thompson V, Chmiel JF, et al. Effect of treatment of cystic fibrosis pulmonary exacerbations on systemic inflammation. Ann Am Thorac Soc 2015;12:708–17.

77. Ratjen F, Saiman L, Mayer-Hamblett N, et al. Effect of azithromycin on systemic markers of inflammation in patients with cystic fibrosis uninfected with *Pseudomonas aeruginosa*. Chest 2012;142:1259–66.

78. Rowe SM, Heltshe SL, Gonska T, et al. Clinical mechanism of the cystic fibrosis transmembrane conductance regulator potentiator ivacaftor in G551D-mediated cystic fibrosis. Am J Respir Crit Care Med 2014;190:175–84.

79. Chmiel JF, Konstan MW, Accurso FJ, et al. Use of ibuprofen to assess inflammatory biomarkers in induced sputum: Implications for clinical trials in cystic fibrosis. J Cyst Fibros 2015. http://dx.doi.org/10.1016/j.jcf.2015.03.007.

80. Aldallal N, McNaughton EE, Manzel LJ, et al. Inflammatory response in airway epithelial cells isolated from patients with cystic fibrosis. Am J Respir Crit Care Med 2002;166:1248–56.

81. Lovewell RR, Patankar YR, Berwin B. Mechanisms of phagocytosis and host clearance of *Pseudomonas aeruginosa*. Am J Physiol Lung Cell Mol Physiol 2014;306:L591–603.

82. Buchanan PJ, Ernst RK, Elborn JS, et al. Role of CFTR, Pseudomonas aeruginosa and Toll-like receptors in cystic fibrosis lung inflammation. Biochem Soc Trans 2009;37:863–7.

83. Chattoraj SS, Murthy R, Ganesan S, et al. *Pseudomonas aeruginosa* alginate promotes *Burkholderia cenocepacia* persistence in cystic fibrosis transmembrane conductance regulator knockout mice. Infect Immun 2010;78:984–93.

84. Konstan MW, Vargo KM, Davis PB. Ibuprofen attenuates the inflammatory response to *Pseudomonas aeruginosa* in a rat model of chronic pulmonary infection. Implications for antiinflammatory therapy in cystic fibrosis. Am Rev Respir Dis 1990;141:186–92.

85. Konstan MW, Byard PJ, Hoppel CL, et al. Effect of high-dose ibuprofen in patients with cystic fibrosis. N Engl J Med 1995;332:848–54.

86. Konstan MW. Ibuprofen therapy for cystic fibrosis lung disease: revisited. Curr Opin Pulm Med 2008;14:567–73.

87. Lands LC, Stanojevic S. Oral non-steroidal anti-inflammatory drug therapy for lung disease in cystic fibrosis. Cochrane Database Syst Rev 2013;(6):CD001505.

88. Konstan MW, VanDevanter DR, Rasouliyan L, et al. Trends in the use of routine therapies in cystic fibrosis: 1995-2005. Pediatr Pulmonol 2010;45:1167–72.

89. Mogayzel PJ, Naureckas ET, Robinson KA, et al. Cystic fibrosis pulmonary guidelines. Chronic medications for maintenance of lung health. Am J Respir Crit Care Med 2013;187:680–9.

90. Zarogoulidis P, Papanas N, Kioumis I, et al. Macrolides: from in vitro anti-inflammatory and immunomodulatory properties to clinical practice in respiratory diseases. Eur J Clin Pharmacol 2012;68:479–503.

91. Saiman L, Marshall BC, Mayer-Hamblett N, et al. Azithromycin in patients with cystic fibrosis chronically infected with *Pseudomonas aeruginosa*: a randomized controlled trial. JAMA 2003;290:1749–56.

92. Saiman L, Anstead M, Mayer-Hamblett N, et al. Effect of azithromycin on pulmonary function in patients with cystic fibrosis uninfected with *Pseudomonas aeruginosa*: a randomized controlled trial. JAMA 2010;303:1707–15.

93. Saiman L, Mayer-Hamblett N, Anstead M, et al. Open-label, follow-on study of azithromycin in pediatric patients with CF uninfected with *Pseudomonas aeruginosa*. Pediatr Pulmonol 2012;47:641–8.

94. Tramper-Stranders GA, Wolfs TFW, Fleer A, et al. Maintenance azithromycin treatment in pediatric patients with cystic fibrosis: long-term outcomes related to macrolide resistance and pulmonary function. Pediatr Infect Dis J 2007;26: 8–12.

95. Eigen H, Rosenstein BJ, FitzSimmons S, et al. A multicenter study of alternate-day prednisone therapy in patients with cystic fibrosis. Cystic Fibrosis Foundation Prednisone Trial Group. J Pediatr 1995;126:515–23.

96. Balfour-Lynn IM, Welch K. Inhaled corticosteroids for cystic fibrosis. Cochrane Database Syst Rev 2014;(10):CD001915.

97. Stelmach I, Korzeniewska A, Stelmach W, et al. Effects of montelukast treatment on clinical and inflammatory variables in patients with cystic fibrosis. Ann Allergy Asthma Immunol 2005;95:372–80.

98. Konstan MW, Döring G, Heltshe SL, et al. A randomized double blind, placebo controlled phase 2 trial of BIIL 284 BS (an LTB4 receptor antagonist) for the treatment of lung disease in children and adults with cystic fibrosis. J Cyst Fibros 2014;13:148–55.

99. Gaggar A, Chen J, Chmiel JF, et al. Inhaled alpha1-proteinase inhibitor therapy in patients with cystic fibrosis. J Cyst Fibros 2015. http://dx.doi.org/10.1016/j.jcf2015.07.009.

100. Burstein SH, Zurier RB. Cannabinoids, endocannabinoids, and related analogs in inflammation. AAPS J 2009;11:109–19.

Respiratory System Disease

Danielle M. Goetz, MD*, Shipra Singh, MD, MPH

KEYWORDS

- Cystic fibrosis • Bronchiectasis • Lung disease • CFTR • Pulmonary exacerbation
- Lung function

KEY POINTS

- Defects in the cystic fibrosis transmembrane regulator (CFTR) lead to airway surface liquid depletion, abnormal pH, inflammation, and chronic infection, causing the pulmonary symptoms/signs of cystic fibrosis (CF).
- Patients with CF are living longer, although respiratory disease remains as the leading cause of mortality; survival bias exists owing to those with "milder" mutations.
- Early lung disease occurs in children with minimal or absent symptoms; the ideal combination of monitoring with lung function, imaging, and bronchoscopy is controversial.
- Pulmonary exacerbations are a major cause of morbidity and expense, although the definition is debated.
- Chronic treatments with physiotherapy, mucolytic, antiinflammatory, and antimicrobial agents are recommended; CFTR potentiators and correctors may change the face of the disease.

 Video content accompanies this article at http://www.pediatric.theclinics.com.

PATHOPHYSIOLOGY

Cystic fibrosis (CF) is an autosomal recessive disease occurring in approximately 1 in 3500 people and 70,000 people worldwide.[1] The gene for CF was discovered in 1989[2] and encodes the cystic fibrosis transmembrane regulator (CFTR) protein. As of 2015, there are nearly 2000 identified mutations in CFTR, approximately 200 of which are disease causing (see www.CFTR2.org). The cascade of events by which CFTR defects lead to irreversible airway wall damage is shown in **Fig. 1**. Lack of chloride and bicarbonate secretion through CFTR and excessive sodium absorption through the epithelial sodium channel leads to airway surface liquid (ASL) depletion.[3] Deficient

---

Disclosure Statement: The authors have nothing to disclose.
Pediatric Pulmonology, Jacobs School of Medicine, Women & Children's Hospital of Buffalo, State University of New York, 219 Bryant Street, Buffalo, NY 14222, USA
* Corresponding author.
E-mail address: dgoetz@upa.chob.edu

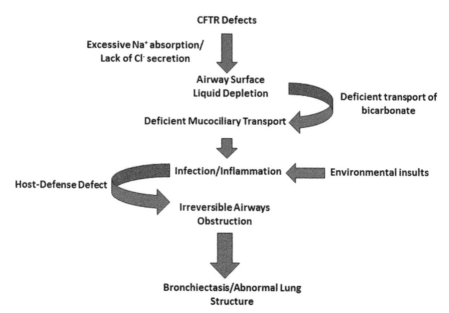

Fig. 1. CFTR defects lead to airway damage and bronchiectasis.

transport of bicarbonate and abnormal pH prevent proper antimicrobial function. The pH in the nasal ASL is lower in CF infants compared with normal infants; in older children and adults, the correlation of pH and genotype is variable, possibly owing to secondary effects of infection and/or inflammation.[4] ASL depletion and abnormal pH contribute to impaired mucociliary clearance. Recent data have suggested that mucociliary transport in piglets with CF is abnormal not only owing to ASL depletion, but also to abnormal adherence of mucus to the submucosal glands[5] and increased mucus viscosity, owing to bicarbonate secretion abnormalities.[6] Reduced MCC effectiveness, amino acid–rich and iron-rich sputum, as well as reduced antimicrobial activity allow typical CF-associated bacteria to grow.[4,7]

Airway inflammation adds to the cycle of excessive mucus production and infection. Neutrophil elastase, a protease released from neutrophils, causes neutrophil transmigration into the airways, mucus secretion, goblet cell hyperplasia, and CFTR degradation.[5] Other proteases such as cathepsins and matrix metalloproteases are involved in the inflammatory cascade. Irreversible airways obstruction leads to bronchiectasis, resulting in loss of lung function. See Video 1 from the CF Foundation (CFF) website demonstrating normal versus abnormal ciliary movement: https://www.youtube.com/watch?feature=player_embedded&v=YzjnxegMWfk.

Lung Disease, Mortality, and Determinants of Lung Disease Severity

The median predicted age of survival in people with CF has steadily increased over the last 25 years from approximately 28 to 39 years of age.[8] These data do not reflect the new corrector/potentiator therapies (see Ong T, Ramsey BW: New Therapeutic Approaches to Modulate and Correct CFTR, in this issue), but reflect earlier diagnosis by newborn screening. In 2014, 64% of new CF diagnoses in the United States were detected by newborn screening.[8] The Wisconsin newborn screening cohort showed that the significant determinants of lung disease were genotype, poor growth, hospitalizations, meconium ileus, and infection with mucoid *Pseudomonas aeruginosa*.[9]

The median age of patients with CF is higher in people who have class IV or V mutations compared with class I, II, or III mutations.[8] However, pulmonary phenotype can be either mild or severe among individuals with the same mutation.[10] On a population level, children with 1 or no copies of the F508del mutation have a slower decline in lung function; low body mass index, female gender, and presence of various organisms on culture are associated with a more rapid decline.[11–13] Hispanic ethnicity is associated with higher mortality in patients with CF.[14]

CLINICAL PRESENTATION
Early Pulmonary Disease

Most infants diagnosed by newborn screening are asymptomatic. Universal adoption of CF newborn screening in the United States[15] has led to earlier diagnosis and treatment. Animal models have shown that structural lung damage occurs in utero and in piglets before symptoms develop.[16,17] Data from the Australian Respiratory Early Surveillance Team for Cystic Fibrosis suggest early lung disease occurs in infants and preschoolers with no symptoms.[3,18–21] Computed tomography (CT) evidence of bronchiectasis was reported in 44% of patients at initial assessment; at the 1-year follow-up, 26% of these findings had resolved. Of the remaining 18%, 74% persisted and 63% progressed.[3] Air trapping was the most common finding, reported in 88% of the scans, and persisted in 81% of subsequent scans.[3] In a longitudinal multicenter observational study in England, volumetric CT scans obtained at 1 year of age in infants with CF showed similar prevalence of bronchiectasis.[22] Air trapping was less common.[19] A study from the Netherlands showed that peripheral bronchiectasis progresses despite normal pulmonary function tests.[23]

The London Cystic Fibrosis Collaboration showed objective measures of decreased lung function in 3-month-old infants with CF diagnosed by newborn screening.[24] These abnormalities indicate the presence of early lung disease in patients with CF compared with normals. Lower infant lung function was also associated with infection from either *Staphylococcus aureus* or *P aeruginosa*.[20] Bronchoalveolar lavage in infants with CF showed neutrophilic inflammation as early as 4 weeks of age,[20,23,25,26] in patients with and without pathogens. Active elastase and increased interleukin-8 levels were present, confirming the presence of inflammation early in life.[25]

Later Pulmonary Disease

Before newborn screening, infants and children were diagnosed clinically with respiratory symptoms such as cough (either dry or productive) in 45% of patients.[27,28] Recurrent bronchiolitis with wheezing or airway reactivity can be seen.[28] Diagnosis may be delayed in patients with milder or rarer mutations, false-negative newborn screens, and birthdate preceding newborn screening implementation in their state of birth. As lung disease progresses, exercise intolerance and shortness of breath develop.[28] Chronic bronchitis progressing to obstructive lung disease and bronchiectasis is the hallmark of CF lung disease. Bronchiectasis (**Fig. 2**) leads to reduced lung function and respiratory failure. Typical physical findings include increased anteroposterior diameter of the chest, seen as hyperinflation on chest radiographs (**Fig. 3**), scattered or localized crackles, and digital clubbing.[28] Other manifestations of CF are listed in **Box 1**.

SINUS DISEASE

The unified airway theory proposes that organisms colonizing the upper airway lead to chronic infection in the lower airways.[29,30] Chronic rhinosinusitis is common in CF and may lead to decreased appetite and cough. Chronic rhinosinusitis is defined in **Box 2**[31]

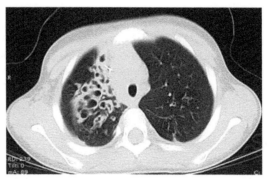

Fig. 2. Bronchiectasis in the right upper lobe in cystic fibrosis.

along with information on treatment of sinusitis and polyps.[29,32–36] In some patients with CF, nasal endoscopy will demonstrate a nose filled with polypoid tissue that bleeds easily; CT of the sinuses is the best imaging modality for diagnosis of anatomic sinus abnormalities in CF,[32] such as sinus hypoplasia, medial bowing of the lateral nasal wall, lower fovea ethmoidalis, and uncinated process reabsorption.[32] Sinus disease in CF can be treated with nonsurgical or surgical measures (**Box 3**).[32]

ASSESSMENT AND MONITORING OF LUNG DISEASE
Lung Function Testing

Spirometry
Spirometry measures the forced expiratory volume in 1 second (FEV_1), using height, gender, and age as standards (FEV_1% predicted). **Box 4**[37–41] describes key points about spirometry. Height changes rapidly during childhood; thus, absolute values for FEV_1 always increase. Predicted values are used to interpret whether the increases are appropriate or show signs of decline. Spirometry is the core measurement of lung function in patients with CF; however, children need to be able to cooperate with the maneuvers. Thus, detection of lung disease in early childhood is challenging. Testing in younger children includes infant lung function testing, preschool spirometry and lung clearance index (**Table 1**).[37,41–59] At present, these tests are not done routinely but are used in research.

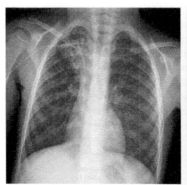
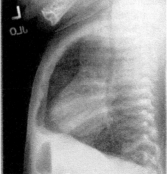

Fig. 3. Hyperinflation and bronchiectasis on chest radiograph in cystic fibrosis (posteroanterior and lateral films).

Box 1
Clinical manifestations of cystic fibrosis

- Bronchiectasis/airways obstruction
- Sinus disease (chronic pansinusitis)
- Pancreatic insufficiency (85%)
- Growth failure
- Pancreatitis
- Digital clubbing
- Infertility
- Meconium ileus/distal intestinal obstructive syndrome
- Cystic fibrosis-related diabetes
- Hepatobiliary disease
- Rectal prolapse

Data from Boat TF, Acton JD. Cystic fibrosis. In: Kliegman B, editor. Nelson textbook of pediatrics. 18th edition: Philadelphia: Elsevier; 2008. p. 1803–16.

Radiology

Chest radiographs and chest computed tomography

The CFF recommends that chest radiographs be done annually. Scoring systems have been developed for objectivity.[60,61] Although less sensitive than chest CT, chest radiographs can detect mucus plugging, atelectasis, consolidation, and bronchial wall thickening. Chest CT scans are not recommended on a routine basis owing to radiation dose, need for sedation, and need to control for volume, especially in young children.[62] However, chest CT may be considered on a case-by-case basis, because it is more sensitive to the presence and severity of disease compared with $FEV_1\%$, shows improvement with therapy, and predicts future disease progression.[20,63] CT also

---

Box 2
Definition of patients with chronic rhinosinusitis

Subjective Symptoms	Objective Symptoms
Mucopurulent nasal drainage	Mucosal inflammation on nasal endoscopy
Nasal congestion	Radiographic findings of mucosal inflammation
Facial pain	
Decreased sense of smell	

- Chronic rhinosinusitis affects 12.5% of the general population; at least 50% of CF patients.[29]

- Ten percent to 36% of CF patients have had sinus surgery.[29]

- Whereas 1 study showed no difference between carriers and the general population,[32] another study showed 36% carriers of a single CFTR mutation reported sinus symptoms compared with 13% of the general population.[33]

Patients must have ≥12 weeks of 2 of the 4 subjective symptoms and 1 of the 2 objective findings.
Abbreviation: CF, cystic fibrosis.

Data from Rosenfeld RM, Andes D, Bhattacharyya N, et al. Clinical practice guideline: adult sinusitis. Otolaryngol Head Neck Surg 2007;137(3 Suppl):S1–31.

Box 3
Treatments for chronic rhinosinusitis and polyposis in CF

Nonsurgical treatment for chronic rhinosinusitis and polyposis in CF

- Saline irrigation (Neti-Pot, saline rinses, etc)
- Topical steroids (nasal steroids)
- Irrigations with 3% hypertonic saline
- Sinusitis treatment with antibiotics for 3 to 6 weeks: penicillins, cephalosporins, quinolones, aminoglycosides
- Irrigations with tobramycin

Surgical treatment for chronic rhinosinusitis and polyposis in CF

- Indications
  - Persistent nasal congestion/obstruction, headache, uncontrolled pain, infection, mucocele, unresolved fevers, awaiting lung transplantation
- Purpose
  - Widen natural sinus ostia to improve drainage, reduced inflammation and to remove nasal polyps
  - Maximize postoperative medical therapy
- Approaches
  - Polypectomy
  - Widening of the natural sinus ostia ("wide antrostomies")
  - Endoscopic medial maxillectomy
  - FESS: chronic sinus disease success rates of 80% to 93%, but with sinonasal polyposis, 40% to 70% resolution of symptoms and recurrence rates are greater than 50%

Abbreviations: CF, cystic fibrosis; FESS, functional endoscopic sinus surgery.
Data from Fundakowski C, Ojo R, Younis R. Rhinosinusitis in the pediatric patient with cystic fibrosis. Curr Pediatr Rev 2014;10(3):198–201.

---

correlates with true endpoints, like survival, pulmonary exacerbations (PEx), quality of life, FEV_1, lung clearance index, and bronchoalveolar lavage inflammatory markers.[64] The role of MRI in the monitoring of lung disease in CF and its response to treatment is being evaluated.[65,66] The clear advantage of MRI over chest CT is the lack of ionizing radiation; however, sedation is needed for most young children.

Airway Cultures

A broad range of bacteria colonize the respiratory tract in patients with CF and are found in throat cultures, sputum, or bronchoalveolar lavage samples. By adulthood,

---

Box 4
Key points about spirometry

- Forced expiratory flow between 25 to 75 of forced vital capacity (FEF_{25-75}) is more variable than FEV_1, but also more sensitive to changes in the small airways.
- FEV_1% predicted predicts future morbidity and mortality.
- Increasing numbers of children have normal spirometry until adolescence.
- Spirometry is useful in those with moderate to severe lung disease, but it is not a sensitive tool for monitoring disease in patients with mild lung disease.

Abbreviations: FEF, forced expiratory flow; FEV_1, forced expiratory volume in 1 second.
Data from Refs.[37–41]

Table 1
Comparison of infant/preschool lung function tests

	Infant Lung Function Testing	Preschool Spirometry	Lung Clearance Index
Technique	Raised volume rapid thoracoabdominal compression	Spirometry	Multiple breath inert gas washout test
Parameter measured	FEF: FEV at 0.5 s ($FEV_{0.5}$) used in infants owing to short time for lung emptying	• Forced expiratory flows: FEV_1, FEF_{25-75} • Modified criteria exist (shorter exhalation, fewer trials)	• High value (>6.8–7.41) indicates ventilation inhomogeneity and small airway dysfunction • Sulfur hexafluoride or nitrogen washout (latter: subject breathes in 100% oxygen to "wash out" nitrogen normally present in the lungs) • Number of lung volume turnovers needed to lower end-tidal tracer gas concentration to 1/40th of the starting concentration
Evidence	Improvement in $FEV_{0.5}$ in CF patients given hypertonic vs normal saline as part of a randomized clinical trial	• Detects early lung disease abnormalities • More sensitive than forced oscillation or inductance plethysmography	• Often correlates inversely with FEV_1% or FEF_{25-75}% • Abnormal in asymptomatic CF babies/preschoolers and patients with normal spirometry • Treatment efficacy in trials of hypertonic saline, DNAse and ivacaftor
Advantages	• Lower in infants with CF • Track into preschool and school-age years	Good reference ranges in people with CF 3–95 y old across the world	• Correlates better with chest CT changes compared with FEV_1% or FEF_{25-75}% predicted • Increased with PE and decreased when treated
Disadvantages	• Sedation required • Time/personnel intensive	50% of children can reliably perform on their first attempt	• Not as useful in infants: lack of correlation with structural changes and infants breathing 100% O_2 have irregular breathing pattern • Lack of FDA-approved devices • Need to ensure repeatable, feasible; establish clinically important differences and use more in patients abnormal FEV_1% predicted

Abbreviations: CF, cystic fibrosis; FDA, Food and Drug Administration; FEF, forced expiratory flow; FEV, forced expiratory volume.
   Data from Refs.[37,41–59]

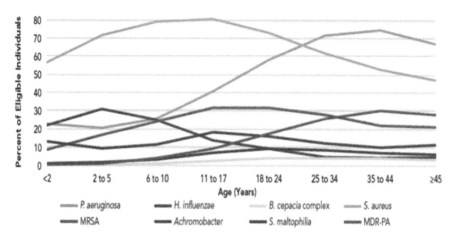

Fig. 4. Prevalence of respiratory microorganisms by age in 2014. The rate of *Pseudomonas aeruginosa* colonization increases significantly with age, whereas *S aureus* and *Haemophilus influenza* rates decrease after early to mid-childhood. Methicillin-resistant *S aureus* and *Stenotrophomonas maltophila* tend to stay relatively stable over the age range. (*Data from* the annual data report 2014, cystic fibrosis foundation patient registry. Available at: https://www.cff.org/About-Us/Assets/2014-Annual-Report. Accessed November 15, 2015.)

50% to 70% of CF patients are chronically infected with *P aeruginosa* (**Fig. 4**),[8] which has negative effects on disease severity, survival and frequency of exacerbations.[5] Methicillin-resistant *Staphylococcus aureus*, *Burkholderia cepacia*, *Stenotrophomonas maltophilia*, and *Mycobacterium abscessus* are associated with deteriorating lung function. The CFF recommends surveillance airway bacterial cultures be obtained in all patients every 3 months and mycobacterial cultures be obtained yearly in some patients. A full review of CF microbiology is found in the article (see Zemanick ET, Hoffman LR: Cystic Fibrosis: Microbiology and Host Response, in this issue).

Bronchoscopy

Bronchoscopy is used to obtain lower airway samples for culture and to assess airway inflammation and look for anatomic abnormalities. However, it requires sedation, which has inherent risks and expense. No improved outcomes or cost benefits have been identified in asymptomatic young patients who underwent bronchoscopy to identify pathogens versus those who did not.[67,68] However, bronchoscopy should be considered in patients who have a decline in FEV$_1$ or have recurrent PEx despite standard therapy.

Pulmonary Exacerbations

PEx are characterized by increased pulmonary symptoms such as cough, dyspnea, sputum production, change in sputum color or consistency, worsening of lung function (>10% decline in FEV$_1$% predicted), and systemic symptoms like fatigue, anorexia, and weight loss. There have been challenges to defining PEx and distinguishing mild, moderate, and severe categories. PEx are associated with poor health-related quality of life,[69] disease progression,[70] and survival.[71] Despite the central role that PEx plays in CF, no consensus diagnostic criteria exist.[72,73] Empiric definitions of PEx have been used in clinical trials evaluating new CF treatments, but they have not been validated formally (**Table 2**).[74–76]

In several studies, symptoms and signs such as increased cough, change in sputum, decreased appetite or weight, change in respiratory examination, and change

Table 2	
Proposed definitions of pulmonary exacerbations	
Study 1	**Study 2**
Pulmonary exacerbation indicated by at least 2 of the following 7 symptoms during the study: • Fever (oral temperature >38°C) • More frequent coughing (increase of 50%) • Sputum volume (increase of 50%) • Loss of appetite • Weight loss of at least 1 kg • Absence from school or work (≥3 or preceding 7 d) owing to illness • Symptoms of upper respiratory tract infection These symptoms had to have been associated with at least one of the following 3 additional criteria: • Decrease in forced vital capacity of at least 10% • An increase in respiratory rate of at least 10 breaths per minute • A peripheral blood neutrophil count of 15,000/mm³ or more	Exacerbation of respiratory symptoms: a patient treated with parental antibiotics for any 4 of 12 signs/symptoms: • Change in sputum • New or increased hemoptysis • Increased cough • Increased dyspnea • Malaise, fatigue or lethargy • Temperature above 38°C • Anorexia or weight loss • Sinus pain or tenderness • Change in sinus discharge • Change in physical examination of the chest • Decrease in pulmonary function by 10% or more from a previously recorded value • Radiographic changes indicative of pulmonary infection

Data from [*Study 1*] Ramsey BW, Pepe MS, Quan JM, et al. Intermittent administration of inhaled tobramycin in patients with cystic fibrosis. Cystic fibrosis inhaled Tobramycin Study Group. N Engl J Med 1999;340:23–30; and [*Study 2*] Fuchs HJ, Borowitz OS, Christiansen DH, et al. Effect of aerosolized recombinant human DNase on exacerbations of respiratory symptoms and on pulmonary function in patients with cystic fibrosis. The Pulmozyme Study Group. N Engl J Med 1994;331(10):637–42.

in respiratory rate were most predictive of PExs[36,77] and were more reliable predictors than laboratory data.[78–80] Although in most cases intensive treatment for PEx leads to significant improvement, 25% to 50% of patients treated for PEx do not return to their baseline lung function.[81]

TREATMENT OF PULMONARY EXACERBATIONS

Although PEx are responsible for one of the largest personal and financial burdens of CF care, there is insufficient evidence in the literature regarding most of the important questions pertaining to treatment.[82–84] The generally accepted basic components are intensified airway clearance therapy, which typically means increasing the frequency of treatments, and antibiotics. Chronic therapies (see below) should be continued during treatment of PEx, although some may need to be held to minimize drug–drug interactions and toxicity.

Site of Treatment: Outpatient Versus Inpatient

There has been 1 randomized control trial[85] and several observations studies[63,86–88] with no difference in the overall outcomes comparing hospital and home antibiotic therapy. The CFF guidelines recommend against delivery of intravenous antibiotics in a nonhospital setting unless resources and support equivalent to the hospital setting can be ensured for the treatment of an acute PEx.[82] Patients who are in distress or "too sick"; those with other comorbidities, that is, CF-related diabetes; and those who require closer drug monitoring or are experiencing side effects of the medications should be managed in the hospital.

Antibiotics

Acute courses of oral antibiotics are used for mild to moderate exacerbations and are tailored to specific organisms on cultures. These exacerbations may be triggered by viruses, but unlike the efforts to minimize use of antibiotics in healthy patients, individuals with CF often need oral antibiotics during what seem to be viral illnesses.

Intravenous antibiotics are the mainstay of the treatment of severe PEx.[64] The choice of antibiotics is usually based on in vitro antibiotic susceptibilities from sputum cultures or throat swabs. However, there is discrepancy between the "in vitro" and the "in vivo" action of the antibiotics; patients may improve on antibiotics that are identified by the microbiology laboratory as "resistant" in vitro.[89,90] The median treatment duration is 13 days for patients less than 18 years compared with 14 days for patients greater than 18 years.[8] There are insufficient data in the literature to recommend an optimal duration of treatment.

Although it is common to use 2 antipseudomonal drugs with different mechanisms of action to enhance activity and reduce resistance,[82] this practice is not well-supported in literature.[89,91,92]

Aminoglycosides

Aminoglycosides are the most common class of antipseudomonals used in the treatment of PEx. They have increased killing as concentration is increased; however, the optimal maximum concentration for treatment of lung infections in CF has not been established.[82] Once-daily dosing increases the concentration. A metaanalysis of single versus multiple dosing of aminoglycosides for the treatment of infection in non-CF patients found that once daily and multiple daily dosing were both equally effective, with once daily dosing having lesser risk of nephrotoxicity.[93] Thus, the CF guidelines recommend once daily dosing of aminoglycosides rather than 3 times daily dosing for treatment of PEx. Patients should receive periodic monitoring of drug concentration with dosage adjustment as necessary, and periodic assessment of toxicity with measurement of creatinine and audiograms.[82]

Beta-lactam antibiotics

Beta-lactam antibiotics demonstrate time-dependent pharmacodynamics properties, that is, maintaining the concentration above the minimum inhibitory concentration for longer portions of the dosing interval is associated with better antibacterial effect, but increasing the concentration does not improve the killing effect. Studies have not shown any statistical difference between continuous and intermittent dosing,[94] thus CF guidelines recommend against continuous infusion of beta-lactam antibiotics for treatment of PEx.

CHRONIC PULMONARY TREATMENT

Chronic therapies are a major component of CF treatment and can prevent declines in lung function. Guidelines are generally for individuals 6 years or older; recommendations for preschoolers will be available soon. In 2014, 65% of patients older than 6 years of age were prescribed hypertonic saline and azithromycin. Most children less than 6 years of age are prescribed bronchodilators. Dornase alfa (recombinant human deoxyribonuclease I, DNAse, or Pulmozyme) is prescribed in 85% of patients younger than 6 years, 42.7% of children younger than 3 years, and in almost 70% of children ages 3 to 5 years.[8]

AIRWAY CLEARANCE THERAPY

A physical method to remove mucus from the airways is a mainstay of daily CF care and intensification of airway clearance therapies is critical during PEx. Various methods are available; none has been shown to be superior to any other[95–102] (**Table 3**[95]). Chest percussion and drainage is the only method that can be used in infants and young children. Adherence to daily treatment can be difficult and it is very important that correct technique is used, no matter what method of airway clearance therapies is used.

MUCUS-MODIFYING AGENTS

Two effective mucus-modifying agents recommended in patients 6 years and older with CF are deoxyribonuclease I (dornase alfa, DNAse) and inhaled 7% hypertonic saline.[3,42,76,103–112] DNAse acts through the digestion of extracellular neutrophil-derived DNA that occurs in the mucus of airways of people with CF. Inhaled hypertonic saline has been proposed to hydrate the ASL, leading to an increase in mucociliary clearance.[108] Use of both therapies in children 6 years of age and older is supported by the literature, in terms of decreased PEx and slower lung function decline.[95] The medications are usually inhaled once to twice daily on a chronic basis.

N-acetylcysteine breaks disulfide bonds in CF mucus and has been used in the past in patients with CF; however, a systematic review confirmed the lack of benefit from or either nebulized or oral N-acetylcysteine.[113]

ANTIINFLAMMATORY DRUGS

Control of inflammation in CF may be important to prevent lung function decline. The goal of azithromycin as a chronic therapy is to reduce inflammation, rather than act as an antibiotic. The medication has mucolytic properties, reduces accumulation of neutrophils by inhibition of intercellular adhesion molecule-1 on epithelial cells, and decreases production of proinflammatory cytokines by neutrophils, monocytes and bronchial epithelial cells. Azithromycin use in those with chronic *P aeruginosa* improved lung function and reduced the rate of PEx. In those without *P aeruginosa*, azithromycin reduced PEx despite no change in lung function.[83,84] Inhaled and oral corticosteroids are not recommended unless asthma or allergic bronchopulmonary aspergillosis is present. Leukotriene receptor antagonists are not recommended owing to a lack of benefit. Ibuprofen reduces the rate of decline of lung function; however, use is limited by gastric and renal toxicities.[114]

ANTIMICROBIAL AGENTS

Eradication of initial *P aeruginosa* growth on airway cultures is thought to prevent irreversible decline in lung function by impairing the development of mucoid colonies. Inhaled tobramycin is used most commonly for 28 days as part of an eradication protocol.[115]

For chronic *P aeruginosa* growth, inhaled antibiotic use is greatest among adolescents and young adults. There are 3 classes of inhaled antibiotics for treatment of *P aeruginosa* infections. Tobramycin is used most frequently, followed by aztreonam and then colistin.[8] Inhaled tobramycin is recommended to reduce exacerbations in patients with CF 6 years and older with persistent growth of *P aeruginosa* in their airway cultures irrespective of lung disease severity. Alternating inhaled antibiotics every month such as tobramycin and aztreonam may decrease the frequency of

Table 3
Summary of ACT

	Percussion and Postural Drainage	PEP	Active Cycle of Breathing Technique	Autogenic Drainage	Oscillatory PEP	High-Frequency Chest Wall Oscillation Vest	Exercise (Aerobic and Anaerobic)
Age	Any	3–4 y, assistance until 8–10 y	3–4 y, assistance until 8–10 y	≥12 y	Adolescents/adults	≥18 mo–3 y	Any
Equipment	• Positioning aids, percussor/vibrator • Caregiver to perform	• Mouthpiece or mask PEP device • Replacement needed	Positioning aids, percussor/vibrator	None	• Assistance required • Specialized equipment (Acapella, Aerobika, Flutter)	• Air pulse generator • Appropriately sized vest	• Assistance required in younger children • Premedicate before exercise with concurrent nebulizer use
Advantages	• Used during PE • Used with nebulizer • Can focus on problem areas • More sputum production compared with no therapy	• Used during PE • Used with nebulizer • Portable	• Used during PE • Inexpensive • Augmented with other therapies	Inexpensive	• Can be used with nebulizer (except Flutter) • Easy to perform, portable, can be used as adjunct to other forms of ACT	• Used during PE • Used with nebulizer • Does not require patient cooperation; can be used in toddlers, provides therapy to large areas of the chest	• May provide multiple health benefits, adjunct to other ACT • Expense depends on type of exercise

Disadvantages	Modified position with GER or increased intracranial pressure	Impair venous return if hemodynamically unstable	Concurrent nebulizer only in upright position	• Not recommended with PE or with nebulizer • Time to learn	• Not recommended with PE • Moderately expensive	Very expensive	• Not recommended with PE • Can cause exercise induced bronchospasm, oxygen desaturations
Contraindications	Patient with chest pain, instability of chest wall or spine	• Sinusitis • Epistaxis • Otitis media • Pneumothorax	Caution with head down position	History of anxiety	Pneumothorax	• Unstable head/ neck injury • Active hemorrhage with hemodynamic instability • Chest tubes, indwelling catheters or other devices in/on chest	Severe hypoxemia or arrhythmias

Abbreviations: ACT, airway clearance therapies; GER, gastroesophageal reflux; PE, pulmonary exacerbation; PEP, positive expiratory pressure.
Data from Refs.[95–99]

PEx in those chronically colonized with *P aeruginosa*.[75,116] Inhaled vancomycin, ciprofloxacin, and levofloxacin are currently under investigation.[8,75,116]

CYSTIC FIBROSIS TRANSMEMBRANE REGULATOR CORRECTORS AND POTENTIATORS

Drugs that can modify the CFTR protein itself and lead to improved expression and function of the CFTR protein have been developed and continue to be explored.[108] They provide a novel therapeutic concept because of their use as preventative medications, ideally used before sinus or lung damage has already been done or to prevent progression of disease (see Ong T, Ramsey BW: New Therapeutic Approaches to Modulate and Correct CFTR, in this issue).

COMPLICATIONS
Hemoptysis

Hemoptysis affects approximately 9.1% of patients; it is usually associated with advanced age and disease (60% with an FEV_1 of <40% predicted).[117] Based on data from the CFF Patient Registry between 1990 and 1999,[117] the annual incidence

Table 4
Suggested management of hemoptysis

	Scant	Mild to Moderate	Massive
Contact health care provider	If first episode or persistent	Yes	Yes
Admitted to hospital	No	Yes	Yes
Antibiotics	Yes, if first episode or persistent bleeding or previous history of increase in bleeding	Yes	Yes
Nonsteroidal antiinflammatory drugs	Continue	Stop	Stop
Airway clearance therapies	Continue	Stop	Stop
Aerosol therapies			
Hypertonic saline or dornase alpha	Continue	Stop	Stop
Inhaled antibiotics	Continue	Continue	Continue
Inhaled bronchodilators	Continue	Continue	Continue
Bilevel positive airway pressure	Continue	Continue	Stop
BAE	No	No	Yes, those who are clinically unstable
Pre BAE testing	N/A	N/A	None: No bronchoscopy, may be CT chest

Abbreviations: BAE, bronchial artery embolization; CT, computed tomography; N/A, not applicable.

Data from Flume PA, Mogayzel PJ Jr, Robinson KA, et al. Cystic fibrosis pulmonary guidelines: pulmonary complications: hemoptysis and pneumothorax. Am J Respir Crit Care Med 2010;182(3):298–306.

of massive hemoptysis in CF is 0.87%. CF accounts for the majority of hemoptysis cases in childhood.[118] Chronic infection and inflammation lead to bronchial artery hypertrophy and proliferation. The thin-walled, tortuous vessels are at increased risk of rupturing into the airways.[119] Categories include: scant (<5 mL), mild to moderate (5–240 mL), and massive (>240 mL in a 24-hr period or recurrent bleeding >100 mL/d over several days).[117,120] Major risk factors are *S aureus* growth and diabetes; *P aeruginosa* and *B cepacia* lowered the risk. Death occurred in 35% within the first year of massive hemoptysis; median survival was 5 years.[117] See **Table 4** for management guidelines.[121]

Pneumothorax

Pneumothorax is defined as air in the pleural cavity. Pneumothorax can be divided into small (<2 cm) versus large (>2 cm).[122] The average annual incidence of pneumothorax 0.64%; it occurs more commonly in older patients, those with *P aeruginosa*, *B cepacia*, or *Aspergillus* growth, and those with severe lung disease (FEV$_1$ <40% predicted). Increased intrapleural pressures owing to airway obstruction lead to a ball–valve phenomenon with mucus retention. Increased morbidity and 2-year mortality rate are observed compared with patients without pneumothorax (49% vs 12%).[123] Clinical manifestations are reviewed in **Box 5**.[121,123] Management is reviewed in **Fig. 5**.[121]

Allergic bronchopulmonary aspergillosis affects 2% to 11% of patients with CF. It involves allergic response (elevated immunoglobulin E, specific immunoglobulin E to *Aspergillus* as well as positive skin test to *Aspergillus*); it causes inflammation, infiltrates, and ultimately fibrosis of the lungs. Clinical symptoms include cough, wheezing, exercise intolerance/asthma, reduced pulmonary function, and increased sputum production. It should always be considered in patients who do not respond

---

Box 5
Clinical manifestations of pneumothorax

- Commonly reported complication in CF:
  ○ Average annual incidence 0.64%; 3.4% of patients overall

- Pathogenesis: increased intrapleural pressures owing to inflammation and obstruction of the airways, leading to ball-valve phenomenon with mucus retention
  ○ More common in
    ■ Older patients (mean age of 22 years)
    ■ Severe lung disease (nearly 75% of patients had FEV$_1$ <40% predicted).

- Increased risk in patients with:
  ○ *Pseudomonas aeruginosa* (OR, 2.3), *Burkholderia cepacia* (OR, 1.8), *Aspergillus fumigatus* (OR, 1.3)
  ○ FEV$_1$ less than 30% predicted (OR, 1.5)
  ○ Enteral feeding (OR, 1.7)
  ○ Pancreatic insufficiency (OR, 1.4)
  ○ Allergic bronchopulmonary aspergillosis (OR, 1.5)
  ○ Massive hemoptysis (OR, 1.4)

- Increased morbidity and 2-year mortality rate compared with patients without pneumothorax (49% vs 12%)

Abbreviations: CF, cystic fibrosis; FEV$_1$, forced expiratory volume in 1 second; OR, odds ratio.
    Data from Flume PA, Mogayzel PJ Jr, Robinson KA, et al. Cystic fibrosis pulmonary guidelines: pulmonary complications: hemoptysis and pneumothorax. Am J Respir Crit Care Med 2010;182(3):298–306; and Flume PA, Strange C, Ye X, et al. Pneumothorax in cystic fibrosis. Chest 2005;128(2):720–8.

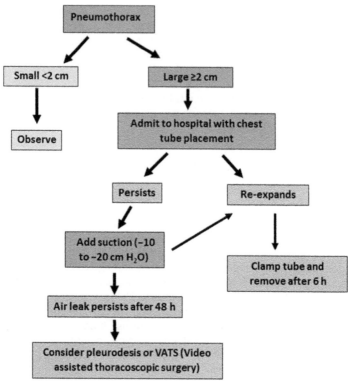

Fig. 5. Pneumothorax management. (*Data from* Flume PA, Mogayzel PJ Jr, Robinson KA, et al. Cystic fibrosis pulmonary guidelines: pulmonary complications: hemoptysis and pneumothorax. Am J Respir Crit Care Med 2010;182:298–306.)

to standard management of PEx. Treatment involves steroids and antifungal medications.[124]

RESPIRATORY INSUFFICIENCY

Noninvasive ventilation in used in patients with CF who have hypercapnic respiratory failure in several situations: infants, patients with a reversible cause of their respiratory failure, those whose underlying disease that was not treated aggressively, and those patients accepted as lung transplant candidates.[125] Surgery for lung disease, such as lobectomy, is done infrequently in rare circumstances with localized bronchiectasis. Lung transplantation is an option for end-stage lung disease (see Faro A, Weymann A: Transplantation, in this issue).

SUMMARY

Sinopulmonary disease in CF can be traced back to CFTR gene defects that cause ASL depletion, abnormal pH, inflammation, and chronic infection. Patients with CF are living longer; however, respiratory disease remains the leading cause of mortality. The presence of early lung disease is now well-recognized, even in the absence of overt symptoms. Assessment and monitoring of early lung disease is thus a topic of continued research. PEx are a major cause of morbidity and expense, despite lack of a precise definition. Chronic therapies help to prevent PEx and lung function decline over time. Future CFTR corrector/potentiator therapies may change the course of the disease.

SUPPLEMENTARY DATA

Supplementary data related to this article can be found at http://dx.doi.org/10.1016/j.pcl.2016.04.007.

REFERENCES

1. Cutting GR. Cystic fibrosis genetics: from molecular understanding to clinical application. Nat Rev Genet 2015;16(1):45–56.
2. Davies JC, Ebdon AM, Orchard C. Recent advances in the management of cystic fibrosis. Arch Dis Child 2014;99(11):1033–6.
3. Grasemann H, Ratjen F. Early lung disease in cystic fibrosis. Lancet Respir Med 2013;1(2):148–57.
4. Stoltz DA, Meyerholz DK, Welsh MJ. Origins of cystic fibrosis lung disease. N Engl J Med 2015;372(16):1574–5.
5. Ong T, Ramsey BW. Update in cystic fibrosis 2014. Am J Respir Crit Care Med 2015;192(6):669–75.
6. Borowitz D. CFTR, bicarbonate, and the pathophysiology of cystic fibrosis. Pediatr Pulmonol 2015;50(Suppl 40):S24–30.
7. Tang AC, Turvey SE, Alves MP, et al. Current concepts: host-pathogen interactions in cystic fibrosis airways disease. Eur Respir Rev 2014;23(133):320–32.
8. CF Foundation (CFF). 2014 patient registry annual data report. 2014. Available at: https://www.cff.org/About-Us/Assets/2014-Annual-Report. Accessed November 15, 2015.
9. Sanders DB, Li Z, Laxova A, et al. Risk factors for the progression of cystic fibrosis lung disease throughout childhood. Ann Am Thorac Soc 2014;11(1): 63–72.
10. Drumm ML, Konstan MW, Schluchter MD, et al. Genetic modifiers of lung disease in cystic fibrosis. N Engl J Med 2005;353(14):1443–53.
11. Cogen J, Emerson J, Sanders DB, et al. Risk factors for lung function decline in a large cohort of young cystic fibrosis patients. Pediatr Pulmonol 2015;50(8): 763–70.
12. Emerson J, Rosenfeld M, McNamara S, et al. Pseudomonas aeruginosa and other predictors of mortality and morbidity in young children with cystic fibrosis. Pediatr Pulmonol 2002;34(2):91–100.
13. Harness-Brumley CL, Elliott AC, Rosenbluth DB, et al. Gender differences in outcomes of patients with cystic fibrosis. J Womens Health (Larchmt) 2014;23(12): 1012–20.
14. Buu MC, Sanders LM, Mayo J, et al. Assessing differences in mortality rates and risk factors between Hispanic and non-Hispanic patients with cystic fibrosis in California. Chest 2016;149(2):380–9.
15. Farrell PM, Rosenstein BJ, White TB, et al. Guidelines for diagnosis of cystic fibrosis in newborns through older adults: cystic fibrosis foundation consensus report. J Pediatr 2008;153(2):S4–14.
16. Adam RJ, Michalski AS, Bauer C, et al. Air trapping and airflow obstruction in newborn cystic fibrosis piglets. Am J Respir Crit Care Med 2013;188(12): 1434–41.

17. Hoegger MJ, Fischer AJ, McMenimen JD, et al. Impaired mucus detachment disrupts mucociliary transport in a piglet model of cystic fibrosis. Science 2014;345(6198):818–22.

18. Pillarisetti N, Williamson E, Linnane B, et al. Infection, inflammation, and lung function decline in infants with cystic fibrosis. Am J Respir Crit Care Med 2011;184(1):75–81.

19. Mott LS, Park J, Murray CP, et al. Progression of early structural lung disease in young children with cystic fibrosis assessed using CT. Thorax 2012;67(6): 509–16.

20. Sly PD, Brennan S, Gangell C, et al. Lung disease at diagnosis in infants with cystic fibrosis detected by newborn screening. Am J Respir Crit Care Med 2009;180(2):146–52.

21. Stick SM, Brennan S, Murray C, et al. Bronchiectasis in infants and preschool children diagnosed with cystic fibrosis after newborn screening. J Pediatr 2009;155(5):623–8.e1.

22. Thia LP, Calder A, Stocks J, et al. Is chest CT useful in newborn screened infants with cystic fibrosis at 1 year of age? Thorax 2014;69(4):320–7.

23. de Jong PA, Lindblad A, Rubin L, et al. Progression of lung disease on computed tomography and pulmonary function tests in children and adults with cystic fibrosis. Thorax 2006;61(1):80–5.

24. Hoo AF, Thia LP, Nguyen TT, et al. Lung function is abnormal in 3-month-old infants with cystic fibrosis diagnosed by newborn screening. Thorax 2012;67(10): 874–81.

25. Khan TZ, Wagener JS, Bost T, et al. Early pulmonary inflammation in infants with cystic fibrosis. Am J Respir Crit Care Med 1995;151(4):1075–82.

26. Armstrong DS, Grimwood K, Carlin JB, et al. Lower airway inflammation in infants and young children with cystic fibrosis. Am J Respir Crit Care Med 1997;156(4 Pt 1):1197–204.

27. Accurso FJ, Sontag MK, Wagener JS. Complications associated with symptomatic diagnosis in infants with cystic fibrosis. J Pediatr 2005;147(3 Suppl): S37–41.

28. Boat TF, Acton JD. Cystic fibrosis. In: Kliegman B, editor. Nelson textbook of pediatrics. 18th edition. Philadelphia: Elsevier; 2008. p. 1803–16.

29. Crosby DL, Adappa ND. What is the optimal management of chronic rhinosinusitis in cystic fibrosis? Curr Opin Otolaryngol Head Neck Surg 2014;22(1):42–6.

30. Aanaes K. Bacterial sinusitis can be a focus for initial lung colonisation and chronic lung infection in patients with cystic fibrosis. J Cyst Fibros 2013; 12(Suppl 2):S1–20.

31. Rosenfeld RM, Andes D, Bhattacharyya N, et al. Clinical practice guideline: adult sinusitis. Otolaryngol Head Neck Surg 2007;137(3 Suppl):S1–31.

32. Fundakowski C, Ojo R, Younis R. Rhinosinusitis in the pediatric patient with cystic fibrosis. Curr Pediatr Rev 2014;10(3):198–201.

33. Settipane GA. Epidemiology of nasal polyps. Allergy Asthma Proc 1996;17(5): 231–6.

34. Shatz A. Management of recurrent sinus disease in children with cystic fibrosis: a combined approach. Otolaryngol Head Neck Surg 2006;135(2):248–52.

35. Castellani C, Quinzii C, Altieri S, et al. A pilot survey of cystic fibrosis clinical manifestations in CFTR mutation heterozygotes. Genet Test 2001;5(3):249–54.

36. Wang X, Kim J, McWilliams R, et al. Increased prevalence of chronic rhinosinusitis in carriers of a cystic fibrosis mutation. Arch Otolaryngol Head Neck Surg 2005;131(3):237–40.

37. Quanjer PH, Stanojevic S, Cole TJ, et al. Multi-ethnic reference values for spirometry for the 3-95-yr age range: the global lung function 2012 equations. Eur Respir J 2012;40(6):1324–43.

38. Corey M, Edwards L, Levison H, et al. Longitudinal analysis of pulmonary function decline in patients with cystic fibrosis. J Pediatr 1997;131(6):809–14.

39. Que C, Cullinan P, Geddes D. Improving rate of decline of FEV1 in young adults with cystic fibrosis. Thorax 2006;61(2):155–7.

40. Aurora P, Stanojevic S, Wade A, et al. Lung clearance index at 4 years predicts subsequent lung function in children with cystic fibrosis. Am J Respir Crit Care Med 2011;183(6):752–8.

41. Ramsey KA, Ranganathan S. Interpretation of lung function in infants and young children with cystic fibrosis. Respirology 2014;19(6):792–9.

42. Rosenfeld M, Ratjen F, Brumback L, et al. Inhaled hypertonic saline in infants and children younger than 6 years with cystic fibrosis: the ISIS randomized controlled trial. JAMA 2012;307(21):2269–77.

43. VanDevanter DR, Pasta DJ. Evidence of diminished FEV1 and FVC in 6-year-olds followed in the European cystic fibrosis patient registry, 2007-2009. J Cyst Fibros 2013;12(6):786–9.

44. Rosenfeld M, Allen J, Arets BH, et al. An official American thoracic society workshop report: optimal lung function tests for monitoring cystic fibrosis, bronchopulmonary dysplasia, and recurrent wheezing in children less than 6 years of age. Ann Am Thorac Soc 2013;10(2):S1–11.

45. Vilozni D, Bentur L, Efrati O, et al. Spirometry in early childhood in cystic fibrosis patients. Chest 2007;131(2):356–61.

46. Kozlowska WJ, Bush A, Wade A, et al. Lung function from infancy to the preschool years after clinical diagnosis of cystic fibrosis. Am J Respir Crit Care Med 2008;178(1):42–9.

47. Kerby GS, Rosenfeld M, Ren CL, et al. Lung function distinguishes preschool children with CF from healthy controls in a multi-center setting. Pediatr Pulmonol 2012;47(6):597–605.

48. Gaffin JM, Shotola NL, Martin TR, et al. Clinically useful spirometry in preschool-aged children: evaluation of the 2007 American thoracic society guidelines. J Asthma 2010;47(7):762–7.

49. Kent L, Reix P, Innes JA, et al. Lung clearance index: evidence for use in clinical trials in cystic fibrosis. J Cyst Fibros 2014;13(2):123–38.

50. Subbarao P, Milla C, Aurora P, et al. Multiple-breath washout as a lung function test in cystic fibrosis. A cystic fibrosis foundation workshop report. Ann Am Thorac Soc 2015;12(6):932–9.

51. Aurora P, Bush A, Gustafsson P, et al. Multiple-breath washout as a marker of lung disease in preschool children with cystic fibrosis. Am J Respir Crit Care Med 2005;171(3):249–56.

52. Amin R, Subbarao P, Jabar A, et al. Hypertonic saline improves the LCI in paediatric patients with CF with normal lung function. Thorax 2010;65(5):379–83.

53. Amin R, Subbarao P, Lou W, et al. The effect of dornase alfa on ventilation inhomogeneity in patients with cystic fibrosis. Eur Respir J 2011;37(4):806–12.

54. Ratjen F, Sheridan H, Lee PS, et al. Lung clearance index as an endpoint in a multicenter randomized control trial of ivacaftor in subjects with cystic fibrosis who have mild lung disease. Am J Respir Crit Care Med 2012;47:350.

55. Ellemunter H, Fuchs SI, Unsinn KM, et al. Sensitivity of lung clearance Index and chest computed tomography in early CF lung disease. Respir Med 2010; 104(12):1834–42.

56. Gustafsson PM, De Jong PA, Tiddens HA, et al. Multiple-breath inert gas washout and spirometry versus structural lung disease in cystic fibrosis. Thorax 2008;63(2):129–34.

57. Owens CM, Aurora P, Stanojevic S, et al. Lung clearance index and HRCT are complementary markers of lung abnormalities in young children with CF. Thorax 2011;66(6):481–8.

58. Vermeulen F, Proesmans M, Boon M, et al. Lung clearance index predicts pulmonary exacerbations in young patients with cystic fibrosis. Thorax 2014; 69(1):39–45.

59. Horsley AR, Davies JC, Gray RD, et al. Changes in physiological, functional and structural markers of cystic fibrosis lung disease with treatment of a pulmonary exacerbation. Thorax 2013;68(6):532–9.

60. Koscik RE, Kosorok MR, Farrell PM, et al. Wisconsin cystic fibrosis chest radiograph scoring system: validation and standardization for application to longitudinal studies. Pediatr Pulmonol 2000;29(6):457–67.

61. Brasfield D, Hicks G, Soong S, et al. The chest roentgenogram in cystic fibrosis: a new scoring system. Pediatrics 1979;63(1):24–9.

62. Brody AS, Molina PL, Klein JS, et al. High-resolution computed tomography of the chest in children with cystic fibrosis: support for use as an outcome surrogate. Pediatr Radiol 1999;29(10):731–5.

63. Yi MS, Tsevat J, Wilmott RW, et al. The impact of treatment of pulmonary exacerbations on the health-related quality of life of patients with cystic fibrosis: does hospitalization make a difference? J Pediatr 2004;144(6):711–8.

64. CF Foundation (CFF). Treatment of pulmonary exacerbations of cystic fibrosis. Clinical practice guidelines for cystic fibrosis. Bethesda (MD): 1997.

65. Eichinger M, Optazaite DE, Kopp-Schneider A, et al. Morphologic and functional scoring of cystic fibrosis lung disease using MRI. Eur J Radiol 2012; 81(6):1321–9.

66. Wielputz MO, Puderbach M, Kopp-Schneider A, et al. Magnetic resonance imaging detects changes in structure and perfusion, and response to therapy in early cystic fibrosis lung disease. Am J Respir Crit Care Med 2014;189(8): 956–65.

67. Wainwright CE, Vidmar S, Armstrong DS, et al. Effect of bronchoalveolar lavage-directed therapy on pseudomonas aeruginosa infection and structural lung injury in children with cystic fibrosis: a randomized trial. JAMA 2011;306(2): 163–71.

68. Moodie M, Lal A, Vidmar S, et al. Costs of bronchoalveolar lavage-directed therapy in the first 5 years of life for children with cystic fibrosis. J Pediatr 2014; 165(3):564–9.e5.

69. Britto MT, Kotagal UR, Hornung RW, et al. Impact of recent pulmonary exacerbations on quality of life in patients with cystic fibrosis. Chest 2002;121(1): 64–72.

70. Smyth A, Elborn JS. Exacerbations in cystic fibrosis: 3–management. Thorax 2008;63(2):180–4.

71. Liou TG, Adler FR, Fitzsimmons SC, et al. Predictive 5-year survivorship model of cystic fibrosis. Am J Epidemiol 2001;153(4):345–52.

72. Ramsey BW, Boat TF. Outcome measures for clinical trials in cystic fibrosis. Summary of a cystic fibrosis foundation consensus conference. J Pediatr 1994;124(2):177–92.

73. Marshall BC. Pulmonary exacerbations in cystic fibrosis: it's time to be explicit! Am J Respir Crit Care Med 2004;169(7):781–2.

74. Goss CH, Burns JL. Exacerbations in cystic fibrosis. 1: Epidemiology and pathogenesis. Thorax 2007;62(4):360–7.

75. Ramsey BW, Pepe MS, Quan JM, et al. Intermittent administration of inhaled tobramycin in patients with cystic fibrosis. Cystic Fibrosis Inhaled Tobramycin Study Group. N Engl J Med 1999;340(1):23–30.

76. Fuchs HJ, Borowitz DS, Christiansen DH, et al. Effect of aerosolized recombinant human DNase on exacerbations of respiratory symptoms and on pulmonary function in patients with cystic fibrosis. The Pulmozyme Study Group. N Engl J Med 1994;331(10):637–42.

77. Ferkol T, Rosenfeld M, Milla CE. Cystic fibrosis pulmonary exacerbations. J Pediatr 2006;148(2):259–64.

78. Rabin HR, Butler SM, Wohl ME, et al. Pulmonary exacerbations in cystic fibrosis. Pediatr Pulmonol 2004;37(5):400–6.

79. Rosenfeld M, Emerson J, Williams-Warren J, et al. Defining a pulmonary exacerbation in cystic fibrosis. J Pediatr 2001;139(3):359–65.

80. Dakin C, Henry RL, Field P, et al. Defining an exacerbation of pulmonary disease in cystic fibrosis. Pediatr Pulmonol 2001;31(6):436–42.

81. Tiddens HA, Stick SM, Wild JM, et al. Respiratory tract exacerbations revisited: ventilation, inflammation, perfusion, and structure (VIPS) monitoring to redefine treatment. Pediatr Pulmonol 2015;50(Suppl 40):S57–65.

82. Flume PA, Mogayzel PJ Jr, Robinson KA, et al. Cystic fibrosis pulmonary guidelines: treatment of pulmonary exacerbations. Am J Respir Crit Care Med 2009; 180(9):802–8.

83. Gold R, Carpenter S, Heurter H, et al. Randomized trial of ceftazidime versus placebo in the management of acute respiratory exacerbations in patients with cystic fibrosis. J Pediatr 1987;111(6 Pt 1):907–13.

84. Wientzen R, Prestidge CB, Kramer RI, et al. Acute pulmonary exacerbations in cystic fibrosis. A double-blind trial of tobramycin and placebo therapy. Am J Dis Child 1980;134(12):1134–8.

85. Wolter JM, Bowler SD, Nolan PJ, et al. Home intravenous therapy in cystic fibrosis: a prospective randomized trial examining clinical, quality of life and cost aspects. Eur Respir J 1997;10(4):896–900.

86. Bosworth DG, Nielson DW. Effectiveness of home versus hospital care in the routine treatment of cystic fibrosis. Pediatr Pulmonol 1997;24(1):42–7.

87. Nazer D, Abdulhamid I, Thomas R, et al. Home versus hospital intravenous antibiotic therapy for acute pulmonary exacerbations in children with cystic fibrosis. Pediatr Pulmonol 2006;41(8):744–9.

88. Thornton J, Elliott R, Tully MP, et al. Long term clinical outcome of home and hospital intravenous antibiotic treatment in adults with cystic fibrosis. Thorax 2004; 59(3):242–6.

89. Smith AL, Doershuk C, Goldmann D, et al. Comparison of a beta-lactam alone versus beta-lactam and an aminoglycoside for pulmonary exacerbation in cystic fibrosis. J Pediatr 1999;134(4):413–21.

90. Smith AL, Fiel SB, Mayer-Hamblett N, et al. Susceptibility testing of pseudomonas aeruginosa isolates and clinical response to parenteral antibiotic administration: lack of association in cystic fibrosis. Chest 2003;123(5):1495–502.

91. Flume P, VanDevanter D. Pulmonary exacerbations. In: Bush A, Bilton D, Hodson M, editors. Hodson and Geddes cystic fibrosis. 4th edition. Boca Raton (FL): CRC Press; 2016. p. 221–35.

92. Doring G, Conway SP, Heijerman HG, et al. Antibiotic therapy against pseudomonas aeruginosa in cystic fibrosis: a European consensus. Eur Respir J 2000; 16(4):749–67.

93. Barza M, Ioannidis JP, Cappelleri JC, et al. Single or multiple daily doses of aminoglycosides: a meta-analysis. BMJ 1996;312(7027):338–45.

94. Bosso JA, Bonapace CR, Flume PA, et al. A pilot study of the efficacy of constant-infusion ceftazidime in the treatment of endobronchial infections in adults with cystic fibrosis. Pharmacotherapy 1999;19(5):620–6.

95. Flume PA, Robinson KA, O'Sullivan BP, et al. Cystic fibrosis pulmonary guidelines: airway clearance therapies. Respir Care 2009;54(4):522–37.

96. Davidson AG, McIlwaine PM, Wong LTK, et al. Comparative trial of positive expiratory pressure, autogenic drainage and conventional percussion and drainage techniques (abstract). Pediatr Pulmonol 1988;5:132.

97. Giles DR, Wagener JS, Accurso FJ, et al. Short-term effects of postural drainage with clapping vs autogenic drainage on oxygen saturation and sputum recovery in patients with cystic fibrosis. Chest 1995;108(4):952–4.

98. Konstan MW, Stern RC, Doershuk CF. Efficacy of the Flutter device for airway mucus clearance in patients with cystic fibrosis. J Pediatr 1994;124(5 Pt 1): 689–93.

99. Kluft J, Beker L, Castagnino M, et al. A comparison of bronchial drainage treatments in cystic fibrosis. Pediatr Pulmonol 1996;22(4):271–4.

100. Warwick WJ, Wielinski CL, Hansen LG. Comparison of expectorated sputum after manual chest physical therapy and high-frequency chest compression. Biomed Instrum Technol 2004;38(6):470–5.

101. Kraig R, Kirkpatrick KR, Howard D, et al. A direct comparison of manual chest percussion with acoustic percussion, an experimental treatment for cystic fibrosis [abstract]. Am J Respir Crit Care Med Suppl 1995;151:A738.

102. Cerny FJ. Relative effects of bronchial drainage and exercise for in-hospital care of patients with cystic fibrosis. Phys Ther 1989;69(8):633–9.

103. Konstan MW, Ratjen F. Effect of dornase alfa on inflammation and lung function: potential role in the early treatment of cystic fibrosis. J Cyst Fibros 2012;11(2): 78–83.

104. Suri R, Marshall LJ, Wallis C, et al. Effects of recombinant human DNase and hypertonic saline on airway inflammation in children with cystic fibrosis. Am J Respir Crit Care Med 2002;166(3):352–5.

105. Quan JM, Tiddens HA, Sy JP, et al. A two-year randomized, placebo-controlled trial of dornase alfa in young patients with cystic fibrosis with mild lung function abnormalities. J Pediatr 2001;139(6):813–20.

106. Konstan MW, Wagener JS, Pasta DJ, et al. Clinical use of dornase alpha is associated with a slower rate of FEV1 decline in cystic fibrosis. Pediatr Pulmonol 2011;46(6):545–53.

107. Fitzgerald DA, Hilton J, Jepson B, et al. A crossover, randomized, controlled trial of dornase alfa before versus after physiotherapy in cystic fibrosis. Pediatrics 2005;116(4):e549–54.

108. Pittman JE, Ferkol TW. The evolution of cystic fibrosis care. Chest 2015;148(2): 533–42.

109. Robinson M, Hemming AL, Regnis JA, et al. Effect of increasing doses of hypertonic saline on mucociliary clearance in patients with cystic fibrosis. Thorax 1997;52(10):900–3.

110. Elkins MR, Robinson M, Rose BR, et al. A controlled trial of long-term inhaled hypertonic saline in patients with cystic fibrosis. N Engl J Med 2006;354(3): 229–40.

111. Eng PA, Morton J, Douglass JA, et al. Short-term efficacy of ultrasonically nebulized hypertonic saline in cystic fibrosis. Pediatr Pulmonol 1996;21(2):77–83.

112. Wark PA, McDonald V, Jones AP. Nebulised hypertonic saline for cystic fibrosis. Cochrane Database Syst Rev 2005;(3):CD001506.

113. Duijvestijn YC, Brand PL. Systematic review of N-acetylcysteine in cystic fibrosis. Acta Paediatr 1999;88(1):38–41.

114. Konstan MW. Ibuprofen therapy for cystic fibrosis lung disease: revisited. Curr Opin Pulm Med 2008;14(6):567–73.

115. Treggiari MM, Retsch-Bogart G, Mayer-Hamblett N, et al. Comparative efficacy and safety of 4 randomized regimens to treat early pseudomonas aeruginosa infection in children with cystic fibrosis. Arch Pediatr Adolesc Med 2011; 165(9):847–56.

116. Maiz L, Giron RM, Olveira C, et al. Inhaled antibiotics for the treatment of chronic bronchopulmonary pseudomonas aeruginosa infection in cystic fibrosis: systematic review of randomised controlled trials. Expert Opin Pharmacother 2013;14(9):1135–49.

117. Flume PA, Yankaskas JR, Ebeling M, et al. Massive hemoptysis in cystic fibrosis. Chest 2005;128(2):729–38.

118. Barben JU, Ditchfield M, Carlin JB, et al. Major haemoptysis in children with cystic fibrosis: a 20-year retrospective study. J Cyst Fibros 2003;2(3):105–11.

119. Hurt K, Simmonds NJ. Cystic fibrosis: management of haemoptysis. Paediatr Respir Rev 2012;13(4):200–5.

120. Schidlow DV, Taussig LM, Knowles MR. Cystic fibrosis foundation consensus conference report on pulmonary complications of cystic fibrosis. Pediatr Pulmonol 1993;15(3):187–98.

121. Flume PA, Mogayzel PJ Jr, Robinson KA, et al. Cystic fibrosis pulmonary guidelines: pulmonary complications: hemoptysis and pneumothorax. Am J Respir Crit Care Med 2010;182(3):298–306.

122. MacDuff A, Arnold A, Harvey J, et al. Management of spontaneous pneumothorax: British thoracic society pleural disease guideline 2010. Thorax 2010; 65(Suppl 2):ii18–31.

123. Flume PA, Strange C, Ye X, et al. Pneumothorax in cystic fibrosis. Chest 2005; 128(2):720–8.

124. Stevens DA, Moss RB, Kurup VP, et al. Allergic bronchopulmonary aspergillosis in cystic fibrosis–state of the art: Cystic Fibrosis Foundation Consensus Conference. Clin Infect Dis 2003;37(Suppl 3):S225–64.

125. Bright-Thomas RJ, Johnson SC. What is the role of noninvasive ventilation in cystic fibrosis? Curr Opin Pulm Med 2014;20(6):618–22.

Nutrition and Growth in Cystic Fibrosis

Sarah Lusman, MD[a], Jillian Sullivan, MD, MSCS[b],*

KEYWORDS

- Cystic fibrosis • Nutrition • Growth • Body mass index • Anthropometrics
- Enteral feeding • Fat-soluble vitamins

KEY POINTS

- Close monitoring of nutrition and growth is essential to the care of children with cystic fibrosis (CF). Growth and nutrition should be assessed at every visit to the CF care center.
- Body mass index (BMI) percentile is the most commonly used marker of nutritional status. Nutritional status is directly associated with pulmonary function.
- It is recommended that children with CF achieve growth and nutritional status comparable with that of well-nourished children without CF. Specifically, this means weight-for-length greater than the 50th percentile in children less than 2 years of age and BMI greater than the 50th percentile in children older than 2 years.
- Barriers to attaining and maintaining nutritional status include decreased caloric intake, gastrointestinal dysfunction, increased caloric expenditure, and psychosocial issues.
- Methods used to optimize nutritional status include intensive dietary and behavioral counseling, use of oral supplements, and enteral tube feedings.

IMPORTANCE OF ADEQUATE NUTRITION AND GROWTH

Close attention to nutrition and growth is integral to the care of patients with cystic fibrosis (CF).[1] The Cystic Fibrosis Foundation (CFF) recommends that children with CF achieve nutritional status comparable with that of healthy children. Growth and nutritional status should be assessed at every visit. Despite multiple advances in the digestive care of patients with CF, appropriate nutritional status remains difficult to attain. In this article the authors discuss the assessment of growth and nutrition, nutritional goals and challenges, and optimization of nutritional status.

Dr Dorothy Andersen wrote the original reference to CF as a new entity in 1938. She described CF causing early death in infants because of extreme malnutrition.

Disclosure Statement: The authors have nothing to disclose.
[a] Department of Pediatrics, Columbia University Medical Center, 622 West 168th Street, PH 17 East 105L, New York, NY 10032, USA; [b] Department of Pediatrics, University of Vermont College of Medicine, 111 Colchester Avenue, Burlington, VT 05401, USA
* Corresponding author.
E-mail address: jillian.sullivan@uvmhealth.org

Pediatr Clin N Am 63 (2016) 661–678
http://dx.doi.org/10.1016/j.pcl.2016.04.005
0031-3955/16/$ – see front matter

Autopsies revealed destruction of the pancreas, and eventually the role of maldigestion as a cause of malnutrition in CF was understood. Dr Harry Shwachman encouraged patients to follow a low-fat or fat-free diet to minimize the symptoms of steatorrhea, resulting in worsening malnutrition and a characteristic physical appearance including a swollen abdomen, lack of subcutaneous fat and muscle mass, and overall wasting. Later, comparisons of 2 large CF programs with differing approaches to dietary fat restriction showed that those on a high-fat diet had better growth and survival contributing to the current recommendations for a high-calorie, fat-unrestricted diet.[2] Important advances in the nutritional management of patients with CF include the development of pancreatic enzyme replacement therapy, the availability of nutritional supplements, and the use of enteral tube feedings.[2,3]

Body mass index (BMI) and BMI percentile for age are important measures of nutritional status in children with CF. It is recommended that height and weight be measured and BMI calculated by dividing the weight in kilograms by the height in meters squared at least every 3 months (**Table 1**). The 2000 edition of the growth charts issued by the Centers for Disease Control and Prevention (CDC) should be used to compare each patient's BMI percentile to age- and sex-matched norms. The goal is a weight-for-length at or greater than the 50th percentile in children less than 2 years of age and a BMI at or greater than the 50th percentile for children older than 2 years, meaning that nutritional status is comparable with that of well-nourished healthy children. The rationale for this goal is that an association exists between lung function, generally measured by forced expiratory volume in 1 second (FEV_1) percent predicted, and nutritional status (**Fig. 1**).[2,4–6]

BMI is the most widely accepted measure of nutritional status in patients with CF. In the past, percentage of ideal body weight was often used; however, BMI is a more accurate measure of nutritional status.[7,8] Even so, it is essential to remember that some children with short stature may have a BMI at or greater than the 50th percentile but still have suboptimal nutritional status. In fact, it is thought that height is related to lung volume; therefore, the importance of achieving adequate linear growth cannot be overstated.[9,10]

The 2002 consensus report on nutrition for pediatric patients with CF[1] notes that extra attention should be paid to nutrition and growth at 3 specific times: the first 12 months after diagnosis, the first 12 months of life for infants diagnosed prenatally or at birth, and the peripubertal growth period. The establishment of a pattern of normal growth (ie, similar to children without CF) during early childhood sets the stage for continued growth for the remainder of childhood and adolescence. As more and more patients are diagnosed prenatally or at birth (see section on newborn screening and diagnosis), increasing emphasis is being placed on the care of toddlers and preschoolers. New guidelines that pertain to all aspects of care in this age group are forthcoming and are discussed later. In addition, recent research based on data from the CF Patient Registry has shown the importance of early childhood nutrition for pulmonary health and overall outcomes later in life. One important study demonstrated that greater weight at 4 years of age is associated with greater height, better pulmonary function, fewer complications of CF, and better survival through 18 years of age.[11]

ASSESSMENT OF GROWTH AND NUTRITIONAL STATUS

The frequency at which growth parameters should be assessed is described in **Table 1**. Growth is measured in children with CF by the same standards that are used for healthy children. For children less than 2 years of age, the World Health

Table 1
Nutritional assessment in routine cystic fibrosis center care

	At Diagnosis	Every 3 mo Birth to 24 mo	Every 3 mo	Annually
Head circumference	x[a]	x	—	—
Weight (to 0.1 kg)	x	x	x	—
Length (to 0.1 cm)	x	x	—	—
Height (to 0.1 cm)	x	—	x	—
Midarm circumference (to 0.1 cm)	x	—	—	x
TSF (to 1.0 mm)	x[b]	—	—	x
Midarm muscle area, mm² (calculated from MAC and TSF)	x[b]	—	—	x
Midarm fat area, mm² (calculated from MAC and TSF)	x[b]	—	—	x
Biological parents height[c]	x	—	—	—
Pubertal status, female	—	—	—	x[d]
Pubertal status, male	—	—	—	x[e]
24-hour diet recall	—	—	—	x
Nutritional supplement intake[f]	—	—	—	x
Anticipatory dietary and feeding behavior guidance	—	x	x[g]	x

Abbreviations: MAC, mid arm circumference; TSF, triceps skinfold.
  [a] If less than 24 months of age at diagnosis.
  [b] Only in patients more than 1 year of age.
  [c] Record in centimeters and sex-specific height percentile; note patients' target height percentile on all growth charts.
  [d] Starting at 9 years of age, annual pubertal self-assessment form (patients or parent and patient) or physician examination for breast and pubic hair Tanner stage determination; annual question as to menarchal status. Record month and year of menarche on all growth charts.
  [e] Starting at 10 years of age, annual pubertal self-assessment form (patients or parent and patient) or physician examination for genital development and pubic hair Tanner stage determination.
  [f] A review of enzymes, vitamins, minerals, oral or enteral formulas, herbal, botanical, and other complementary and alternative medicine products.
  [g] Routine surveillance may be done informally by other team members, but the annual assessment and every 3 monthly visits in the first 2 years of life and every 3 monthly visits for patients at nutritional risk should be done by the center dietician.
  From Borowitz D, Baker RD, Stallings V. Consensus report on nutrition for pediatric patients with cystic fibrosis. J Pediatr Gastroenterol Nutr 2002;35(3):247; with permission.

Organization's growth standards are used to track weight, recumbent length, head circumference, and weight-for-length.[12] For patients greater than 2 years of age, weight, height, and BMI are tracked using the CDC standard curves.[13,14] Given the importance of height, growth velocity should be interpreted based on the child's genetic potential for height. This velocity may be estimated using a variety of methods, including the midparental target height prediction.[15]

In addition to anthropometrics, other components of the clinical evaluation may be used to assess nutritional status. Pubertal development is often delayed in patients with CF and can be due to poor nutrition (see section on endocrine disorders). Pubertal status may be assessed by patient or parent report or by physical examination with Tanner staging. Bone health may be evaluated by history, physical examination,

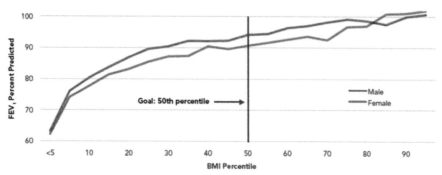

Fig. 1. FEV$_1$ percent predicted versus BMI percentile for children aged 6 to 19 years, 2012 CFF Registry. (*From* Cystic Fibrosis Foundation Patient Registry. Annual report to the center directors. Cystic Fibrosis Foundation. Bethesda (MD). 2012; with permission.)

laboratory, or radiologic studies (see section on endocrine disorders). Laboratory monitoring of nutritional status is discussed later (**Table 2**).

NUTRITIONAL GOALS
Calories

Optimal energy intake is critical to the overall health of individuals with CF. A variety of factors contribute to an individual's specific energy needs, including nutrient maldigestion and/or malabsorption, presence of a pulmonary exacerbation, pulmonary function, fat free mass, sex, pubertal status, CF transmembrane conductance regulator (CFTR) mutation, age, and other medical complications, such as liver disease and CF-related diabetes.[16] Recommendations for calculating energy requirements for individuals with CF are included (**Table 3**).

Enzyme Administration

Pancreatic enzyme replacement therapy (PERT) should be initiated once pancreatic insufficiency (PI) has been determined.[1] PERT should be administered with all food and milk products (including formula and breast milk). Numerous formulations of pancreatic enzymes are available commercially in various strengths. Each brand of enzymes contains United States Pharmacopeia (USP) units of lipase, amylase, and protease.

Dosage of PERT is based on USP units of lipase.

- Infants
  - 2000 to 4000 lipase units per 120 mL of human milk or formula[17]
- Children greater than 12 months of age
  - No more than 2500 lipase units per kilogram per meal and half of a meal dose with snacks, with a daily maximum of 10,000 lipase units per kilogram of body weight per day[1]

Fat-Soluble Vitamins

Individuals with CF are at risk for fat-soluble vitamin deficiency (vitamins A, D, E, and K) because of PI, liver disease, and intestinal malabsorption. The CFF recommends monitoring of fat-soluble vitamin levels and fat-soluble vitamin supplementation in all infants and children with CF (even those with normal laboratory values and those with pancreatic sufficiency), beginning at the time of diagnosis (see **Table 2**; **Table 4**).[1]

Table 2
Laboratory monitoring of nutritional status

Nutrient	At Diagnosis (Including At Newborn Screen)	Annually	Other	Test
		How Often to Monitor		
Beta carotene	—	—	At physician's discretion	Serum levels
Vitamin A	x	x	—	Vitamin A (retinol)
Vitamin D	x	x	—	25-OH vitamin D
Vitamin E	x	x	—	α-tocopherol
Vitamin K	x	—	Monitor in patients with hemoptysis, hematemesis, and/or liver disease	PIVKA-II (preferably) or prothrombin time
Essential fatty acids	—	—	Consider checking in infants or those with FTT	Triene/tetraene
Calcium/bone status	—	—	Age >8 y if risk factors are present[a]	Calcium, phosphorus, ionized PTH, DEXA scan
Iron	x	x	Consider in-depth evaluation for patients with poor appetite	Hemoglobin, hematocrit
Zinc	—	—	Consider 6-mo supplementation trial and follow growth[b]	—
Sodium	—	—	Infants should be started on 0.125 tsp salt supplementation at diagnosis if <6 mo; increase to 0.25 tsp salt daily at 6 mo Consider checking if patients are exposed to heat stress and become dehydrated	Serum sodium; spot urine sodium if total body sodium depletion suspected
Protein stores	x	x	Check in patients with nutritional failure or those at risk	Albumin

Abbreviations: DEXA, dual-energy x-ray absorptiometry; FTT, failure to thrive; PIVKA-II, proteins induced by vitamin k absence; PTH, parathyroid hormone.
[a] Risk factors for poor bone health include candidate for organ transplant, after transplantation, end-stage lung disease, bone fracture associated with low-impact activity, chronic steroid use, delayed pubertal development, nutritional failure.
[b] Particularly in infants not adequately growing despite adequate caloric intake and pancreatic enzyme replacement therapy.
Adapted from Borowitz D, Baker RD, Stallings V. Consensus report on nutrition for pediatric patients with cystic fibrosis. J Pediatr Gastroenterol Nutr 2002;35(3):246–59; and Cystic Fibrosis Foundation, Borowitz D, Robinson KA, et al. Cystic Fibrosis Foundation evidence-based guidelines for management of infants with cystic fibrosis. J Pediatr 2009;155(6 Suppl):S73–93.

Table 3
Determination of energy requirements according to the US Cystic Fibrosis Foundation

Calculate BMR in Kilocalories from Body Weight in Kilograms Using World Health Organization Equations[a]

Age Range (y)	Females	Males
0–3	61.0 wt − 51	60.9 wt − 54
3–10	22.5 wt + 499	22.7 wt + 495
10–18	12.2 wt + 746	17.5 wt + 651
18–30	14.7 wt + 496	15.3 wt + 679

Calculate the DEE by Multiplying the BMR by Activity Plus Disease Coefficients

AC	Disease Coefficients	DEE
Confined to bed: BMR × 1.3	FEV_1 >80% predicted: 0	BMR × (AC + 0)
Sedentary: BMR × 1.5	FEV_1 40%−79% predicted: 0.2	BMR × (AC + 0.2)
Active: BMR × 1.7	FEV_1 <40% predicted: 0.3 to 0.5[b]	BMR × (AC + 0.3)

Calculate Total DERs From DEE and Degree of Steatorrhea

If a stool collection is not available to determine the fraction of fat intake, an approximate value of 0.85 may be used in the calculation. For PS patients and PI patients with a COA >93% of intake, DER = DEE. For example: a patient with a COA of 0.78, the factor is 0.93/0.78 or 1.2. If the COA is not known the factor is 1.1.

Example: 10-year-old boy, weight = 32 kg; AC = active; FEV_1% predicted = 85%; COA = not available.

12.2 (32) + 746 = 1136

1136 × (1.7 + 0) = 1931

1931 × 1.1 = 2124 calories per day

Abbreviations: AC, activity coefficients; BMR, basal metabolic rate; COA, coefficient of fat absorption; DEE, daily energy expenditure; DER, daily energy requirement; PI, pancreatic insufficiency; PS, pancreatic sufficient; wt, weight.
[a] *From* World Health Organization. Energy and protein requirements [appendix B]. World Health Organ Tech Rep Ser 1985;924(724):115–6.
[b] May range up to 0.5 with very severe lung disease.
From Michel SH, Maqbool A, Hanna MD, et al. Nutrition management of pediatric patients who have cystic fibrosis. Pediatr Clin North Am 2009;56(5):1127; with permission; and *Data from* Ramsey BW, Farrell PM, Pencharz P. Nutritional assessment and management in cystic fibrosis: a consensus report. Am J Clin Nutr 1992;55:108–16.

Table 4
Recommendations for vitamin supplementation

	Individual Vitamin Daily Supplementation			
	Vitamin A (IU)	Vitamin E (IU)	Vitamin D (IU)	Vitamin K (mg)
0–12 mo	1500	40–50	400	0.3–0.5[a]
1–3 y	5000	80–150	400–800	0.3–0.5[a]
4–8 y	5000–1,00,000	100–200	400–800	0.3–0.5[a]
>8 y	10,000	200–400	400–800	0.3–0.5[a]

[a] Currently, commercially available products do not have ideal doses for supplementation. In a recent review, no adverse effects have been reported at any dosage level of vitamin K. Clinicians should try to follow these recommendations as closely as possible until better dosage forms are available. Prothrombin time or, ideally, PIVKA-II levels should be checked in patients with liver disease and vitamin K dose titrated as indicated.
From Borowitz D, Baker RD, Stallings V. Consensus report on nutrition for pediatric patients with cystic fibrosis. J Pediatr Gastroenterol Nutr 2002;35(3):251; with permission.

Vitamin A

- Function
  - It is important for vision, epithelial cell integrity, immune function, and growth.
- Deficiency
  - Deficiency can cause night blindness, skin changes, and impaired immune response.[18]
- Metabolism
  - It is ingested as retinol (preformed) or as carotenoids (provitamin A).
  - Provitamin A is metabolized to retinol, stored in the liver as retinol esters, and exported bound to retinol binding protein and to transthyretin.
- Toxicity
  - Excessive vitamin A intake can result in bone mineral loss and hepatotoxicity.
  - There are several reports of elevated serum retinol levels in individuals with CF.[19] This finding is difficult to interpret given that serum retinol is a better marker of vitamin A deficiency than vitamin A excess. In response to these concerns, several CF-specific multivitamins now have lower retinol content (**Table 5**).[16]

The CFF recommends annual monitoring of vitamin A status through measurement of serum retinol in all individuals with CF (see **Table 2**).[1] Serum retinol binding protein and retinol esters should be measured in individuals with liver disease.

Vitamin D

- Function
  - It is important for calcium metabolism and bone mineralization as well as in innate immunity and muscle function.[20]
- Deficiency
  - Deficiency can result in osteoporosis and increased risk of infection.
  - It is common among individuals with CF as well as in the general US population.[20,21]
  - Despite the CFF's recommendations, however, deficiencies in vitamin D remain common in individuals with CF.[20,21]
- Metabolism
  - Vitamin D2 and vitamin D3 are hydroxylated in the liver to 25-hydroxyvitamin D (calcidiol) and then converted in the kidney to 1, 25-dihydroxyvitamin D (active form).
  - Vitamin D3 (cholecalciferol) is a common over-the-counter supplement and is the recommended form of vitamin D supplementation for people with CF as opposed to vitamin D2 (ergocalciferol).

Vitamin E

- Function
  - It is an antioxidant in cell membranes.
- Deficiency
  - Deficiency can cause cognitive defects, peripheral neuropathy, ataxia, retinopathy, hemolytic anemia, and reduced immunity.
- Toxicity
  - Excess vitamin E is rare; but because high doses of vitamin E may inhibit platelet aggregation, coagulopathy and hemorrhagic stroke may occur.

Table 5
Comparison of cystic fibrosis-specific vitamin and mineral supplements in United States to non-cystic fibrosis-specific products

Age	MVW Complete Formulation (Drops, Chewables, Softgels)	AquADEKs (Drops, Chewables, Softgels)	Vitamax (Drops and Chewables)	ChoiceFul (Chewables, Softgels)	Libertas Abdek (Drops, Chewables, Softgels)	Poly-Vi-Sol Drops and Centrum Chewables and Tablets
Vitamin A (IU): retinol and beta carotene						
0–12 mo	4627 (1 mL)	5751 (1 mL)	3170 (1 mL)	—	4627 (1 mL)	1500 (1 mL)
1–3 y	9254 (2 mL)	11,502 (2 mL)	6340 (2 mL)	—	9254 (2 mL)	3000 (2 mL)
4–8 y	16,000 (1 chewable)	18,167 (2 chewables)	5000 (1 chewable)	13,000 (1 chewable)	16,000 (1 chewable)	3500 (1 chewable)
>9 y	32,000 (2 softgels)	36,334 (2 softgels)	10,000 (2 chewables)	28,000 (2 softgels)	32,000 (2 softgels)	7000 (2 tablets)
Vitamin E (IU)						
0–12 mo	50 (0.5 mL)	50 (1 mL)	50 (1 mL)	—	50 (1 mL)	5 (1 mL)
1–3 y	100 (1 mL)	100 (2 mL)	100 (2 mL)	—	100 (2 mL)	10 (2 mL)
4–8 y	200 (1 chewable)	100 (2 chewables)	200 (1 chewable)	180 (1 chewable)	200 (1 chewable)	30 (1 chewable)
>9 y	400 (2 softgels)	300 (2 softgels)	400 (2 chewables)	340 (2 softgels)	400 (2 softgels)	60 (2 tablets)
Vitamin D (IU)						
0–12 mo	750 (0.5 mL)	600 (1 mL)	400 (1 mL)	—	500 (1 mL)	400 (1 mL)
1–3 y	1500 (1 mL)	1200 (2 mL)	800 (2 mL)	—	1000 (2 mL)	800 (2 mL)

4–8 y	1500 (1 chewable)	1200 (2 chewables)	400 (1 chewable)	800 (1 chewable)	1000 (1 chewable)	400 (1 chewable)
>9 y	3000 (2 softgels)	2400 (2 softgels)	800 (2 chewables)	2000 (2 softgels)	2000 (2 softgels)	800 (2 tablets)
Vitamin K (µg)						
0–12 mo	500 (0.5 mL)	400 (1 mL)	300 (1 mL)	—	400 (1 mL)	0
1–3 y	1000 (1 mL)	800 (2 mL)	600 (2 mL)	—	800 (2 mL)	0
4–8 y	1000 (1 chewable)	700 (2 chewables)	200 (chewable)	600 (1 chewable)	800 (1 chewable)	10 (1 chewable)
>9 y	1600 (2 softgels)	1400 (2 softgels)	400 (2 chewables)	1400 (2 softgels)	1600 (2 softgels)	50 (2 tablets)
Zinc (mg)						
0–12 mo	5 (0.5 mL)	5 (1 mL)	7.5 (1 mL)	—	5 (1 mL)	0
1–3 y	10 (1 mL)	10 (2 mL)	15 (2 mL)	—	10 (2 mL)	0
4–8 y	15 (1 chewable)	10 (2 chewables)	7.5 (1 chewable)	15 (1 chewable)	15 (1 chewable)	1 (1 chewable)
>9 y	20 (2 softgels)	20 (2 softgels)	15 (2 chewables)	30 (2 softgels)	30 (2 softgels)	22 (2 tablets)

Adapted from Michel SH, Maqbool A, Hanna MD, et al. Nutrition management of pediatric patients who have cystic fibrosis. Pediatr Clin North Am 2009;56(5):1124–25; with permission.

Vitamin K

- Function
  - Important cofactor required for the activity of many proteins, including pro-thrombin and bone metabolism-related proteins
- Deficiency
  - Coagulopathy, poor bone health
- Toxicity
  - No reported toxicities of vitamin K excess[22]
- Metabolism
  - Vitamin K is found in dietary sources, including green leafy vegetables, and produced by intestinal bacteria. Therefore, fat malabsorption and intestinal dysbiosis increase the risk for vitamin K deficiency in individuals with CF.

The CFF recommends monitoring if an individual has symptoms of hemoptysis or hematemesis or a history of liver disease; additional supplementation may be needed (see **Tables 2** and **4**).[1]

Minerals and Trace Elements

Sodium

"An excessively salty taste to the skin" is one of the earliest descriptions of CF.[23] Sodium chloride (table salt) is important in the management of CF. Individuals with CF lose salt excessively through the skin; thus, hyponatremic dehydration may occur.[24–26] The CFF recommends sodium chloride supplementation in infancy (0.125 tsp daily for infants <6 months of age, increased to 0.25 tsp daily at 6 months of age).[27] Older patients are encouraged to eat a high-salt diet and active individuals in warm environments should consider adding 0.25 tsp of salt to 12 oz of electrolyte sports drinks.[16,28]

Fluoride

Children with CF have similar fluoride requirements as the general population in order to prevent and control dental caries. Prevention of dental caries is important as individuals with CF experience tooth enamel defects more commonly than individuals without CF.[29,30] Similar to the general population, fluoride should be prescribed in children who drink fluoride-deficient water beginning at 6 months of age.[31]

Zinc

Zinc is important in many enzymatic reactions and particularly in growth, lung health, and immunity. Deficiency can result in poor appetite, growth failure, and impaired immune function. Individuals with CF are at increased risk for zinc deficiency, as fat malabsorption negatively affects zinc absorption.[32,33] Because zinc deficiency can occur with normal plasma zinc levels, the CFF recommends empirical zinc supplementation for 6 months in individuals with CF who have short stature or failure to thrive.[27,34]

Iron

Anemia is seen in individuals with CF, usually caused by anemia of chronic disease or iron deficiency anemia.[35] Iron deficiency in CF may be multifactorial and due in part to poor dietary intake of iron and increased iron losses in sputum and in the gastrointestinal (GI) tract.[16,36] The CFF recommends annual screening for anemia with hemoglobin and hematocrit.[1]

Essential Fatty Acids

Linoleic acid (an omega-6 fatty acid) and alpha-linolenic acid (an omega-3 fatty acid) cannot be synthesized by humans and, thus, are termed essential fatty acids (EFAs).

Diets rich in EFAs include vegetable oils and cold-water fish. Linoleic acid and alpha-linolenic acid are further metabolized to arachidonic acid (proinflammatory) and docosahexaenoic acid (antiinflammatory), respectively. Although the CFF does not recommend for routine supplementation or screening for EFA deficiency, EFA deficiency should be considered and treated, if present, in individuals with failure to thrive.[1,27]

DIFFICULTY OF ATTAINING APPROPRIATE NUTRITIONAL STATUS

Despite close monitoring and appropriate anticipatory guidance, BMI greater than the 50th percentile can be difficult to attain and maintain. Overall nutritional status in children with CF has been improving over time[37] (**Fig. 2**); however, on average BMI percentile decreases with advancing age (**Fig. 3**). Similar to failure to thrive in the general pediatric population, malnutrition in CF is best understood as an imbalance between energy input and output. Malnutrition results from discrepancy between energy and micronutrient requirements and food intake modified by malabsorption. Energy needs in children with CF are 110% to 200% of the energy needs for the healthy population of similar age, sex, and size.

The cause of malnutrition in CF is often multifactorial:

Insufficient Caloric Intake

Poor appetite
Poor appetite is related to increased work of breathing and to both pulmonary and GI dysfunction. Nasal polyps may diminish the sense of smell and, hence, appetite. CF leads to a multitude of GI problems (see section on GI system) that affect nutritional status. Gastroesophageal reflux disease and gastroparesis may affect appetite or lead to loss of calories through vomiting or early satiety. Distal intestinal obstruction syndrome and constipation may similarly affect caloric intake and lead to hospitalization and/or periods of time when a child is unable to eat by mouth. CF-related liver disease may lead to development of ascites and organomegaly, which decrease appetite.

Malabsorption
Eighty-five percent to 90% of patients with CF have pancreatic insufficiency, leading to malabsorption of nutrients, especially fat and fat-soluble vitamins (see section on GI

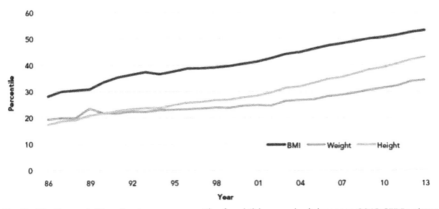

Fig. 2. Median nutritional outcome percentiles for children and adolescents, 2013 CFF Registry. (*From* LMS parameters for boys and LMS parameters for girls: height for age. National Health and Nutrition Survey (NHANES); CDC/National Center for Health Statistics.)

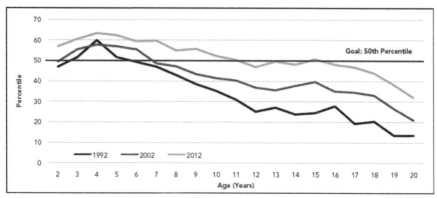

Fig. 3. Median BMI percentile for children and teens, 2013 CFF Registry. (*From* Cystic Fibrosis Foundation Patient Registry. Annual report to the center directors. Cystic Fibrosis Foundation, Bethesda (MD). 2012; with permission.)

system). Even with pancreatic enzyme replacement therapy, fat absorption is only 85% to 90% of that of healthy individuals, possibly because of altered intestinal pH.[38,39] A history of bowel resection, that is, for meconium ileus, may lead to further malabsorption. Small bowel bacterial overgrowth may impair absorption due to diarrhea. CF-related liver disease may exacerbate fat-soluble vitamin deficiencies and affect bone health. Decreased bile acid production and subsequent impaired micelle formation may adversely affect absorption of nutrients.[40]

Psychosocial concerns

Children with complex family or social situations may not have sufficient access to food, enteral supplements, or medications (see section on psychosocial challenges). Body image affects eating behaviors, particularly in adolescent girls. Female patients with CF tend to overestimate their weight, whereas male patients with CF tend to underestimate their weight.[41] Many female patients express contentment with their weight and have a fear of gaining weight if told to increase caloric intake.

Increased Caloric Expenditure

Pulmonary disease

Increased work of breathing leads to increased caloric expenditure. Chronic pulmonary infection and inflammation lead to cytokine-induced catabolism.

Other systemic disease

CF-related diabetes mellitus and impaired glucose tolerance may affect energy metabolism due to muscle catabolism and glucosuria (see section on endocrine disorders). CF-related diabetes is related to decreased weight z score and pulmonary function.

Cystic fibrosis transmembrane conductance regulator mutations

CFTR dysfunction and other genetic factors, such as gene modifiers, may affect metabolism to varying degrees.

HOW TO OPTIMIZE NUTRITIONAL STATUS

Children with CF not meeting their nutritional goals (weight/length >50th percentile in children <2 years of age and BMI >50th percentile in children older than 2 years) should be evaluated for other comorbidities (see *Difficulty of attaining appropriate nutritional status*) and assessed by a multidisciplinary team, to include a pulmonologist, primary care provider (PCP), gastroenterologist, endocrinologist, dietician, social worker, nurse, and behavioral therapist.[8,27,42,43] It is important for PCPs to support these goals despite the emphasis on preventing overweight in the general population.

A variety of options are available for management of suboptimal nutritional status, including nutritional therapy, behavioral therapy, pharmacotherapy, and the use of enteral feedings. Each of these therapeutic options should be discussed with the family and child at the onset of suboptimal nutritional status.[42,43]

Nutritional Therapy

Caloric deficits are a common cause for suboptimal nutritional status in individuals with CF; thus, increasing caloric intake using high-fat additives and foods is often a first step. A thorough dietary history and food record should be assessed and appropriate nutritional education provided. Although proprietary oral supplementation is recommended, it may not be sufficient to improve nutritional status.[8,44,45]

Behavioral Treatment

Behavioral feeding problems are commonly seen in preschool and school-aged children with CF.[46–48] A recent randomized clinical trial in preschoolers with CF demonstrated improvement in height for age z score and caloric intake in subjects receiving behavioral therapy compared with general nutritional and anticipatory care education.[49] Thus, the CFF recommends parents to[8,27]

- Consistently and specifically compliment appropriate eating behaviors.
- Pay minimal attention to behavior not compatible with eating.
- Limit mealtimes to 15 minutes for toddlers, and use snack times as mini-meals.

Pharmacotherapy

Appetite stimulants
Appetite stimulants may be considered to improve caloric intake once other causes of malnutrition have been considered.

- Cyproheptadine
  - It is a first-generation antihistamine with a secondary effect of appetite stimulation. The mechanism of action of appetite stimulation is unknown.[50]
  - Aside from transient drowsiness at the time of initiation of drug therapy, cyproheptadine is generally well tolerated.
  - Weight gain is generally modest and occurs within the first few months of use.[50,51]
- Megestrol acetate
  - It is a derivative of progesterone with a secondary effect of weight gain and appetite stimulation. The mechanism of action of appetite stimulation is unknown.
  - Small studies in CF have reported weight gain; however, other effects, including adrenal suppression and diabetes, were reported with long-term use.[50]
- Dronabinol
  - It is the oral form of delta-9-tetrahydrocannabinol and is the principal psychoactive substance present in marijuana.
  - A small study of 11 (primarily adult) patients with CF noted an improvement in weight, with one patient experiencing euphoria, hallucinations, and lethargy.

Growth hormone

A recent meta-analysis of 4 studies in patients with CF demonstrate improvement in height, weight, and lean tissue mass, with one study demonstrating an improvement in forced vital capacity percent predicted.[52] Longer-term studies are recommended before routinely using growth hormone in patients with CF.[52]

Cystic fibrosis transmembrane conductance regulator modulators

Ivacaftor, an oral CFTR potentiator, has recently been studied in patients with at least one G551D CFTR mutation. Nutritional status improved (weight z score, BMI z score) after 48 weeks in subjects receiving ivacaftor compared with placebo.[53]

Enteral Nutrition

Enteral nutrition (specifically enteral nutrition administered via nasogastric, gastrostomy, or jejunal tubes) improves nutritional and growth status in children and adults with CF.[54–57]

- Nasogastric tubes
  - They may be appropriate for short-term use.
  - They may be used chronically; but many patients will not tolerate chronic use because of discomfort, cough, or presence of nasal polyps.
- Gastrostomy tubes
  - Considered first line for most patients with CF
  - May be placed surgically, endoscopically, or via interventional radiology
  - Allows for both bolus and continuous feeds
- Jejunal or gastro-jejunal tubes
  - May be considered for patients with severe gastroesophageal reflux disease or gastroparesis
  - Require continuous feeds and may be cumbersome to manage

The option to use enteral feeds should not be thought of as a last resort or failure but rather should be considered early as a means to attain growth and nutrition goals in patients with CF.[42]

The CFF recommends use of enteral tube feedings in patients with CF who are unable to attain caloric requirements to meet growth/weight maintenance goals despite evaluation by a multidisciplinary team.[42]

Formula

- Infants
  - Human milk is recommended as the initial type of feeding.
  - Standard infant formulas should be used unless intolerance is documented.
  - Caloric density of formula or human milk may be increased if nutritional status is suboptimal.[27]
- In children older than 2 years, formula choice should be determined based on the individual patient with CF, as there is insufficient evidence to support use of one specific type of formula (polymeric, semielemental, elemental).[42,57,58] Generally, overnight continuous feeds are recommended to allow children with CF to eat as desired during the day.

Enzyme administration

Observational reports describe various methods of administering PERT with enteral nutrition. Although no evidence-based recommendations exist,[42] methods have been described, including use of semielemental formula,[59] dissolving PERT microspheres in nectar thick fruit juice,[60] dissolving PERT in bicarbonate solution,[61] and (most commonly observed) giving PERT before and after enteral feeds as well as in the middle of enteral feeds if patients wake at night.[62]

SUMMARY

Close attention to nutrition and growth is essential in caring for children with CF. Growth and nutritional status should be monitored as part of routine CF care, including measurement of anthropometrics (weight, length or height, and BMI percentile) and pubertal status. It is recommended that children with CF achieve growth and nutritional status comparable with that of well-nourished children without CF. A variety of tools, including oral supplementation (vitamin and mineral supplementation and calorie-dense liquids), behavioral treatment, pharmacotherapy (including appetite stimulants and CFTR modulators), and enteral nutrition, may be used to help achieve this goal.

REFERENCES

1. Borowitz D, Baker RD, Stallings V. Consensus report on nutrition for pediatric patients with cystic fibrosis. J Pediatr Gastroenterol Nutr 2002;35(3):246–59.
2. Corey M, McLaughlin FJ, Williams M, et al. A comparison of survival, growth, and pulmonary function in patients with cystic fibrosis in Boston and Toronto. J Clin Epidemiol 1988;41(6):583–91.
3. Robberecht E, De Clercq D, Genetello M. Historical overview and update on nutrition in cystic fibrosis: zooming in on small. Acta Sci Pol Technol Aliment 2011;10(3):407–14.
4. Cystic fibrosis foundation patient registry. Annual report to the center directors, Cystic Fibrosis Foundation. Bethesda (MD). 2012.
5. Kraemer R, Rudeberg A, Hadorn B, et al. Relative underweight in cystic fibrosis and its prognostic value. Acta Paediatr Scand 1978;67(1):33–7.
6. Dalzell AM, Shepherd RW, Dean B, et al. Nutritional rehabilitation in cystic fibrosis: a 5 year follow-up study. J Pediatr Gastroenterol Nutr 1992;15(2):141–5.
7. Hirche TO, Hirche H, Jungblut S, et al. Statistical limitations of percent ideal body weight as measure for nutritional failure in patients with cystic fibrosis. J Cyst Fibros 2009;8(4):238–44.
8. Stallings VA, Stark LJ, Robinson KA, et al. Evidence-based practice recommendations for nutrition-related management of children and adults with cystic fibrosis and pancreatic insufficiency: results of a systematic review. J Am Diet Assoc 2008;108(5):832–9.
9. Vieni G, Faraci S, Collura M, et al. Stunting is an independent predictor of mortality in patients with cystic fibrosis. Clin Nutr 2013;32(3):382–5.
10. Beker LT, Russek-Cohen E, Fink RJ. Stature as a prognostic factor in cystic fibrosis survival. J Am Diet Assoc 2001;101(4):438–42.
11. Yen EH, Quinton H, Borowitz D. Better nutritional status in early childhood is associated with improved clinical outcomes and survival in patients with cystic fibrosis. J Pediatr 2013;162(3):530–5.e1.
12. WHO Multicentre Growth Reference Study Group. WHO child growth standards: growth velocity based on weight, length, and head circumference: methods and development. Geneva: World Health Organization; 2009. p. 242.
13. Kuczmarski RJ, Ogden CL, Guo SS, et al. 2000 CDC growth charts for the United States: methods and development. Vital Health Stat 11 2002;246:1–190.

14. Machogu E, Cao Y, Miller T, et al. Comparison of WHO and CDC growth charts in predicting pulmonary outcomes in cystic fibrosis. J Pediatr Gastroenterol Nutr 2015;60(3):378–83.
15. Kuczmarski RJ, Ogden CL, Guo SS, et al. 2000 CDC growth charts for the United States: Methods and development. Vital Health Stat 11 2002;(246):1–190.
16. Michel SH, Maqbool A, Hanna MD, et al. Nutrition management of pediatric patients who have cystic fibrosis. Pediatr Clin North Am 2009;56(5):1123–41.
17. Borowitz D, Gelfond D, Maguiness K, et al. Maximal daily dose of pancreatic enzyme replacement therapy in infants with cystic fibrosis: a reconsideration. J Cyst Fibros 2013;12(6):784–5.
18. American Academy of Pediatrics. Committee on Nutrition, Barness LA. Pediatric nutrition handbook. 6th edition. Elk Grove Village (IL): American Academy of Pediatrics; 2009.
19. Maqbool A, Graham-Maar RC, Schall JI, et al. Vitamin A intake and elevated serum retinol levels in children and young adults with cystic fibrosis. J Cyst Fibros 2008;7(2):137–41.
20. Maqbool A, Stallings VA. Update on fat-soluble vitamins in cystic fibrosis. Curr Opin Pulm Med 2008;14(6):574–81.
21. Bertolaso C, Groleau V, Schall JI, et al. Fat-soluble vitamins in cystic fibrosis and pancreatic insufficiency: efficacy of a nutrition intervention. J Pediatr Gastroenterol Nutr 2014;58(4):443–8.
22. Conway SP. Vitamin K in cystic fibrosis. J R Soc Med 2004;97(Suppl 44):48–51.
23. Taussig LM. Cystic fibrosis: an overview. New York: Thieme-Stratton; 1984.
24. Kessler WR, Andersen DH. Heat prostration in fibrocystic disease of the pancreas and other conditions. Pediatrics 1951;8(5):648–56.
25. Guimaraes EV, Schettino GC, Camargos PA, et al. Prevalence of hyponatremia at diagnosis and factors associated with the longitudinal variation in serum sodium levels in infants with cystic fibrosis. J Pediatr 2012;161(2):285–9.
26. Nussbaum E, Boat TF, Wood RE, et al. Cystic fibrosis with acute hypoelectrolytemia and metabolic alkalosis in infancy. Am J Dis Child 1979;133(9):965–6.
27. Cystic Fibrosis Foundation, Borowitz D, Robinson KA, et al. Cystic Fibrosis Foundation evidence-based guidelines for management of infants with cystic fibrosis. J Pediatr 2009;155(6 Suppl):S73–93.
28. Kriemler S, Wilk B, Schurer W, et al. Preventing dehydration in children with cystic fibrosis who exercise in the heat. Med Sci Sports Exerc 1999;31(6):774–9.
29. Narang A, Maguire A, Nunn JH, et al. Oral health and related factors in cystic fibrosis and other chronic respiratory disorders. Arch Dis Child 2003;88(8):702–7.
30. Chi DL. Dental caries prevalence in children and adolescents with cystic fibrosis: a qualitative systematic review and recommendations for future research. Int J Paediatr Dent 2013;23(5):376–86.
31. American Academy of Pediatric D. Guideline on fluoride therapy. Pediatr Dent 2013;35(5):E165–8.
32. Krebs NF, Sontag M, Accurso FJ, et al. Low plasma zinc concentrations in young infants with cystic fibrosis. J Pediatr 1998;133(6):761–4.
33. Krebs NF. Overview of zinc absorption and excretion in the human gastrointestinal tract. J Nutr 2000;130(5S Suppl):1374S–7S.
34. Burke MS, Ragi JM, Karamanoukian HL, et al. New strategies in nonoperative management of meconium ileus. J Pediatr Surg 2002;37(5):760–4.
35. von Drygalski A, Biller J. Anemia in cystic fibrosis: incidence, mechanisms, and association with pulmonary function and vitamin deficiency. Nutr Clin Pract 2008; 23(5):557–63.

36. Reid DW, Withers NJ, Francis L, et al. Iron deficiency in cystic fibrosis: relationship to lung disease severity and chronic pseudomonas aeruginosa infection. Chest 2002;121(1):48–54.
37. Cystic Fibrosis Foundation Patient Registry. Annual report to the center directors. Bethesda (MD): Cystic Fibrosis Foundation; 2013.
38. Wouthuyzen-Bakker M, Bodewes FA, Verkade HJ. Persistent fat malabsorption in cystic fibrosis; lessons from patients and mice. J Cyst Fibros 2011;10(3):150–8.
39. Gelfond D, Ma C, Semler J, et al. Intestinal pH and gastrointestinal transit profiles in cystic fibrosis patients measured by wireless motility capsule. Dig Dis Sci 2013;58(8):2275–81.
40. Rowland M, Gallagher CG, O'Laoide R, et al. Outcome in cystic fibrosis liver disease. Am J Gastroenterol 2011;106(1):104–9.
41. Tierney S. Body image and cystic fibrosis: a critical review. Body Image 2012; 9(1):12–9.
42. Schwarzenberg SJ, Hempstead SE, McDonald CM, et al. Enteral tube feeding for individuals with cystic fibrosis: Evidence-informed guidelines. J Cystic Fibrosis, in press.
43. Lahiri T, Hempstead SE, Brady C, et al. Clinical Practice Guidelines From the Cystic Fibrosis Foundation for Preschoolers with Cystic Fibrosis. Pediatrics 2016;137(4):e20151784.
44. Smyth RL, Rayner O. Oral calorie supplements for cystic fibrosis. Cochrane Database Syst Rev 2014;(11):CD000406.
45. Poustie VJ, Russell JE, Watling RM, et al. Oral protein energy supplements for children with cystic fibrosis: CALICO multicentre randomised controlled trial. BMJ 2006;332(7542):632–6.
46. Stark LJ, Jelalian E, Powers SW, et al. Parent and child mealtime behavior in families of children with cystic fibrosis. J Pediatr 2000;136(2):195–200.
47. Powers SW, Patton SR, Byars KC, et al. Caloric intake and eating behavior in infants and toddlers with cystic fibrosis. Pediatrics 2002;109(5):E75.
48. Sanders MR, Turner KM, Wall CR, et al. Mealtime behavior and parent-child interaction: a comparison of children with cystic fibrosis, children with feeding problems, and nonclinic controls. J Pediatr Psychol 1997;22(6):881–900.
49. Powers SW, Stark LJ, Chamberlin LA, et al. Behavioral and nutritional treatment for preschool-aged children with cystic fibrosis: a randomized clinical trial. JAMA Pediatr 2015;169(5):e150636.
50. Nasr SZ, Drury D. Appetite stimulants use in cystic fibrosis. Pediatr Pulmonol 2008;43(3):209–19.
51. Homnick DN, Homnick BD, Reeves AJ, et al. Cyproheptadine is an effective appetite stimulant in cystic fibrosis. Pediatr Pulmonol 2004;38(2):129–34.
52. Thaker V, Haagensen AL, Carter B, et al. Recombinant growth hormone therapy for cystic fibrosis in children and young adults. Cochrane Database Syst Rev 2015;(5):CD008901.
53. Borowitz D, Lubarsky B, Wilschanski M, et al. Nutritional status improved in cystic fibrosis patients with the G551D mutation after treatment with ivacaftor. Dig Dis Sci 2016;61(1):198–207.
54. Vandeleur M, Massie J, Oliver M. Gastrostomy in children with cystic fibrosis and portal hypertension. J Pediatr Gastroenterol Nutr 2013;57(2):245–7.
55. White H, Morton AM, Conway SP, et al. Enteral tube feeding in adults with cystic fibrosis; patient choice and impact on long term outcomes. J Cyst Fibros 2013; 12(6):616–22.

56. Bradley GM, Carson KA, Leonard AR, et al. Nutritional outcomes following gastrostomy in children with cystic fibrosis. Pediatr Pulmonol 2012;47(8):743–8.
57. Oliver MR, Heine RG, Ng CH, et al. Factors affecting clinical outcome in gastrostomy-fed children with cystic fibrosis. Pediatr Pulmonol 2004;37(4):324–9.
58. Rosenfeld M, Casey S, Pepe M, et al. Nutritional effects of long-term gastrostomy feedings in children with cystic fibrosis. J Am Diet Assoc 1999;99(2):191–4.
59. Erskine JM, Lingard CD, Sontag MK, et al. Enteral nutrition for patients with cystic fibrosis: comparison of a semi-elemental and nonelemental formula. J Pediatr 1998;132(2):265–9.
60. Ferrie S, Graham C, Hoyle M. Pancreatic enzyme supplementation for patients receiving enteral feeds. Nutr Clin Pract 2011;26(3):349–51.
61. Nicolo M, Stratton KW, Rooney W, et al. Pancreatic enzyme replacement therapy for enterally fed patients with cystic fibrosis. Nutr Clin Pract 2013;28(4):485–9.
62. O'Brien CE, Harden H, Com G. A survey of nutrition practices for patients with cystic fibrosis. Nutr Clin Pract 2013;28(2):237–41.

Gastrointestinal, Pancreatic, and Hepatobiliary Manifestations of Cystic Fibrosis

Meghana Nitin Sathe, MD[a], Alvin Jay Freeman, MD[b],*

KEYWORDS

- CF and GI manifestations • CF pancreas • CFLD (CF liver disease)
- PERT (pancreatic enzyme replacement therapy)

KEY POINTS

- Gastrointestinal (GI) and hepatic manifestations of cystic fibrosis (CF) deserve special attention, as essentially all patients with CF will experience at least one such complaint during their lifetime.
- GI, pancreatic, and hepatic manifestations of CF are known to have significant effects on growth and nutrition, pulmonary function, and patient-perceived wellness.
- Defects in the CF transmembrane receptor protein affect fluid viscosity, flow, and pH, resulting in the clinical GI, pancreatic, and hepatobiliary manifestations of CF.
- Recognizing and managing GI manifestations is part of a comprehensive, multisystem approach to care.
- Clinicians should be aware of conditions in which diagnostic tests need to be interpreted differently in patients with CF than in the general population.

Pulmonary disease is the primary cause of morbidity and mortality in people with cystic fibrosis (CF), but significant involvement within gastrointestinal (GI), pancreatic, and hepatobiliary systems occurs as well.[1] GI, pancreatic, and hepatic manifestations of CF deserve special attention, as essentially all patients with CF will experience at least 1 such complaint during their lifetime. Additionally, many GI, pancreatic, and hepatic manifestations of CF are known to have significant effects on disease outcomes, including but not limited to (1) growth and nutrition, (2) pulmonary function, and (3) patient-perceived wellness.[1,2]

Disclosure Statement: The authors have nothing to disclose.
a Division of Pediatric Gastroenterology and Nutrition, Children's Health, University of Texas Southwestern, F4.06, 1935 Medical District Drive, Dallas, TX 75235, USA; b Division of Pediatric Gastroenterology, Hepatology and Nutrition, Children's Healthcare of Atlanta, Emory University, 2015 Uppergate Drive, Northeast, Atlanta, GA 30322, USA
* Corresponding author.
E-mail address: afreem6@emory.edu

The CF transmembrane regulator protein (CFTR) is expressed on the apical epithelium of the intestines and pancreatic and biliary duct systems where it regulates chloride and bicarbonate secretion.[3] Homozygosity of the mutant CFTR gene results in viscous and acidic secretions secondary to deficient surface fluid and bicarbonate efflux. This leads to partial or complete obstruction in the various hollow epithelial-lined structures of the GI tract and is responsible for most GI, pancreatic, and hepatobiliary manifestations of CF.[1,4] The associated increase in local and systemic inflammation is also detrimental to nutrition and growth (**Fig. 1**).

PANCREAS

Severe CFTR mutations (class I–III) are associated with dramatically decreased pancreatic ductal flow and absent digestive enzymes (pancreatic insufficiency [PI]), whereas milder mutations (class IV and V) tend to be associated with decreased flow but to an extent that allows digestive enzymes to flow into the duodenum (pancreatic sufficiency [PS]).[5] The bicarbonate milieu created by pancreatic fluid is essential to neutralize gastric acid so as to optimize the function of pancreatic enzymes, promote micelle formation, and dissolve the enteric coating on exogenous pancreatic enzyme replacement therapy (PERT).[6] The result of alterations in fluid volume, viscosity, and flow is that proenzymes get trapped within the pancreatic ducts, leading to early activation of pancreatic enzymes that inflame and damage the pancreas. Damage begins in utero as early as 17 weeks gestation.[6] Destruction of the pancreas leads to PI in most patients.

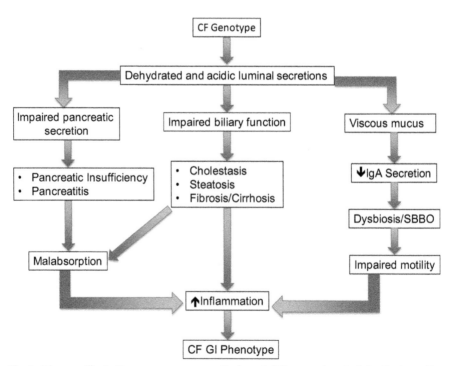

Fig. 1. Diagram illustrating common pancreatic, hepatobiliary, and gastrointestinal manifestations of CF that result in a common end pathway of increased systemic inflammation and CF phenotype.

Diagnosis of Pancreatic Insufficiency

PI can be diagnosed by calculating the coefficient of fat absorption from a collection of feces produced during a 3-day diet containing 100 g of fat per day. PI is presumed if less than 93% of fat is absorbed or greater than 7 g of fat is excreted during this time period.[7,8] In practice, this test has been replaced by the more efficient fecal elastase test, which measures the absence of endogenous elastase. Fecal elastase has a sensitivity of 72% and specificity of 90% for severe PI, but may not be as effective in diagnosis of mild to moderate PI.[7,9] False positives are seen in the setting of watery diarrhea and diabetes (levels are noted to decrease with increased duration of diabetes).[10] More invasive testing with secretin stimulation of the pancreas and direct collection and analysis of pancreatic juice is available but not often used. Patients do not have maldigestion until less than 10% of exocrine pancreatic function remains.[10]

Management of Pancreatic Insufficiency

PI is managed with exogenous PERT before every meal and snack and with fat-soluble vitamin supplementation. Presently, all PERT is formulated from porcine extracts that contain amylase (digests carbohydrates), protease (digests proteins), and lipase (digests fat). Dosing is based on lipase units/kg per meal or grams of fat ingested (**Table 1**).[11]

For infants and those unable to swallow, PERT capsules can be opened and the enteric-coated beads can be mixed in applesauce or another acidic medium. The enteric-coated beads cannot be crushed. Acid-suppressing medications are often used to increase the pH of gastric fluid delivered to the proximal duodenum to allow the enteric coating to dissolve.[12]

The efficacy of PERT is determined by monitoring weight, height, weight-for-length, and body mass index. Dose may be increased if there are symptoms of malabsorption. If PERT is at the recommended upper limit and growth is still lacking or malabsorption is still present, assessment for comorbid conditions should be initiated[7] (**Fig. 2**).

PANCREATITIS

Patients with milder mutations (class IV and V) are likely to be PS and are much more likely to develop pancreatitis than those with PI (10.3% vs 0.5%).[13] There is good correlation between genotype and pancreatic functional status but not between genotype and which patients with PS will develop pancreatitis. Pancreatitis is most frequently seen in patients with recurrent pulmonary exacerbations, viral infections, or after surgery. Patients with PS who have chronic recurrent pancreatitis are at high risk for developing PI as well as cystic fibrosis related diabetes (CFRD) due to ongoing damage within the

Table 1		
Guidelines for dosing PERT based on weight doses and grams of fat consumed		
Lipase units/kg/meal	**Lipase units/kg/g of Fat Eaten**	
<4 y of age: 1000–2500 lipase units/kg/meal [a]1/2 for snack	Infant formula or breast milk: 2000–4000 lipase units/120 mL	
>4 y of age: 500–2500 lipase units/kg/meal [a]1/2 for snack	Beyond infancy: 500–4000 lipase units/g of fat eaten	

[a] *Adapted from* CF Foundation Consensus Guidelines 1995; with permission.

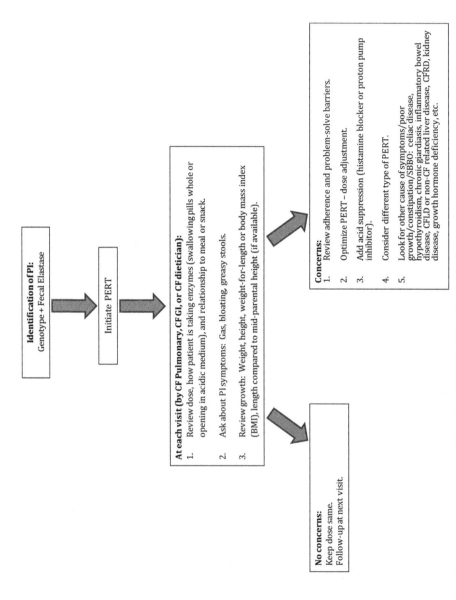

Identification of PI:
Genotype + Fecal Elastase

Initiate PERT

At each visit (by CF Pulmonary, CF GI, or CF dietician):

1. Review dose, how patient is taking enzymes (swallowing pills whole or opening in acidic medium), and relationship to meal or snack.

2. Ask about PI symptoms: Gas, bloating, greasy stools.

3. Review growth: Weight, height, weight-for-length or body mass index (BMI), length compared to mid-parental height (if available).

No concerns:
Keep dose same.
Follow-up at next visit.

Concerns:
1. Review adherence and problem-solve barriers.
2. Optimize PERT – dose adjustment.
3. Add acid suppression (histamine blocker or proton pump inhibitor).
4. Consider different type of PERT.
5. Look for other cause of symptoms/poor growth/constipation/SBBO: celiac disease, hypothyroidism, chronic giardiasis, inflammatory bowel disease, CFLD or non-CF related liver disease, CFRD, kidney disease, growth hormone deficiency, etc.

Fig. 2. Algorithm for management and maximization of PERT in CF patient with PI.

pancreas. Pancreatitis can be the initial presentation of CF and therefore patients with recurrent pancreatitis should be investigated for CF.[14]

MONITORING OF PANCREATIC SUFFICIENCY TO PANCREATIC INSUFFICIENCY

Infants may be PS at diagnosis but convert to PI during the first year of life due to ongoing pancreatic damage.[15] Even in the absence of pancreatitis, some older patients will progress from PS to PI. For this reason, in patients with CF and PS, fecal elastase should be considered as part of the annual evaluation.

GASTROESOPHAGEAL REFLUX DISEASE

Patients with CF experience an increased number of transient lower esophageal sphincter relaxations and may have delayed gastric emptying.[2] In patients with CF, the combination of these physiologic processes as well as a number of secondary pathophysiologic mechanisms (**Fig. 3**) increases the risk to develop gastroesophageal reflux disease (GERD).[16,17] Therefore, it is not surprising that reflux is one of the most common GI manifestations of CF, with its prevalence reported as high as 25% in infants and up to 85% in children and adults.[17,18]

Recent pH-impedance data suggest that reflux is present in more than half of children with CF, with nearly two-thirds of those patients reporting no clinical signs or symptoms of GERD. More than 75% of reflux episodes were acidic and more than 40% of episodes were "full-column," reaching the proximal esophagus.[19] GERD may be asymptomatic or may present as abdominal or chest pain, dysphasia, odynophagia, food impaction, and/or cough.[20] Although the impact of asymptomatic GERD is unclear in patients with CF, symptomatic GERD has been associated with worse pulmonary outcomes in CF but its severity is poorly correlated with objective measures of pulmonary function.[2]

The therapeutic approach for uncomplicated GERD in patients with CF is no different than for the general population; proton-pump inhibitors (PPIs) are

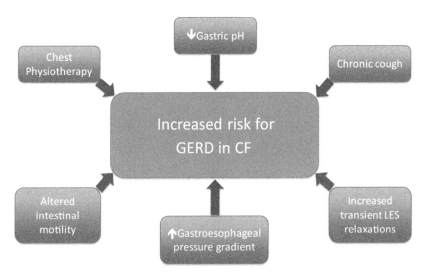

Fig. 3. Primary and secondary factors that increase the risk for a patient with CF developing GERD.

preferentially used for acid suppression. Improved lung function parameters are seen in patients on PPI therapy but long-term adverse effects have been described in people without CF. Both benefits and risks have been seen in people with CF treated with PPIs, yet no adequately powered randomization trials have been conducted. For patients with more complicated GERD, fundoplication has been reported to decrease the reflux-cough sequence, decrease the number of pulmonary exacerbations, slow pulmonary function decline, and aid in weight gain.[21] However, the rate of complications postoperatively may be higher than in non-CF patient populations and should be reserved for high-risk patients in consultation with a gastroenterologist familiar with CF.

INTESTINAL MOTILITY

A number of CF-associated variables, such as frequent antibiotic use, intestinal inflammation, and small bowel bacterial overgrowth (SBBO), have all been shown to impact gut motility in CF animal models.[22,23] Additionally, poor glycemic control, fat-rich and/or carbohydrate-rich meals, previous surgery, and hydration may affect gut motility.[24,25] Clinical studies have shown inconsistent results (normal, delayed, and rapid transit times all reported) and are hampered by small study sizes and a lack of standard outcome measures.

Gastric Emptying

Delayed gastric emptying has been reported in as many as one-third of adults with CF.[18,26] Others have reported both normal[25,27] and increased gastric emptying in children and adults.[24] Gastric emptying may be influenced by glycemic control and whether patients with PI are adherent to PERT.[24,28] Thus, the potential benefits of prokinetics on gastric emptying must be evaluated on a patient-by-patient basis.

Small Bowel Transit

Delayed small bowel transit has consistently been observed in patients with CF and may be up to twice as long as that seen in healthy controls.[2,25,27] The impact of delayed transit time on PERT effectiveness and common CF-associated GI conditions, including abdominal pain, bloating, and SBBO, is unclear.

Total Gastrointestinal Transit

Despite slow small bowel transit time, total GI and colonic transit time are not significantly different in patients with CF compared with healthy controls.[2,27] These findings are surprising, as constipation is common and some patients develop distal intestinal obstruction syndrome (DIOS).[29] Retained mucofeculent material adherent to the bowel wall with a liquid central channel could explain this discrepancy.

PEPTIC ULCER DISEASE/HELICOBACTER PYLORI

Despite reduced bicarbonate secretion in patients with CF, normal or even decreased prevalence rates of peptic ulcer disease (PUD) and *Helicobacter pylori* infections are seen.[30] This "CF paradox" may be due to retained bicarbonate within the enterocyte cytoplasm, which prevents injury and ulcer formation.[31] Alternatively, gastric metaplasia as a host defense mechanism in conjunction with frequent antibiotic use may prevent PUD and duodenal ulcerations in CF.[30]

Use of fecal immunoassay to detect *H pylori* in the CF population may be compromised due to cross-reactivity with anti-*Pseudomonas* antibodies.[32,33] Urea breath test (UBT) in the CF population is also problematic, as the test cannot differentiate SBBO or malabsorption from *H pylori* infection and there is discordance between stool antigen detection and UBT test results.[34] Therefore, indirect *H pylori* testing in the pediatric CF population must be interpreted with caution. Endoscopic evaluation can provide definitive diagnosis, but risks of anesthesia must be considered in the context of the patient's medical needs and underlying pulmonary status.

SMALL BOWEL BACTERIAL OVERGROWTH

SBBO is defined as greater than 10^5 colony-forming units per milliliter in the small intestine with a predominance of colonic/anaerobic species.[35] SBBO defined by breath testing has a prevalence of 30% to 55% in the CF population.[36] Delayed small bowel transit time, frequent antibiotics, prolonged use of acid suppression medications, PI, intestinal inflammation, and high rates of constipation increase the risk of developing SBBO.[37]

The presentation of SBBO can vary widely from direct consequences of the excessive bacterial burden (eg, bloating and abdominal pain) to secondary effects of intestinal damage (eg, anemia, malabsorption, malnutrition).[16,37] Failure to adequately treat SBBO can also result in a "positive feedback" that ultimately leads to worsening of the overgrowth and further consequences of intestinal inflammation/damage, as outlined in **Fig. 4**.

Consensus about diagnostic modalities and treatment is lacking.[38] A high index of suspicion should be maintained for SBBO among patients with CF with prolonged GI symptoms or persistent fat malabsorption, especially those with a history of intestinal surgery.[39] Antibiotics covering gram-negative anaerobic bacteria should be used (ie, metronidazole, amoxicillin-clavulanate, fluoroquinolones, gentamicin, rifamycin). Due to high reoccurrence rates, rotating oral antibiotic treatment strategies may be required.[40] However, these regimens, especially if required over long periods of time, carry a theoretic risk of bacterial resistance and increased *Clostridium difficile* infections.[16] Probiotics have been shown to be safe and efficacious in CF patient populations and may be considered as supplemental therapy.[41,42] Probiotics should be used with caution in any patient with indwelling port-a-caths, due to lactobacillus sepsis having been reported in patients with compromised gut motility and permeability.[43]

MUCOSAL DISEASES
Celiac Disease

Scandinavian population studies have shown a 2 to 3 times higher risk of developing celiac disease in patients with CF compared with the general population.[44] Diagnosis may be challenging given the varied and nonspecific presentations of celiac disease. Additionally, tissue transglutaminase immunoglobulin (Ig)A, which is used as a screening marker for celiac tissue, is often falsely elevated in patients with CF due to nonspecific intestinal inflammation.[45] As in the general population, duodenal biopsy is required for diagnosis. Assistance from a skilled CF dietician is critical to ensure that appropriate nutritional status is maintained if a gluten-free diet is required.

Inflammatory Bowel Disease

Initial reports suggested a seven-fold increase in Crohn disease among the CF population, but subsequent studies have come to different conclusions. Bresso and colleagues[46] determined in a European cohort that F508del mutant CFTR might exert a protective effect against the development of inflammatory bowel disease (IBD), whereas Bahmanyar and colleagues[47] reported no association between CFTR gene mutations and IBD using the Swedish national registry.[48] Calprotectin may be

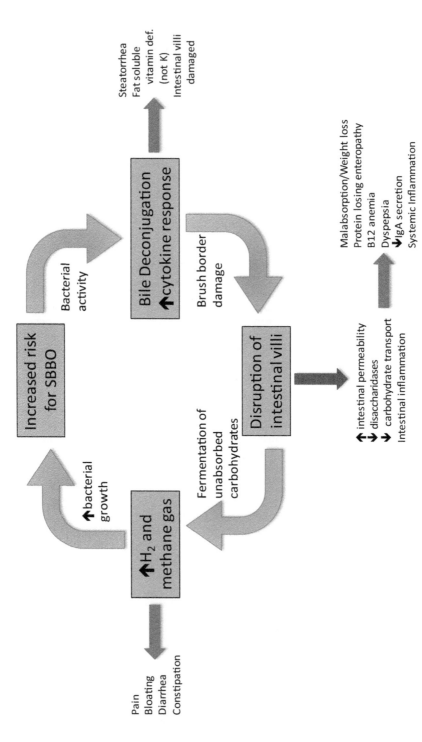

Fig. 4. Sequela of SBBO that predisposes the patient with CF to a variety of clinical manifestations and provides a feedback loop, which may lead to worsening SBBO and increases in both local and systemic inflammation.

elevated in patients with CF due to nonspecific intestinal inflammation and is not useful in screening for IBD.[49] Thus, endoscopic evaluation with biopsy is warranted for any patient with CF presenting with signs and/or symptoms of IBD.

APPENDICEAL FINDINGS

The appendix of children with CF is more distended than is seen in the general population.[50] However, patients with CF are largely asymptomatic or have symptoms inconsistent with acute appendicitis.[51,52] Despite the distention, the prevalence of appendicitis in the CF population is only 1% to 2% as compared with 7% in the general population.[53] Distention of the appendix with mucin, which appears as a mucoid appendix or a mucocele on imaging and is difficult to distinguish from acute appendicitis, in addition to frequent antibiotic use, may serve to protect the patient with CF from appendicitis.[54] When appendicitis does occur, it is often misdiagnosed due to its relatively low incidence and propensity to present with nonclassic symptoms (often mistaken for DIOS). This results in an increased risk for appendiceal perforation and abscess formation.[53]

INTUSSUSCEPTION

The prevalence of intussusception is 1% in the CF population, a rate that is 10-fold greater than the general population.[55] Intussusception in an older child should prompt a diagnostic evaluation for CF. Children with CF present with acute abdominal pain, similar to that seen in the general population. However, adolescents and adults with CF often present with insidious, colicky abdominal pain that spontaneously resolves and reoccurs and may be confused with DIOS.[1,16] Up to 25% of patients with CF can present with obstruction in addition to typical symptoms associated with intussusception (emesis, abdominal pain, palpable mass, and rectal bleeding): radiographic findings are the same as other patient populations.[53,56] The most common location is ileocolonic, although appendiceal and small bowel intussusception have been reported. Inspissated secretions, lymphoid hyperplasia, altered motility, and chronically distended appendix may all serve as lead points.[1,53] Although computed tomography (CT) or abdominal ultrasound may be required to distinguish intussusception from appendicitis, DIOS, or other causes of abdominal pain, air-enema reduction remains the treatment of choice in uncomplicated patients, although recurrence rates are high.[51]

PNEUMATOSIS INTESTINALIS

Pneumatosis intestinalis is a rare radiographic finding of linear foci of air in the dependent portion of the bowel on CT.[1] Its development typically coincides with the advancement of obstructive lung disease and is thought to be caused by dissection of air from the pulmonary interstitium.[51] It is usually discovered incidentally during workup of abdominal pain but has no clinical significance; no intervention is needed beyond management of lung disease.[1] If present, other causes of abdominal pain should be sought.

MECONIUM ILEUS

Meconium ileus (MI) is a neonatal intestinal obstruction caused by inspissated intraluminal meconium in the terminal ileum. Between 10% and 20% of neonates with CF will present with MI, and its presence in full-term infants is strongly suggestive of CF, with an odds ratio of 13 for infants homozygous for F508del.[57,58] Most infants with MI will have a negative newborn screen, so sweat testing and genetic evaluation should be obtained. Clinically, 2 distinct forms of MI exist: (1) simple obstruction with failure to pass meconium during the first 48 hours of life, and (2) complex disease, which occurs in 40% of patients with MI with manifestations such as perforation, meconium peritonitis, and/or volvulus. Simple obstruction may be relieved with hyperosmolar enemas, intravenous (IV) hydration, and nasogastric decompression. Surgical intervention is required in infants with complex MI or if obstruction does not resolve with repeated hyperosmolar enemas in infants with simple MI.[59] Meconium plug syndrome presents similar to MI with inspissated meconium failing to pass in the first 48 hours, but occurs in the colon rather than the terminal ileum and is not as highly associated with CF.[60]

DISTAL INTESTINAL OBSTRUCTION SYNDROME

DIOS is a condition unique to CF that occurs at all ages and is characterized by complete or incomplete fecal obstruction in the ileocecum.[61] Intestinal dysmotility, intestinal inflammation, fat malabsorption, and defective ion and water secretion into the gut lumen may all contribute to the development of DIOS.[52] More than 90% of patients with DIOS are PI, 50% have a history of MI, and it is 7 times more likely to occur in adults.[1]

Patients may present with acute or recurrent episodes of colicky abdominal pain, emesis, and abdominal distention, often with a palpable mass in the right lower quadrant. Anorexia and flatulence may be present, and the continued passage of stool can be seen if obstruction is incomplete.[2] DIOS can be diagnosed by history and radiographic imaging of the abdomen (**Fig. 5**), but CT is often used to distinguish DIOS from surgical causes of abdominal pain, including appendicitis.[52]

Medical management with IV hydration, polyethylene glycol solutions, and oral laxatives usually suffice to treat incomplete DIOS. If obstruction is complete (repeated emesis, absent bowel sounds), a nasogastric tube should be placed to decompress the stomach and treatment should be from below with Gastrografin enemas. In severe, complete DIOS, surgical consultation is appropriate, but surgery should be reserved as a last resort.[2] Adherence to PERT should be reviewed in all patients who experience DIOS and the importance of routine osmotic laxatives should be emphasized to minimize recurrence.[52] Patients with DIOS are often coaffected with chronic constipation.

CONSTIPATION

Constipation is one of the most common GI manifestations among patients with CF, affecting nearly one-half of pediatric and most adult patients.[29] Similar to DIOS, constipation is associated with PI, a history of MI, and fat malabsorption. Most patients with CF with chronic constipation experience daily bowel movements and therefore the consistency of stool should be considered in addition to the frequency; however, the most common symptoms include abdominal pain, flatulence, and decreased appetite. Constipation begins distally in the colon and extends proximally as the condition worsens as opposed to DIOS in which the opposite is true, although both conditions often occur together.[2] History alone should be enough for diagnosis, with radiographic imaging reserved for special instances in which other etiologies need to be excluded. Therapy focuses on the use of osmotic laxatives. The use of fiber is not emphasized, as it may add to the bulkiness of stools and lead to worsening of the constipation.

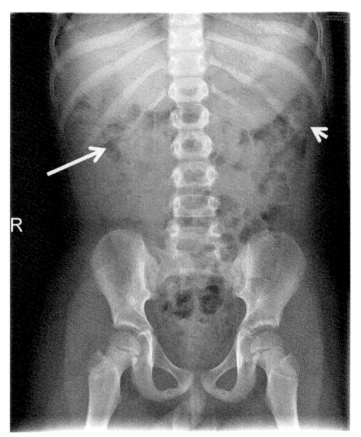

Fig. 5. Solid arrow indicates "bubbly-granular" mass in right colon suggestive of DIOS. Constipation often co-occurs with DIOS as evident by scybala of stool present on radiograph (*arrowhead*). (*Courtesy of* Drucy Borowitz, MD, Buffalo, NY.)

CLOSTRIDIUM DIFFICILE

Studies of adults with CF show *Clostridium difficile* carrier rates approaching 50% versus 3% in the general population. However, despite frequent hospitalizations, rotating antibiotic therapies, intestinal inflammation, and prolonged use of acid suppression medications, which should increase the risk for developing *C difficile* and colonic dysbiosis in patients with CF, symptomatic disease is rare in nontransplanted patients.[62] Only 1% to 2% of hospitalized patients with CF are affected. This number increases to nearly 30% in patients who have undergone lung transplantation.[63] Classic presentation with hematochezia, as well as atypical presentations that mimic constipation and/or DIOS may be seen. Recurrence is common and is associated with an increased risk of death in the CF population.[64] Treatment is the same as in the non-CF population.

FIBROSING COLONOPATHY

Fibrosing colonopathy was first described in 1994 and subsequently was directly associated with high doses of PERT, a history of GI complications, and use of some medications.[65] Patients often presented with colitis-like symptoms or failed to respond to standard DIOS therapy.[56] Patients develop concentric fibrous rings beneath the submucosa of the proximal colon that may span the length of the entire colon. Hypertrophy of muscularis mucosa, as well as denudation and reepithelialization of the mucosa are seen, suggesting recurrent ischemia rather than an inflammatory pattern of injury.[66]

When present, fibrosing colonopathy may progress to complete obstruction, most commonly in the ascending colon. In these cases, surgical resection is necessary (**Fig. 6**).[1]

In response to the epidemic of fibrosing colonopathy, guidelines limited lipase exposure to no more than 2500 lipase units/kg per meal.[11] Additionally, in 2004 the Food and Drug Administration mandated that enzymes go through a New Drug Application process and ensure standardization of doses; before this time, PERT capsules may have been overfilled with up to 200% of what was stated on the package label. Subsequently, a decreased incidence of fibrosing colonopathy has been seen.

RECTAL PROLAPSE

Recent studies suggest less than 5% of patients with CF will experience rectal prolapse, which is far less than the previously reported incidence of 20%.[67,68] This is likely due to earlier diagnosis of CF by newborn screening, attention to preventing constipation, and improved PERT formulations. When present, rectal prolapse is likely secondary to increased abdominal pressures from cough and constipation. Conservative management focuses on decreasing straining during defecation and use of stool softeners.[1] Although in most cases of rectal prolapse CF is not the cause, it should be included in the differential diagnosis.

GASTROINTESTINAL MALIGNANCY

Patients with CF carry a 23-fold increased lifetime risk of digestive tract malignancy, most commonly occurring at sites where CFTR is expressed, including the intestines, pancreas, and biliary tree.[69] This rate increases further in patients who have

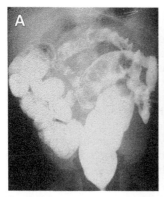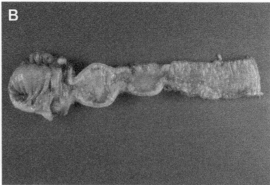

Fig. 6. (A) Barium enema with findings suggestive of fibrosing colonopathy, including a diminished caliber colon with a shortened ascending segment and abnormal haustra throughout the colon. (B) Surgically resected fibrosing colonopathy segment reveals a narrow caliber colon with loss of anatomic markings. Additionally, thickened muscularis layer can be seen, resulting in thickening of the colonic wall. (*Courtesy of* John Stevens, MD.)

undergone lung transplantation.[70] Curiously, the increased cancer risk is not seen in the lungs or vas deferens.[56] Screening recommendations will be available soon. Until then, patients with CF should be made aware of the increased risk of malignancies and these should be considered in patients with GI complaints in whom routine workup has failed to elicit a diagnosis.

SPECTRUM OF HEPATOBILIARY DISEASE

CFTR is located on the apical surface of cholangiocytes and in the gallbladder epithelium, but is not on hepatocytes.[71] Chloride and bicarbonate regulation via CFTR is essential to bile formation with impaired flow resulting in a wide range of CF-associated hepatobiliary presentations.[72]

Biliary Tract

The 2 most common findings within the biliary tract are microgallbladder and cholelithiasis. The presence of gallstones is often seen in the absence of clinical symptoms of right upper quadrant pain, fever, and jaundice. Cholecystectomy should be pursued only if there is evidence of clinical complications, including cholecystitis or bile duct obstruction.

Liver

Transient elevation of liver transaminases is seen frequently. This is often idiopathic or due to antibiotics metabolized within the liver that are used to treat pulmonary exacerbations.

Hepatic steatosis is the most common hepatic finding in CF.[73] This can be related to malnutrition as well as altered phospholipid metabolism.[74] Alterations in bile acid metabolism can lead to impaired lipogenesis contributing to steatosis and lipotoxicity.[75] Treatment focuses on optimizing PERT and caloric intake to improve nutritional status. Hepatic steatosis can also be present in poorly controlled CF-related diabetes, which can present indolently and should be considered if steatosis is present.[76]

Neonatal cholestasis affects less than 2% of infants with CF, likely due to obstruction of bile ducts by thickened secretions. In infancy, the presence of microgallbladder or absent gallbladder can be confused with biliary atresia.[77,78] Meconium ileus is a risk factor for the development of cholestasis. Although cholestasis usually resolves within 3 months, use of PERT in patients with PI, nutritional support, and short-term ursodeoxycholic acid, a synthetic bile acid, can help improve bile flow. Time is key to resolution.[73]

CYSTIC FIBROSIS–ASSOCIATED LIVER DISEASE

The term CF-associated liver disease (CFLD) has been used to describe a wide range of findings from transient elevation of transaminases with no clinical consequences to focal biliary cirrhosis (FBC) seen on autopsy to cirrhosis with portal hypertension, which is present in 5% to 10% of patients with CF.[79] CFLD is the third leading cause of mortality in CF. Unlike PI, CFLD does not have direct genotypic:phenotypic correlation. Risk factors for the development of CFLD include severe CFTR mutation (class I–III) with PI and male gender.

Despite the multitude of articles published on the pathophysiology of CFLD, a cohesive mechanism has not yet been proposed. Transforming growth factor β polymorphism and modifier genes, such as SERPINA-1Z-allele, which codes for alpha-1-antitrypsin deficiency, have been implicated.[80,81] Disruption of bile acid homeostasis results in increased concentrations of cholic acid, which is associated with hepatic fibrosis, inflammation, and limiting plate disruption.[82] A recent pilot study provided evidence that alterations in the gut microbiome, intestinal permeability, and intestinal transit time trigger hepatic inflammation and fibrosis.[72]

Diagnosis of Cystic Fibrosis–Associated Liver Disease

Decreased platelet count or hepatosplenomegaly suggest CFLD. Signs of chronic liver disease (clubbing, spider angiomata, jaundice, ascites) are uncommon unless a patient has advanced cirrhosis.[80] Once CFLD is suspected, diagnostic workup involves exclusion of other common causes of pediatric liver disease (**Fig. 7**).

Other diagnostic tools include imaging and liver biopsy. A recent large multicenter study of young children with CF is in progress by the Cystic Fibrosis Liver Disease Network to look at the role of ultrasound as an early predictor of patients at risk to develop cirrhosis.[83] This study found a 3.3% incidence of ultrasound findings suggestive of cirrhosis on initial ultrasound performed in asymptomatic patients, implying that cirrhosis occurs very early in life. However, the study was unable to conclusively make universal recommendation regarding use of ultrasounds as a tool to screen for CFLD. Portal hypertension can be detected by Doppler measurement of blood flow through the portal vein or a recanalized umbilical vein. The role of MRI for evaluation and conformation of CFLD is being explored. Fibroscan and acoustic radiation force impulse imaging are noninvasive means to evaluate liver stiffness and have shown some promise in evaluating CFLD.[84]

The role of liver biopsy remains controversial due to the patchy nature of FBC and the risk of anesthesia and pneumothorax in patients with underlying CF lung disease. Those who advocate for liver biopsy think that pathologic and histologic findings are vital in the assessment of disease progression and prognosis.[85] Those who advocate against liver biopsy reason that all end-stage liver disease is managed similarly: emphasizing liver health and avoiding hepatotoxic drugs, optimizing nutritional status, and managing complications of portal hypertension, including ascites and varices.

Management of Cystic Fibrosis–Associated Liver Disease

Management of CFLD emphasizes optimizing nutritional status via PERT, caloric intake, and fat-soluble vitamin supplementation, and avoiding hepatotoxic drugs. Gastrostomy tube feedings are safe and can contribute to improvement in nutritional status and lung function.[86] A Cochrane review found insufficient evidence to recommend routine use of ursodeoxycholic acid (UDCA) in CFLD.[87] Studies in patients with primary sclerosing cholangitis using high-dose UDCA noted an increased risk of colon cancer. The relationship between UDCA and colon cancer in patients with CF needs to be evaluated further due to the increased risk of colon cancer in these patients, especially after lung transplantation.[1,70]

Esophageal or gastric variceal bleeding is the most serious, life-threatening complication of portal hypertension. However, primary prophylaxis is not considered standard practice. The gold standard in management of esophageal variceal bleeding is sclerotherapy or variceal banding. However, even with serial endoscopic management, esophageal varices have a high rate of recurrence. Beta-blockers can be used safely in patients with CF, as recently shown in treatment of hemoptysis; however, they tend to be underused due to concern of bronchospasm.[88] Options for gastric varices are limited. Life-threatening gastric varices can be tamponaded, and patients should be immediately shunted with either transjugular intrahepatic portosystemic shunt or distal splenorenal shunt.[89,90]

Patients with CF who have significant cirrhosis usually maintain good hepatic synthetic function and many remain stable for years even in the presence of severe

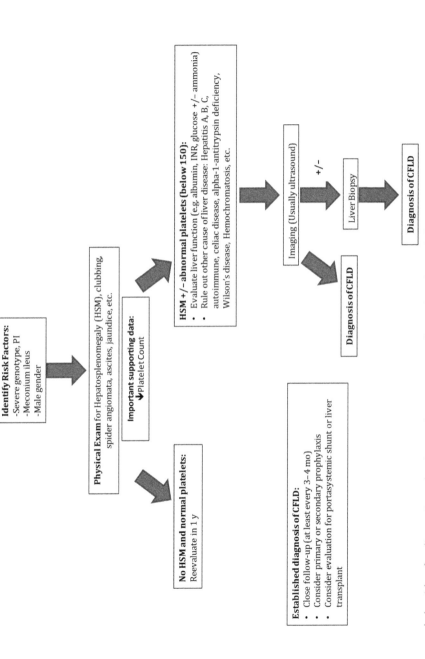

Identify Risk Factors:
- Severe genotype, PI
- Meconium ileus
- Male gender

Physical Exam for Hepatosplenomegaly (HSM), clubbing, spider angiomata, ascites, jaundice, etc.

Important supporting data:
→ Platelet Count

No HSM and normal platelets: Reevaluate in 1 y

HSM +/– abnormal platelets (below 150):
- Evaluate liver function (e.g. albumin, INR, glucose +/– ammonia)
- Rule out other cause of liver disease: Hepatitis A, B, C, autoimmune, celiac disease, alpha-1-antitrypsin deficiency, Wilson's disease, Hemochromatosis, etc.

Imaging (Usually ultrasound)

Diagnosis of CFLD

+/–

Liver Biopsy

Diagnosis of CFLD

Established diagnosis of CFLD:
- Close follow-up (at least every 3–4 mo)
- Consider primary or secondary prophylaxis
- Consider evaluation for portasystemic shunt or liver transplant

Fig. 7. Proposed algorithm for diagnosis, evaluation, and management of CFLD based on risk factors, clinical examination, and platelet count.

cirrhosis. Patients should be referred for liver transplantation when there is intractable variceal bleeding that is not adequately controlled by other means, marked ascites and jaundice, hepatopulmonary syndrome, portopulmonary hypertension, hypoalbuminemia with coagulopathy, deteriorating pulmonary function, or severe malnutrition.[91]

SUMMARY

Patients with CF may experience a vast array of GI and hepatic manifestations throughout their lifetime. Recognition and management of these is part of a comprehensive, multisystem approach to care and contributes to improved survival and quality of life.

REFERENCES

1. Kelly T, Buxbaum J. Gastrointestinal manifestations of cystic fibrosis. Dig Dis Sci 2015;60(7):1903–13.
2. Gelfond D, Borowitz D. Gastrointestinal complications of cystic fibrosis. Clin Gastroenterol Hepatol 2013;11(4):333–42 [quiz: 30–1].
3. Rowe SM, Miller S, Sorscher EJ. Cystic fibrosis. N Engl J Med 2005;352(19): 1992–2001.
4. De Lisle RC, Borowitz D. The cystic fibrosis intestine. Cold Spring Harb Perspect Med 2013;3(9):a009753.
5. Ahmed N, Corey M, Forstner G, et al. Molecular consequences of cystic fibrosis transmembrane regulator (CFTR) gene mutations in the exocrine pancreas. Gut 2003;52(8):1159–64.
6. Gibson-Corley KN, Meyerholz DK, Engelhardt JF. Pancreatic pathophysiology in cystic fibrosis. J Pathol 2016;238(2):311–20.
7. Fieker A, Philpott J, Armand M. Enzyme replacement therapy for pancreatic insufficiency: present and future. Clin Exp Gastroenterol 2011;4:55–73.
8. Walkowiak J, Sands D, Nowakowska A, et al. Early decline of pancreatic function in cystic fibrosis patients with class 1 or 2 CFTR mutations. J Pediatr Gastroenterol Nutr 2005;40(2):199–201.
9. Lankisch PG, Schmidt I, König H, et al. Faecal elastase 1: not helpful in diagnosing chronic pancreatitis associated with mild to moderate exocrine pancreatic insufficiency. Gut 1998;42(4):551–4.
10. Hahn J-U, Kerner W, Maisonneuve P, et al. Low fecal elastase 1 levels do not indicate exocrine pancreatic insufficiency in type-1 diabetes mellitus. Pancreas 2008;36(3):274–8.
11. Borowitz DS, Grand RJ, Durie PR. Use of pancreatic enzyme supplements for patients with cystic fibrosis in the context of fibrosing colonopathy. Consensus Committee. J Pediatr 1995;127:681–4.
12. Vecht J, Symersky T, Lamers CBHW, et al. Efficacy of lower than standard doses of pancreatic enzyme supplementation therapy during acid inhibition in patients with pancreatic exocrine insufficiency. J Clin Gastroenterol 2006;40(8):721–5.
13. De Boeck K, Weren M, Proesmans M, et al. Pancreatitis among patients with cystic fibrosis: correlation with pancreatic status and genotype. Pediatrics 2005;115(4):e463–9.
14. Ooi CY, Dorfman R, Cipolli M, et al. Type of CFTR mutation determines risk of pancreatitis in patients with cystic fibrosis. Gastroenterology 2011;140(1):153–61.

15. Bronstein MN, Sokol RJ, Abman SH, et al. Pancreatic insufficiency, growth, and nutrition in infants identified by newborn screening as having cystic fibrosis. J Pediatr 1992;120(4 Pt 1):533–40.
16. Haller W, Ledder O, Lewindon PJ, et al. Cystic fibrosis: an update for clinicians. Part 1: nutrition and gastrointestinal complications. J Gastroenterol Hepatol 2014; 29(7):1344–55.
17. Pauwels A, Blondeau K, Dupont LJ, et al. Mechanisms of increased gastroesophageal reflux in patients with cystic fibrosis. Am J Gastroenterol 2012;107(9): 1346–53.
18. Pauwels A, Blondeau K, Mertens V, et al. Gastric emptying and different types of reflux in adult patients with cystic fibrosis. Aliment Pharmacol Ther 2011;34(7): 799–807.
19. Dziekiewicz MA, Banaszkiewicz A, Urzykowska A, et al. Gastroesophageal reflux disease in children with cystic fibrosis. Adv Exp Med Biol 2015;873:1–7 [Chapter: 154].
20. Sabati AA, Kempainen RR, Milla CE, et al. Characteristics of gastroesophageal reflux in adults with cystic fibrosis. J Cyst Fibros 2010;9(5):365–70.
21. Sheikh SI, Ryan-Wenger NA, McCoy KS. Outcomes of surgical management of severe GERD in patients with cystic fibrosis. Pediatr Pulmonol 2013;48(6): 556–62.
22. De Lisle RC, Meldi L, Roach E, et al. Mast cells and gastrointestinal dysmotility in the cystic fibrosis mouse. PLoS One 2009;4(1):e4283.
23. de Lisle RC, Sewell R, Meldi L. Enteric circular muscle dysfunction in the cystic fibrosis mouse small intestine. Neurogastroenterol Motil 2010;22(3):341-e87.
24. Kuo P, Stevens JE, Russo A, et al. Gastric emptying, incretin hormone secretion, and postprandial glycemia in cystic fibrosis–effects of pancreatic enzyme supplementation. J Clin Endocrinol Metab 2011;96(5):E851–5.
25. Rovner AJ, Schall JI, Mondick JT, et al. Delayed small bowel transit in children with cystic fibrosis and pancreatic insufficiency. J Pediatr Gastroenterol Nutr 2013;57(1):81–4.
26. Bodet-Milin C, Querellou S, Oudoux A, et al. Delayed gastric emptying scintigraphy in cystic fibrosis patients before and after lung transplantation. J Heart Lung Transplant 2006;25(9):1077–83.
27. Hedsund C, Gregersen T, Joensson IM, et al. Gastrointestinal transit times and motility in patients with cystic fibrosis. Scand J Gastroenterol 2012;47(8–9): 920–6.
28. Perano S, Rayner CK, Couper J, et al. Cystic fibrosis related diabetes–a new perspective on the optimal management of postprandial glycemia. J Diabet Complications 2014;28(6):904–11.
29. van der Doef HPJ, Kokke FTM, Beek FJA, et al. Constipation in pediatric cystic fibrosis patients: an underestimated medical condition. J Cyst Fibros 2010;9(1): 59–63.
30. Ramos AFP, de Fuccio MB, Moretzsohn LD, et al. Cystic fibrosis, gastroduodenal inflammation, duodenal ulcer, and H. pylori infection: the "cystic fibrosis paradox" revisited. J Cyst Fibros 2013;12(4):377–83.
31. Akiba Y, Jung M, Ouk S, et al. A novel small molecule CFTR inhibitor attenuates HCO3-secretion and duodenal ulcer formation in rats. Am J Physiol Gastrointest Liver Physiol 2005;289(4):G753–9.
32. Rocha GA, Oliveira AM, Queiroz DM, et al. Immunoblot analysis of humoral immune response to Helicobacter pylori in children with and without duodenal ulcer. J Clin Microbiol 2000;38(5):1777–81.

33. Israel NR, Khanna B, Cutler A, et al. Seroprevalence of *Helicobacter pylori* infection in cystic fibrosis and its cross-reactivity with anti-pseudomonas antibodies. J Pediatr Gastroenterol Nutr 2000;30(4):426–31.

34. Drzymała-Czy S, Stawinska-Witoszynska B, Mądry E, et al. Non-invasive detection of *Helicobacter pylori* in cystic fibrosis–the fecal test vs. the urea breath test. Eur Rev Med Pharmacol Sci 2014;18(16):2343–8.

35. Vaishnava S, Yamamoto M, Severson KM, et al. The antibacterial lectin RegIII-gamma promotes the spatial segregation of microbiota and host in the intestine. Science 2011;334(6053):255–8.

36. Fridge JL, Conrad C, Gerson L, et al. Risk factors for small bowel bacterial overgrowth in cystic fibrosis. J Pediatr Gastroenterol Nutr 2007;44(2):212–8.

37. Miazga A, Osiński M, Cichy W, et al. Current views on the etiopathogenesis, clinical manifestation, diagnostics, treatment and correlation with other nosological entities of SIBO. Adv Med Sci 2015;60(1):118–24.

38. Schneider ARJ, Klueber S, Posselt H-G, et al. Application of the glucose hydrogen breath test for the detection of bacterial overgrowth in patients with cystic fibrosis–a reliable method? Dig Dis Sci 2009;54(8):1730–5.

39. Wouthuyzen-Bakker M, Bodewes FAJA, Verkade HJ. Persistent fat malabsorption in cystic fibrosis; lessons from patients and mice. J Cyst Fibros 2011;10(3):150–8.

40. Malik BA, Xie YY, Wine E, et al. Diagnosis and pharmacological management of small intestinal bacterial overgrowth in children with intestinal failure. Can J Gastroenterol 2011;25(1):41–5.

41. del Campo R, Garriga M, Pérez-Aragón A, et al. Improvement of digestive health and reduction in proteobacterial populations in the gut microbiota of cystic fibrosis patients using a *Lactobacillus reuteri* probiotic preparation: a double blind prospective study. J Cyst Fibros 2014;13(6):716–22.

42. Bruzzese E, Callegari ML, Raia V, et al. Disrupted intestinal microbiota and intestinal inflammation in children with cystic fibrosis and its restoration with Lactobacillus GG: a randomised clinical trial. PLoS One 2014;9(2):e87796.

43. Kunz AN, Fairchok MP, Noel JM. Lactobacillus sepsis associated with probiotic therapy. Pediatrics 2005;116(2):517 [author reply: 517–8].

44. Fluge G, Olesen HV, Gilljam M, et al. Co-morbidity of cystic fibrosis and celiac disease in Scandinavian cystic fibrosis patients. J Cyst Fibros 2009;8(3):198–202.

45. Hasosah M, Davidson G, Jacobson K. Persistent elevated tissue-transglutaminase in cystic fibrosis. J Paediatr Child Health 2009;45(4):172–3.

46. Bresso F, Askling J, Astegiano M, et al. Potential role for the common cystic fibrosis DeltaF508 mutation in Crohn's disease. Inflamm Bowel Dis 2007;13(5):531–6.

47. Bahmanyar S, Ekbom A, Askling J, et al. Cystic fibrosis gene mutations and gastrointestinal diseases. J Cyst Fibros 2010;9(4):288–91.

48. Lloyd-Still JD. Crohn's disease and cystic fibrosis. Dig Dis Sci 1994;39(4):880–5.

49. Dhaliwal J, Leach S, Katz T, et al. Intestinal inflammation and impact on growth in children with cystic fibrosis. J Pediatr Gastroenterol Nutr 2015;60(4):521–6.

50. Lardenoye SW, Puylaert JB, Smit MJ, et al. Appendix in children with cystic fibrosis: US features. Radiology 2004;232(1):187–9.

51. Robertson MB, Choe KA, Joseph PM. Review of the abdominal manifestations of cystic fibrosis in the adult patient. Radiographics 2006;26(3):679–90.

52. Colombo C, Ellemunter H, Houwen R, et al. Guidelines for the diagnosis and management of distal intestinal obstruction syndrome in cystic fibrosis patients. J Cyst Fibros 2011;10(Suppl 2):S24–8.

53. Lavelle LP, McEvoy SH, Ni Mhurchu E, et al. Cystic fibrosis below the diaphragm: abdominal findings in adult patients. Radiographics 2015;35(3):680–95.
54. Chaudry G, Navarro OM, Levine DS, et al. Abdominal manifestations of cystic fibrosis in children. Pediatr Radiol 2006;36(3):233–40.
55. Nash EF, Stephenson A, Helm EJ, et al. Intussusception in adults with cystic fibrosis: a case series with review of the literature. Dig Dis Sci 2011;56(12): 3695–700.
56. Wilschanski M, Durie PR. Patterns of GI disease in adulthood associated with mutations in the CFTR gene. Gut 2007;56(8):1153–63.
57. Blackman SM, Deering-Brose R, McWilliams R, et al. Relative contribution of genetic and nongenetic modifiers to intestinal obstruction in cystic fibrosis. Gastroenterology 2006;131(4):1030–9.
58. Gorter RR, Karimi A, Sleeboom C, et al. Clinical and genetic characteristics of meconium ileus in newborns with and without cystic fibrosis. J Pediatr Gastroenterol Nutr 2010;50(5):569–72.
59. Karimi A, Gorter RR, Sleeboom C, et al. Issues in the management of simple and complex meconium ileus. Pediatr Surg Int 2011;27(9):963–8.
60. Cuenca AG, Ali AS, Kays DW, et al. "Pulling the plug–"management of meconium plug syndrome in neonates. J Surg Res 2012;175(2):e43–6.
61. Houwen RH, van der Doef HP, Sermet I, et al. Defining DIOS and constipation in cystic fibrosis with a multicentre study on the incidence, characteristics, and treatment of DIOS. J Pediatr Gastroenterol Nutr 2010;50(1):38–42.
62. Com G, Cetin N, O'Brien CE. Complicated *Clostridium difficile* colitis in children with cystic fibrosis: association with gastric acid suppression? J Cyst Fibros 2014;13(1):37–42.
63. Theunissen C, Knoop C, Nonhoff C, et al. *Clostridium difficile* colitis in cystic fibrosis patients with and without lung transplantation. Transpl Infect Dis 2008; 10(4):240–4.
64. Egressy K, Jansen M, Meyer KC. Recurrent *Clostridium difficile* colitis in cystic fibrosis: an emerging problem. J Cyst Fibros 2013;12(1):92–6.
65. FitzSimmons SC, Burkhart GA, Borowitz D, et al. High-dose pancreatic-enzyme supplements and fibrosing colonopathy in children with cystic fibrosis. N Engl J Med 1997;336(18):1283–9.
66. Smyth RL, van Velzen D, Smyth AR, et al. Strictures of ascending colon in cystic fibrosis and high-strength pancreatic enzymes. Lancet 1994;343(8889):85–6.
67. El-Chammas KI, Rumman N, Goh VL, et al. Rectal prolapse and cystic fibrosis. J Pediatr Gastroenterol Nutr 2015;60(1):110–2.
68. Wyllie R. Gastrointestinal manifestations of cystic fibrosis. Clin Pediatr (Phila) 1999;38(12):735–8.
69. Maisonneuve P, Marshall BC, Knapp EA, et al. Cancer risk in cystic fibrosis: a 20-year nationwide study from the United States. J Natl Cancer Inst 2013;105(2): 122–9.
70. Meyer KC, Francois ML, Thomas HK, et al. Colon cancer in lung transplant recipients with CF: increased risk and results of screening. J Cyst Fibros 2011;10(5): 366–9.
71. Cohn JA, Strong TV, Picciotto MR, et al. Localization of the cystic fibrosis transmembrane conductance regulator in human bile duct epithelial cells. Gastroenterology 1993;105(6):1857–64.
72. Flass T, Tong S, Frank DN, et al. Intestinal lesions are associated with altered intestinal microbiome and are more frequent in children and young adults with cystic fibrosis and cirrhosis. PLoS One 2015;10(2):e0116967.

73. Flass T, Narkewicz MR. Cirrhosis and other liver disease in cystic fibrosis. J Cyst Fibros 2012;12(2):116–24.

74. Staufer K, Halilbasic E, Trauner M, et al. Cystic fibrosis related liver disease–another black box in hepatology. Int J Mol Sci 2014;15(8):13529–49.

75. Trauner M, Claudel T, Fickert P, et al. Bile acids as regulators of hepatic lipid and glucose metabolism. Dig Dis 2010;28(1):220–4.

76. Moran A, Brunzell C, Cohen RC, et al. Clinical care guidelines for cystic fibrosis-related diabetes: a position statement of the American Diabetes Association and a clinical practice guideline of the Cystic Fibrosis Foundation, endorsed by the Pediatric Endocrine Society. Diabetes Care 2010;33(12):2697–708.

77. Perkins WG, Klein GL, Beckerman RC. Cystic fibrosis mistaken for idiopathic biliary atresia. Clin Pediatr (Phila) 1985;24(2):107–9.

78. Eminoglu TF, Polat E, Gökçe S, et al. Cystic fibrosis presenting with neonatal cholestasis simulating biliary atresia in a patient with a novel mutation. Indian J Pediatr 2013;80(6):502–4.

79. Lamireau T, Monnereau S, Martin S, et al. Epidemiology of liver disease in cystic fibrosis: a longitudinal study. J Hepatol 2004;41(6):920–5.

80. Colombo C, Battezzati PM, Crosignani A, et al. Liver disease in cystic fibrosis: a prospective study on incidence, risk factors, and outcome. Hepatology 2002; 36(6):1374–82.

81. Bartlett JR, Friedman KJ, Ling SC, et al. Genetic modifiers of liver disease in cystic fibrosis. JAMA 2009;302(10):1076–83.

82. Smith JL, Lewindon PJ, Hoskins AC, et al. Endogenous ursodeoxycholic acid and cholic acid in liver disease due to cystic fibrosis. Hepatology 2004;39(6): 1673–82.

83. Safak AA, Simsek E, Bahcebasi T. Sonographic assessment of the normal limits and percentile curves of liver, spleen, and kidney dimensions in healthy school-aged children. J Ultrasound Med 2005;24(10):1359–64.

84. Behrens CB, Langholz JH, Eiler J, et al. A pilot study of the characterization of hepatic tissue strain in children with cystic-fibrosis-associated liver disease (CFLD) by acoustic radiation force impulse imaging. Pediatr Radiol 2013;43(5): 552–7.

85. Lewindon PJ, Shepherd RW, Walsh MJ, et al. Importance of hepatic fibrosis in cystic fibrosis and the predictive value of liver biopsy. Hepatology 2011;53(1): 193–201.

86. Vandeleur M, Massie J, Oliver M. Gastrostomy in children with cystic fibrosis and portal hypertension. J Pediatr Gastroenterol Nutr 2013;57(2):245–7.

87. Cheng K, Ashby D, Smyth RL. Ursodeoxycholic acid for cystic fibrosis-related liver disease. Cochrane Database Syst Rev 2014;(12):CD000222.

88. Moua J, Nussbaum E, Liao E, et al. Beta-blocker management of refractory hemoptysis in cystic fibrosis: a novel treatment approach. Ther Adv Respir Dis 2013;7(4):217–23.

89. Pozler O, Krajina A, Vanicek H, et al. Transjugular intrahepatic portosystemic shunt in five children with cystic fibrosis: long-term results. Hepatogastroenterology 2003;50(52):1111–4.

90. Debray D, Kelly D, Houwen R, et al. Best practice guidance for the diagnosis and management of cystic fibrosis-associated liver disease. J Cyst Fibros 2011; 10(Suppl 2):S29–36.

91. Fridell JA, Bond GJ, Mazariegos GV, et al. Liver transplantation in children with cystic fibrosis: a long-term longitudinal review of a single center's experience. J Pediatr Surg 2003;38(8):1152–6.

Endocrine Disorders in Cystic Fibrosis

Scott M. Blackman, MD, PhD[a],*, Vin Tangpricha, MD, PhD[b]

KEYWORDS

- Diabetes • Osteoporosis • Short stature • Hypogonadism • Hypoglycemia

KEY POINTS

- Endocrine complications of cystic fibrosis (CF) tend to occur more frequently in older individuals and thus can be expected to become more common as CF medical care improves and the population grows older.
- It is unknown to what degree that these complications may be affected by treatment with CF transmembrane conductance regulator (CFTR) modulator medications.
- It is essential to detect and treat endocrine complications as part of high-quality medical care for people with CF.

INTRODUCTION

CF is caused by defects in the CF transmembrane conductance regulator (*CFTR*) gene, an epithelial chloride channel that is widely expressed. The most common complications of CF are exocrine pancreatic insufficiency (PI) and progressive lung disease, which is the most common cause of death from CF. In addition, people with CF have several important endocrine abnormalities, which are the focus of this review, including diabetes (CF-related diabetes [CFRD]), bone disease, poor linear growth, and hypogonadism.

S.M. Blackman is supported by the Cystic Fibrosis Foundation, the Gilead Research Scholars in CF program (Gilead Sciences), the Jaeb Center for Health Research, and the Johns Hopkins Institute for Clinical and Translational Research (ICTR), which is funded in part by Grant Number UL1TR001079 from the National Center for Advancing Translational Sciences (NCATS), a component of the National Institutes of Health (NIH), and NIH Roadmap for Medical Research. S.M. Blackman participated in an advisory board for Vertex Pharmaceuticals. V. Tangpricha is supported by the NCATS of NIH under Award Number UL1TR000454. The content is solely the responsibility of the authors and does not necessarily represent the official view of the authors' institutions or funding agencies, including ICTR, NCATS, or NIH.
[a] Division of Pediatric Endocrinology, Department of Pediatrics, Johns Hopkins Hospital, Johns Hopkins University, 200 North Wolfe Street, Baltimore, MD 21287, USA; [b] Division of Endocrinology, Metabolism and Lipids, Department of Medicine, Atlanta VA Medical Center, Emory University School of Medicine, 101 Woodruff Circle NE, WMRB1301, Atlanta, GA 30322, USA
* Corresponding author.
E-mail address: sblackman@jhmi.edu

THE RELATIONSHIP OF CYSTIC FIBROSIS TRANSMEMBRANE CONDUCTANCE REGULATOR GENETICS AND COMPLICATIONS OF CYSTIC FIBROSIS

The risks of developing complications of CF depend in part on the level and function of the CFTR protein.[1] Most people (approximately 85%) with CF have 2 mutations resulting in essentially no CFTR function; these individuals almost always develop exocrine PI within the first year of life, and they are at risk of developing all of the endocrine complications of CF, including diabetes and bone disease, as well as the nonendocrine complications, such as lung disease, meconium ileus, and liver disease. The remaining approximately 15% of people with CF have 1 or 2 copies of CFTR with partial function, which confer delayed-onset exocrine PI or pancreatic sufficiency (PS). People with CFTR mutations in this category can have lower risk of some endocrine and nonendocrine complications (diabetes, meconium ileus, and liver disease) but not others (bone disease) and still develop CF lung disease at a high rate.

CYSTIC FIBROSIS–RELATED DIABETES

Individuals with CF are at high risk of developing a form of diabetes over time, which is called CFRD.[2-4] CFRD is distinct from type 1 diabetes mellitus and type 2 diabetes mellitus but has similarities to both. As is the case for all forms of diabetes, people with CFRD have elevated blood glucose (hyperglycemia). In type 1 diabetes mellitus, hyperglycemia is due to complete or near-complete absence of insulin-producing β-cells in the pancreatic islets. In type 2 diabetes mellitus, hyperglycemia is due to a combination of reduced sensitivity to insulin and insufficient production of insulin. People with CFRD tend to have normal insulin sensitivity but have reduced and abnormal production of insulin. In contrast to type 1A diabetes mellitus, in which insulin production declines rapidly and has an abrupt and symptomatic onset, in CFRD, insulin production declines gradually, and diabetes can be asymptomatic.

The main complications of CFRD are worse lung disease, poorer nutritional status, and increased mortality. In addition, CFRD can cause some of the same complications seen for other forms of diabetes, including retinopathy, nephropathy, and neuropathy.[4] All of the CF-specific complications have been shown to improve with treatment of CFRD. Therefore, detection and appropriate treatment of CFRD are key components of the medical care for persons with CF.

Epidemiology

As of 2014, in the US CF Foundation Patient Registry, the prevalence of CFRD among all living patients was 22%, with few prepubertal children with CFRD, approximately 10% to 15% adolescents, and 30% to 40% adults. These prevalence statistics may, however, under-represent the actual risk of CFRD to most people with CF. The risk of CFRD is approximately 5 times higher in people with CFTR genotypes that cause exocrine PI than in those with residual-function mutations that cause PS.[5] The risk of developing CFRD for people with PI CFTR genotypes begins to rise in adolescence and reaches greater than 80% by age 40.[6] Individuals with PS CFTR genotypes do develop CFRD over time at a rate that is still substantially higher than that of type 2 diabetes mellitus in the general population.[6]

Apart from age and CFTR genotype, several other risk factors have been identified. Genes other than CFTR (genetic modifiers) strongly influence the risk of CFRD,[7] and the 5 such risk variants identified so far are responsible for approximately 4-fold variation in CFRD risk.[8,9] Two other potent risk factors are a family history of type 2 diabetes mellitus and CF-related liver disease, both varying the risk by approximately 3-fold.[5,8,10]

Pathophysiology

CFRD is characterized by reduced or delayed insulin secretion with generally normal sensitivity to insulin action. In the fasted state, insulin and C-peptide levels tend to be normal. Reduced early-phase insulin release, prolonged hyperglycemia, and reactive hypoglycemia are all seen in both CFRD and in type 2 diabetes mellitus.[4]

The strong correlation of CFRD with exocrine PI suggests that preexisting PI contributes to causing CFRD, initially thought primarily by a reduction in endocrine pancreatic mass. In CF with PI, lack of CFTR causes abnormally viscous secretions, plugging of pancreatic ducts, and a chronic pancreatitis-like picture with fatty infiltration and fibrosis of the pancreas.[2,4] Pancreatic islets are relatively spared in autopsy studies, but the number and mass of islets are reduced in all patients with CF regardless of whether CFRD was present.[11] Therefore, CFRD did not correlate with islet number or mass. CFRD has been reported, however, to correlate with presence in islets of amyloid, a peptide cosecreted with insulin, also deposited in the setting of type 2 diabetes mellitus and which may be detrimental to islet cells.[11] This finding suggests that factors intrinsic to the islet cell or β-cell also contribute to the development of CFRD.

Other studies have demonstrated defects beyond islet cell mass in development of CFRD. Mice with CF do not have pancreatic insufficiency but are more prone to developing diabetes after a mild β-cell injury,[12] suggesting that the β-cells have an intrinsic defect. In humans, the risk of CFRD is increased in people with a family history of type 2 diabetes mellitus or who have susceptibility gene variants for type 2 diabetes mellitus,[8,9] indicating that some of the same glucose metabolic pathways play a role in both CFRD and in type 2 diabetes mellitus. Insulin production can be both increased and decreased in CF animal models,[13,14] further supporting qualitative rather than quantitative defects in insulin production. Finally, there are recent reports that CFTR is present in islets and affects insulin secretion,[15,16] which could help explain the qualitative alterations in insulin secretion in CF.

With the development of CFTR modulator medications, such as ivacaftor and lumacaftor, the extent to which CFRD is reversible has become a clinically relevant question. So far, 3 small studies have reported improvement of insulin secretion and hyperglycemia after treatment with ivacaftor.[17–19] Anecdotal reports of hypoglycemia in people treated with CFTR modulators suggest the need for caution and perhaps increased blood glucose monitoring after beginning treatment with a CFTR modulator medication.

Diagnosis of Cystic Fibrosis–Related Diabetes

The Cystic Fibrosis Foundation and the American Diabetes Association issued guidelines in 2010, which have been endorsed by the Pediatric Endocrine Society and the International Society for Pediatric and Adolescent Diabetes.[20,21] CFRD may be diagnosed in individuals with classic symptoms of diabetes (polydipsia and polyuria) with plasma glucose greater than or equal to 200 mg/dL (7.0 mmol/L). In asymptomatic individuals, CFRD is diagnosed by elevated glucose on an oral glucose tolerance test or after sufficiently abnormal random glucose measurements or sufficiently elevated hemoglobin A_{1c}. Because CFRD has an impact on the course of CF but may be asymptomatic, the Cystic Fibrosis Foundation and the European Cystic Fibrosis Society guidelines recommend annual screening by 2-hour oral glucose tolerance test starting at age 10 years. Alternative screening and diagnosis strategies using different provocation, identifying high-risk or low-risk groups or continuous glucose monitoring are under investigation.

Treatment of Cystic Fibrosis–Related Diabetes

CFRD is a disease of insulin insufficiency, and the only treatment that has been shown to improve outcomes is insulin. A typical insulin regimen used is basal-bolus, consisting of once-daily or twice-daily long-acting insulin injections plus extra short-acting insulin with a meal or snacks. Use of basal-only regimen has been shown effective in some studies, perhaps in early CFRD. Insulin pumps are effective in CFRD and can simplify the intensive insulin regimen resulting in increased adherence. Tube feedings can be covered by premixed insulin of intermediate duration or with appropriate programming of an insulin pump. Use of continuous subcutaneous insulin infusion (ie, insulin pump) is an effective option for insulin delivery, which can be particularly advantageous if a person with CF is requiring multiple boluses for frequent extra meals; in addition, because of the minimal risk of diabetic ketoacidosis to people with CFRD, continuous subcutaneous insulin infusion is associated with lower risk in CFRD compared with type 1 diabetes mellitus. Continuous glucose sensors have been recommended as a tool to help guide insulin therapy.[21]

There are no general restrictions on quantity of dietary carbohydrates in CFRD, in contrast to the general recommendations for type 2 diabetes mellitus. Pure sugar, such as sweet sodas, are not recommended, but otherwise, the same dietary recommendations for people with CF without CFRD (eg, high-calorie, high-fat, and high-protein diet) stand for those with CFRD. It is recommended to avoid large quantities of simple carbohydrate and to spread the daily intake of complex carbohydrate over all meals.

Insulin secretagogues, such as repaglinide, may increase insulin secretion in early CFRD. Studies have failed to demonstrate, however, efficacy of repaglinide in improving body mass index (BMI) or lung function, so this class of oral agents is thought inferior to insulin and recommended only as adjunct to insulin or in cases where insulin cannot be used. Insulin sensitizing agents, such as metformin or thiazolidinediones, are not generally recommended for CFRD, because insulin sensitivity is generally normal, and these medications carry associated side effects and risks as well. Glucagon-like peptide-1 (GLP-1) agonists (eg, sitagliptin) or dipeptidyl peptidase 4 inhibitors, which indirectly increase GLP-1 levels (eg, exenatide), are under investigation in CFRD but are not currently recommended outside of the context of a research study. Acarbose, which prevents absorption of carbohydrate, is not generally recommended for use in CFRD, because carbohydrates plus insulin are necessary for adequate nutrition.

Hypoglycemia

People with CF may experience hypoglycemia even in the absence of CFRD or insulin treatment,[4,22] occurring either postprandially or otherwise. There are no consistent data relating hypoglycemia to later CFRD or to other CF outcomes. It is recommended that CF practitioners become familiar with symptoms of hypoglycemia and alert people with CF to the possibility of hypoglycemia. Individuals with symptoms that might be due to hypoglycemia may benefit from point-of-care (glucometer) testing at the time of symptoms.

LINEAR GROWTH ABNORMALITIES IN CYSTIC FIBROSIS

Reduced linear growth has been reported in several studies in CF (reviewed by Wong and colleagues[23]) with a prevalence of short stature (defined by height z score <-2 SDs below the Centers for Disease Control mean) found in approximately 20% of all people with CF in 1993.[24] A clear likely contributor to poor growth is fat and micronutrient malabsorption, which may not always be completely treated using pancreatic enzyme replacement therapy. Other factors include chronic inflammation, chronic infection, and treatment with inhaled and systemic glucocorticoid medications. Inhaled glucocorticoids even at moderate doses (eg, budesonide, 400 μg/d, in 5–13 year olds), when given consistently and daily, can suppress growth.[25] It has been proposed that chronic insufficiency of insulin, which itself is an anabolic hormone, may also contribute to poor linear growth in CF.[26–28] Growth can seem poorer when parents' heights are below average or puberty is late to normal or delayed in CF.[29] On the other hand, at birth, average length (with or without adjustment for gestational age) and levels of insulin-like growth factor 1 (IGF-1) levels in CF are reduced in humans[30,31] and animal models,[32,33] suggesting that intrauterine growth abnormalities may occur before many of these factors likely play a role.

The extent to which abnormalities in the growth hormone (GH)/IGF-1 axis play a role is unclear. Like insulin, GH and IGF-1 have anabolic effects and could theoretically have beneficial effects in people with CF. Many studies have associated IGF-1 levels with reduced nutrition in CF and reduced lean body mass, with 1 study also finding IGF-1 to predict worse nutrition in 1 year.[34] A possible confounder is that fasting and malnutrition cause both GH resistance and reduced IGF-1 levels (reviewed by Wong and colleagues[23]). Studies of recombinant human GH (rhGH) in CF have been summarized in 2 recent meta-analyses[35,36] and a recent review.[23] In meta-analysis, rhGH was found to increase height by approximately 0.2 to 0.6 SDs and to increase lean body mass in people with CF with short stature. Also, GH has been reported to increase bone mineral content,[37] increase forced vital capacity, and reduce hospitalization rate (see Thaker and colleagues[35] and Phung and colleagues[36]), but outcomes were not consistent across studies, and other key outcomes, such as forced expiratory volume in 1 second and rate of pulmonary exacerbation, were not affected. More research is needed to determine whether treatment with rhGH might have clinical benefit in some people with CF and growth failure, who do not have GH deficiency.

Recommendations

At each clinic visit, height, weight, and BMI percentiles should be calculated using World Health Organization (for age <2 y) and Centers for Disease Control (for age 2–20 y) growth charts. Assessment of growth should be made considering the context of parental heights and of pubertal stage (because delayed puberty can mimic growth failure). Poor linear growth can manifest either as low absolute height or as abnormal height trajectory (eg, low growth velocity causing downward crossing of height percentiles on a growth chart). When growth failure is identified, treatable causes should be considered. CF disease treatments should be optimized. Inhaled and systemic glucocorticoid medications should be reduced to the lowest dose necessary to achieve therapeutic goals. Adherence and effectiveness of pancreatic enzyme replacement therapy should be monitored. Screening for CFRD should be performed. Non–CF-related diagnoses may also be considered, such as thyroid dysfunction, GH deficiency, or celiac or inflammatory bowel disease. Treatment should be directed to the cause identified.

CYSTIC FIBROSIS–RELATED BONE DISEASE
Prevalence and Pathogenesis

The causes of CF-related bone disease (CFBD) are multifactorial and include nutritional deficiencies of vitamin D, vitamin K, and calcium; glucocorticoid use; sex steroid deficiency; an altered GH axis; inflammation and the mutation of the *CFTR* gene itself.[38] The prevalence of fractures in children and adults with CF have been reported to occur in up to a third of patients.[39,40] A recent systematic review of adults with CF found a pooled prevalence of low bone mineral density (BMD) (T score <-1 and >-2.5) of 38% and osteoporosis (T score <-2.5) of 23.5% by dual-energy x-ray absorptiometry (DEXA)[41] and of vertebral fractures by lateral spine radiograph of 14% and nonvertebral fractures by self-report of 19.7%. More recent advanced imaging studies with high-resolution peripheral quantitative CT in adults with CF demonstrate compromised cortical and trabecular bone microarchitecture compared with matched non-CF controls.[42] Lower bone strength and quality not only increase the risk of clinical fractures but also are associated with lower lung function in cross-sectional studies.[43,44] Furthermore, lower BMD has been associated with recurrent pulmonary exacerbations and mortality in children with CF.[45,46]

Mutations in the *CFTR* may directly impair bone formation in rodent models.[47] Primary cultured human osteoblast cells indicate a potential deficit in the production of osteoprotegerin.[48–50] Recent studies in rodent models suggest that correction of the CFTR function may prevent deterioration of bone microarchitecture associated with CFBD.[51] CTFR correctors hold promise to improve the bone disease associated with CF; however, no data on humans have been reported.[52]

Approach to Screening and Treatment of Cystic Fibrosis—Related Bone Disease

The European Cystic Fibrosis Society recommends an initial BMD test by DEXA starting at approximately 8 years to 10 years of age with repeat testing every 1 year or 2 years if the z scores are less than -2 and -1, respectively.[53] In adults, the European Cystic Fibrosis Society recommends DEXA testing every 5 years if the BMD z score is greater than -1, every 2 years if the z score is -1 to -2, and every year if the z score is greater than -2.[53] The Cystic Fibrosis Foundation has similar recommendations with annual BMD testing if the z score is less than or equal to -2, every 2 to 4 years if the z score is between -1 and -2, and every 5 years if the z score is greater than or equal to -1.[54]

All patients with CF, especially those with CFBD, should have adequate vitamin D status with a serum 25-hydroxyvitamin D (25[OH]D) greater than 30 ng/mL.[55] All children and adults should take at least 400 IU to 800 IU of vitamin D initially, with stepwise increases in vitamin D dosing to achieve a 25(OH)D in the optimal range.[55] Typically, most children and adults with CF require 1000 IU to 2000 IU of vitamin D or more to maintain optimal vitamin D status.[56] In contrast to vitamin D, intestinal absorption of calcium does not seem altered in CF.[57] Children and adults with CF should consume 1000 mg to 1500 mg of elemental calcium in divided doses, preferably from the diet or supplemented with pills to ensure adequate mineralization of the skeleton. Other nutrients, such as vitamin K, magnesium, and phosphorus, are also important for optimal skeletal health.[58] Excessive alcohol[59] and vitamin A intake[60] should be avoided, which may have a negative impact on bone.

Adults and adolescents at highest risk for fragility fractures should be considered for pharmacologic therapy for treatment of osteoporosis/CFBD.[53] A Cochrane review of 9 randomized controlled trials conducted in individuals with CF found that oral and intravenous bisphosphonates significantly increase BMD.[61] Despite the increase in BMD, there was insufficient data to demonstrate a reduction in fractures.[61] Teriparatide, a Food and Drug Administration–approved anabolic treatment of severe osteoporosis, has been reported to improve BMD in a case series of adults with CF.[62] Another promising therapy that has not been well studied in CF is denosumab, which is a Food and Drug Administration–approved therapy for osteoporosis whose mechanism of action is preventing the action of receptor activator of nuclear factor κB on osteoclasts, thus preventing their maturation.[63]

MALE HYPOGONADISM IN CYSTIC FIBROSIS

In a cross-sectional study of young men with CF, approximately 25% had low levels of testosterone.[64] Testosterone levels positively correlate with BMD and its deficiency has been associated with the presence of vertebral fractures documented by spine radiograph.[64,65] There are no screening guidelines for hypogonadism in adult men with CF. In addition, there are no prospective randomized controlled trials evaluating treatment of hypogonadism in men with CF. Screening for low testosterone should be considered in men with symptoms of hypogonadism and as part of the evaluation of osteoporosis in men with CF. Testosterone measurements should be done in the morning and not during an acute illness. A low testosterone level should be confirmed twice before committing a patient to testosterone therapy. Finally, prior to the initiation of testosterone, patients should be advised that testosterone therapy diminishes spermatogenesis and has an adverse impact on reproductive potential.

SUMMARY

Endocrine complications of CF tend to occur more frequently in older individuals and thus can be expected to become more common as CF medical care improves and the population grows older. It is unknown to what degree that these complications may be affected by treatment with CFTR modulator medications. It is essential to detect and treat endocrine complications as part of high-quality medical care for people with CF.

REFERENCES

1. Hamosh A, Corey M. Correlation between genotype and phenotype in patients with cystic fibrosis. The cystic fibrosis genotype-phenotype consortium. N Engl J Med 1993;329:1308–13.
2. Barrio R. Management of endocrine disease: cystic fibrosis-related diabetes: novel pathogenic insights opening new therapeutic avenues. Eur J Endocrinol 2015;172:R131–41.
3. Moran A, Becker D, Casella SJ, et al. Epidemiology, pathophysiology, and prognostic implications of cystic fibrosis-related diabetes: a technical review. Diabetes Care 2010;33:2677–83.
4. Kelly A, Moran A. Update on cystic fibrosis-related diabetes. J Cyst Fibros 2013; 12:318–31.
5. Marshall BC, Butler SM, Stoddard M, et al. Epidemiology of cystic fibrosis-related diabetes. J Pediatr 2005;146:681–7.
6. Lewis C, Blackman SM, Nelson A, et al. Diabetes-related mortality in adults with cystic fibrosis. Role of genotype and sex. Am J Respir Crit Care Med 2015;191: 194–200.
7. Blackman SM, Hsu S, Vanscoy LL, et al. Genetic modifiers play a substantial role in diabetes complicating cystic fibrosis. J Clin Endocrinol Metab 2009;94:1302–9.
8. Blackman SM, Hsu S, Ritter SE, et al. A susceptibility gene for type 2 diabetes confers substantial risk for diabetes complicating cystic fibrosis. Diabetologia 2009;52:1858–65.
9. Blackman SM, Commander CW, Watson C, et al. Genetic modifiers of cystic fibrosis-related diabetes. Diabetes 2013;62:3627–35.
10. Minicucci L, Lorini R, Giannattasio A, et al. Liver disease as risk factor for cystic fibrosis-related diabetes development. Acta Paediatr 2007;96:736–9.
11. Couce M, O'Brien TD, Moran A, et al. Diabetes mellitus in cystic fibrosis is characterized by islet amyloidosis. J Clin Endocrinol Metab 1996;81:1267–72.

12. Stalvey MS, Muller C, Schatz DA, et al. Cystic fibrosis transmembrane conductance regulator deficiency exacerbates islet cell dysfunction after beta-cell injury. Diabetes 2006;55:1939–45.

13. Olivier AK, Yi Y, Sun X, et al. Abnormal endocrine pancreas function at birth in cystic fibrosis ferrets. J Clin Invest 2012;122:3755–68.

14. Uc A, Olivier AK, Griffin MA, et al. Glycaemic regulation and insulin secretion are abnormal in cystic fibrosis pigs despite sparing of islet cell mass. Clin Sci (Lond) 2015;128:131–42.

15. Edlund A, Esguerra JL, Wendt A, et al. CFTR and Anoctamin 1 (ANO1) contribute to cAMP amplified exocytosis and insulin secretion in human and murine pancreatic beta-cells. BMC Med 2014;12:87.

16. Guo JH, Chen H, Ruan YC, et al. Glucose-induced electrical activities and insulin secretion in pancreatic islet beta-cells are modulated by CFTR. Nat Commun 2014;5:4420.

17. Bellin MD, Laguna T, Leschyshyn J, et al. Insulin secretion improves in cystic fibrosis following ivacaftor correction of CFTR: a small pilot study. Pediatr Diabetes 2013;14:417–21.

18. Hayes D Jr, McCoy KS, Sheikh SI. Resolution of cystic fibrosis-related diabetes with ivacaftor therapy. Am J Respir Crit Care Med 2014;190:590–1.

19. Tsabari R, Elyashar HI, Cymberknowh MC, et al. CFTR potentiator therapy ameliorates impaired insulin secretion in CF patients with a gating mutation. J Cyst Fibros 2015. [Epub ahead of print].

20. Moran A, Brunzell C, Cohen RC, et al. Clinical care guidelines for cystic fibrosis-related diabetes: a position statement of the American Diabetes Association and a clinical practice guideline of the cystic fibrosis foundation, endorsed by the pediatric endocrine society. Diabetes Care 2010;33:2697–708.

21. Moran A, Pillay K, Becker DJ, et al. ISPAD clinical practice consensus guidelines 2014. Management of cystic fibrosis-related diabetes in children and adolescents. Pediatr Diabetes 2014;15(Suppl 20):65–76.

22. Hirsch IB, Janci MM, Goss CH, et al. Hypoglycemia in adults with cystic fibrosis during oral glucose tolerance testing. Diabetes Care 2013;36:e121–2.

23. Wong SC, Dobie R, Altowati MA, et al. Growth and the growth hormone-insulin like growth factor 1 axis in children with chronic inflammation: current evidence, gaps in knowledge, and future directions. Endocr Rev 2016;37:62–110.

24. Lai HC, Kosorok MR, Sondel SA, et al. Growth status in children with cystic fibrosis based on the National Cystic Fibrosis Patient Registry data: evaluation of various criteria used to identify malnutrition. J Pediatr 1998;132:478–85.

25. Kelly HW, Sternberg AL, Lescher R, et al. Effect of inhaled glucocorticoids in childhood on adult height. N Engl J Med 2012;367:904–12.

26. Ripa P, Robertson I, Cowley D, et al. The relationship between insulin secretion, the insulin-like growth factor axis and growth in children with cystic fibrosis. Clin Endocrinol (Oxf) 2002;56:383–9.

27. Cheung MS, Bridges NA, Prasad SA, et al. Growth in children with cystic fibrosis-related diabetes. Pediatr Pulmonol 2009;44:1223–5.

28. Bizzarri C, Montemitro E, Pedicelli S, et al. Glucose tolerance affects pubertal growth and final height of children with cystic fibrosis. Pediatr Pulmonol 2015; 50:144–9.

29. Woestenenk JW, Hoekstra T, Hesseling C, et al. Comparison of height for age and height for bone age with and without adjustment for target height in pediatric patients with CF. J Cyst Fibros 2011;10:272–7.

30. Haeusler G, Frisch H, Waldhor T, et al. Perspectives of longitudinal growth in cystic fibrosis from birth to adult age. Eur J Pediatr 1994;153:158–63.

31. Festini F, Taccetti G, Repetto T, et al. Gestational and neonatal characteristics of children with cystic fibrosis: a cohort study. J Pediatr 2005;147:316–20.

32. Rogan MP, Reznikov LR, Pezzulo AA, et al. Pigs and humans with cystic fibrosis have reduced insulin-like growth factor 1 (IGF1) levels at birth. Proc Natl Acad Sci U S A 2010;107:20571–5.

33. Rosenberg LA, Schluchter MD, Parlow AF, et al. Mouse as a model of growth retardation in cystic fibrosis. Pediatr Res 2006;59:191–5.

34. Sermet-Gaudelus I, Souberbielle JC, Azhar I, et al. Insulin-like growth factor I correlates with lean body mass in cystic fibrosis patients. Arch Dis Child 2003; 88:956–61.

35. Thaker V, Haagensen AL, Carter B, et al. Recombinant growth hormone therapy for cystic fibrosis in children and young adults. Cochrane Database Syst Rev 2015;(5):CD008901.

36. Phung OJ, Coleman CI, Baker EL, et al. Recombinant human growth hormone in the treatment of patients with cystic fibrosis. Pediatrics 2010;126:e1211–26.

37. Hardin DS, Adams-Huet B, Brown D, et al. Growth hormone treatment improves growth and clinical status in prepubertal children with cystic fibrosis: results of a multicenter randomized controlled trial. J Clin Endocrinol Metab 2006;91:4925–9.

38. Stalvey MS, Clines GA. Cystic fibrosis-related bone disease: insights into a growing problem. Curr Opin Endocrinol Diabetes Obes 2013;20:547–52.

39. Henderson RC, Specter BB. Kyphosis and fractures in children and young adults with cystic fibrosis. J Pediatr 1994;125:208–12.

40. Wolfenden LL, Judd SE, Shah R, et al. Vitamin D and bone health in adults with cystic fibrosis. Clin Endocrinol (Oxf) 2008;69:374–81.

41. Paccou J, Zeboulon N, Combescure C, et al. The prevalence of osteoporosis, osteopenia, and fractures among adults with cystic fibrosis: a systematic literature review with meta-analysis. Calcif Tissue Int 2010;86:1–7.

42. Putman MS, Milliren CE, Derrico N, et al. Compromised bone microarchitecture and estimated bone strength in young adults with cystic fibrosis. J Clin Endocrinol Metab 2014;99:3399–407.

43. Rossini M, Del Marco A, Dal Santo F, et al. Prevalence and correlates of vertebral fractures in adults with cystic fibrosis. Bone 2004;35:771–6.

44. Sheikh S, Gemma S, Patel A. Factors associated with low bone mineral density in patients with cystic fibrosis. J Bone Miner Metab 2015;33:180–5.

45. Alicandro G, Bisogno A, Battezzati A, et al. Recurrent pulmonary exacerbations are associated with low fat free mass and low bone mineral density in young adults with cystic fibrosis. J Cyst Fibros 2014;13:328–34.

46. O'Reilly R, Fitzpatrick P, Leen G, et al. Severe bone demineralisation is associated with higher mortality in children with cystic fibrosis. Ir Med J 2009;102:47–9.

47. Le Henaff C, Gimenez A, Haÿ E, et al. The F508del mutation in cystic fibrosis transmembrane conductance regulator gene impacts bone formation. Am J Pathol 2012;180:2068–75.

48. Gimenez-Maitre A, Le Henaff C, Norez C, et al. Deficit of osteoprotegerin release by osteoblasts from a patient with cystic fibrosis. Eur Respir J 2012;39:780–1.

49. Le Heron L, Guillaume C, Velard F, et al. Cystic fibrosis transmembrane conductance regulator (CFTR) regulates the production of osteoprotegerin (OPG) and prostaglandin (PG) E2 in human bone. J Cyst Fibros 2010;9:69–72.

50. Stalvey MS, Clines KL, Havasi V, et al. Osteoblast CFTR inactivation reduces differentiation and osteoprotegerin expression in a mouse model of cystic fibrosis-related bone disease. PLoS One 2013;8:e80098.

51. Le Henaff C, Haÿ E, Velard F, et al. Enhanced F508del-CFTR channel activity ameliorates bone pathology in murine cystic fibrosis. Am J Pathol 2014;184: 1132–41.

52. Jacquot J, Delion M, Gangloff S, et al. Bone disease in cystic fibrosis: new pathogenic insights opening novel therapies. Osteoporos Int 2016;27(4):1401–12.

53. Sermet-Gaudelus I, Bianchi ML, Garabédian M, et al. European cystic fibrosis bone mineralisation guidelines. J Cyst Fibros 2011;10(Suppl 2):S16–23.

54. Aris RM, Merkel PA, Bachrach LK, et al. Guide to bone health and disease in cystic fibrosis. J Clin Endocrinol Metab 2005;90:1888–96.

55. Tangpricha V, Kelly A, Stephenson A, et al. An update on the screening, diagnosis, management, and treatment of vitamin D deficiency in individuals with cystic fibrosis: evidence-based recommendations from the cystic fibrosis foundation. J Clin Endocrinol Metab 2012;97:1082–93.

56. Chesdachai S, Tangpricha V. Treatment of vitamin D deficiency in cystic fibrosis. J Steroid Biochem Mol Biol 2015. [Epub ahead of print].

57. Hillman LS, Cassidy JT, Popescu MF, et al. Percent true calcium absorption, mineral metabolism, and bone mineralization in children with cystic fibrosis: effect of supplementation with vitamin D and calcium. Pediatr Pulmonol 2008;43: 772–80.

58. Alvarez J, Tangpricha V. Vitamin D and bone health in nutrition in cystic fibrosis. In: Leonard A, Yen E, editors. A guide for clinicians. New York: Springer; 2016.

59. Maurel DB, Boisseau N, Benhamou CL, et al. Alcohol and bone: review of dose effects and mechanisms. Osteoporos Int 2012;23:1–16.

60. Maqbool A, Graham-Maar RC, Schall JI, et al. Vitamin A intake and elevated serum retinol levels in children and young adults with cystic fibrosis. J Cyst Fibros 2008;7:137–41.

61. Conwell LS, Chang AB. Bisphosphonates for osteoporosis in people with cystic fibrosis. Cochrane Database Syst Rev 2014;(3):CD002010.

62. Siwamogsatham O, Stephens K, Tangpricha V. Evaluation of teriparatide for treatment of osteoporosis in four patients with cystic fibrosis: a case series. Case Rep Endocrinol 2014;2014:893589.

63. Lacativa PG, Farias ML. Osteoporosis and inflammation. Arq Bras Endocrinol Metabol 2010;54:123–32.

64. Leifke E, Friemert M, Heilmann M, et al. Sex steroids and body composition in men with cystic fibrosis. Eur J Endocrinol 2003;148:551–7.

65. Donovan DS Jr, Papadopoulos A, Staron RB, et al. Bone mass and vitamin D deficiency in adults with advanced cystic fibrosis lung disease. Am J Respir Crit Care Med 1998;157:1892–9.

Transplantation

Albert Faro, MD*, Alexander Weymann, MD

KEYWORDS

- Lung transplantation • Liver transplantation • Rejection • Allograft • Cystic fibrosis

KEY POINTS

- Despite improvement in median life expectancy and overall health, some children with cystic fibrosis (CF) progress to end-stage lung or liver disease and become candidates for transplant.
- Lung and liver transplants have the potential to extend life and improve the quality of life, but require strict adherence to a complex medical regimen.
- Chronic lung allograft dysfunction continues to be a major barrier to the success of lung transplants.
- Determining the optimal time to move forward with a liver transplant in CF remains controversial.

LUNG TRANSPLANTATION

Introduction

In the second decade of the twenty-first century clinicians are witnessing a revolution in the care of patients with cystic fibrosis (CF). The introduction of genetic modulators has for the first time allowed clinicians to directly target the basic defect in CF.[1,2] However, for some children, these therapies have come along too late in the course of the disease to be of significant benefit. In those cases, lung transplant (LTx) is a potential life-extending therapy.

Indications

General indications for LTx in children were published by the American Society of Transplantation in 2007.[3] The transplantation community was quick to recognize the potential utility of survival models to aid in determining appropriate timing for referral and listing for LTx. Kerem and colleagues'[4] criteria were one of the first such models. Patients with a forced expiratory volume in 1 second (FEV_1) less than 30% of predicted, a Pao_2 less than 55 mm Hg, or a $Paco_2$ greater than 50 mm Hg had 2-year mortalities more than 50%, with younger female patients doing the worst for any given

Department of Pediatrics, Washington University in St. Louis, Campus Box 8116, 660 South Euclid Avenue, St Louis, MO 63110, USA
* Corresponding author. Campus Box 8116, 660 South Euclid Avenue, St Louis, MO 63110.
E-mail address: faro_a@kids.wustl.edu

http://dx.doi.org/10.1016/j.pcl.2016.04.010
0031-3955/16/$ – see front matter

FEV_1. Several other investigators have studied models that include more variables,[5,6] but none of these models are any more precise than Kerem and colleagues'[4] criteria.

The number of children and young adults with CF who have received lung or liver transplants are listed in **Table 1**. Consensus criteria have been established for when patients with CF should be referred to a transplant center (**Box 1**).[7] In general, early referral is preferred. Importantly, early referral does not mean early transplant or even early listing, but it does provide the child and family the opportunity to establish a relationship with the transplant team. It gives the patient time to understand the process and commitment required and allows the center to put into place any necessary measures to optimize the posttransplant outcome.

In addition, all candidates should at the least possess:

1. An adequate array of family support, including 2 care providers
2. Adequate access to transplant services and medications
3. Adequate evidence of an ability to adhere to the complex posttransplant regimen

Contraindications

There is a great deal of variability among LTx centers in the contraindications for transplant. The reasons for this variability include:

1. The list of contraindications is not static over time. The introduction of newer techniques or therapies may yield meaningful improvements in outcome to change how a particular condition is viewed.
2. Center-specific experience.
3. Center-specific interpretation of published data.

The common thread is that contraindications place patients at greater risk for a poor outcome. Contraindications are usually divided into absolute versus relative. Among transplant centers, there is variability as to which contraindications are in which category. What is considered an absolute contraindication at one center may only be a relative contraindication at another (**Box 2**).

Of particular interest in patients with CF is the microbiology of the airway. Patients with CF are chronically infected with a variety of pathogens. Some of these microorganisms are known to lead to a more rapid decline in lung function before transplant. However, some of those same organisms are associated with poor outcomes after LTx. The posttransplant management of patients infected with *Burkholderia cenocepacia* highlights this quandary. *B cenocepacia* is associated with higher morbidity and mortality in CF, but, in general, posttransplant survival rates are very poor for those infected with this organism.[8] As a result, most transplant centers view infection with *B cenocepacia* as an absolute contraindication. Importantly, patients infected

Table 1			
Number of lung or liver transplants in patients with CF per year and age group			
	2012	**2013**	**2014**
Age (y)	**Lung/Liver**	**Lung/Liver**	**Lung/Liver**
5–9	0/0	a/5	a/a
10–14	a/a	15/a	6/5
15–19	17/7	23/a	16/7

[a] At least 1, but fewer than 5 patients.
Courtesy of Samar Rizvi, Bethesda, MD. Patient Registry Cystic Fibrosis Foundation.

Box 1
Consensus recommendations for when to refer a patient with CF to a transplant center.

Lung function

- FEV$_1$ less than or equal to 30% predicted
- Rapid rate of lung function decline (especially in a female patient)
- Six-minute walk distance less than 400 m
- Need for noninvasive positive pressure ventilation

Pulmonary hypertension

- Systolic PAP greater than 35 mm Hg on echocardiography
- Or mean PAP greater than 25 mm Hg on cardiac catheterization

Infection

- Increasing antibiotic resistance
- Poor clinical recovery from pulmonary exacerbations

Nutrition

- Worsening nutritional status despite supplementation and appetite stimulants

Other clinical signs or symptoms

- Pneumothorax
- Life-threatening hemoptysis
- Diabetes

Abbreviation: PAP, pulmonary artery pressure.
Adapted from Weill D, Benden C, Corris PA, et al. A consensus document for the selection of lung transplant candidates: 2014–an update from the Pulmonary Transplantation Council of the International Society for Heart and Lung Transplantation. J Heart Lung Transplant 2015;34(1):6–7; with permission.

---

with other *Burkholderia cepacia* complex (BCC) organisms, apart from *Burkholderia dolosa*, have outcomes that are just as acceptable as those of patients not infected with BCC organisms.[8] Other organisms that raise concern in the transplantation community include *Burkholderia gladioli*, a non-BCC organism, and *Mycobacterium abscessus*. For more detail, readers are referred to the excellent review article by Lobo and Noone.[9]

Referring centers must also be aware that documented, refractory nonadherence does not portend a good posttransplant outcome. Referring centers must be transparent with the transplant center and the patient when referring patients for consideration. This requirement is not meant to be punitive, but is meant to optimize the potential for a good outcome, and allows for a dialogue to occur and plans to be put into place to give the patients the best opportunity to succeed.

Timing of Transplant

Timing of the transplant is critically important because 5-year survival rates after pediatric LTx remain at about 50% (**Fig. 1**).[10] Results from mathematical modeling before the advent of the lung allocation score (LAS) in the United States suggested that children with CF derived no survival benefit from LTx.[11] However, the validity of the conclusion has been challenged because the data set used covariates that were obtained well before the transplant.[12]

Box 2
Commonly accepted contraindications for lung transplant (not true for all centers).

Absolute

- Infectious
  - *Burkholderia cenocepacia*
  - *Mycobacterium abscessus*
  - Active tuberculosis
  - Sepsis

- Malignancy
  - Less than 2 years disease free (many centers use up to 5 years)

- Multi-organ dysfunction

- Neurologic
  - Severe neuromuscular disease
  - Poor rehabilitation potential

- Psychosocial
  - Lack of adequate social support system
  - Documented, refractory nonadherence

- Body habitus
  - Severe scoliosis
  - Severe chest wall deformity

Relative

- Infectious
  - Multidrug-resistant organisms

- Previous surgery
  - Pleurodesis
  - Multiple thoracotomies

- Immunologic
  - Sever immunodeficiency syndromes
  - Active collagen vascular disease
  - High circulating human leukocyte antigen antibody titers

There is an optimal window during which patients are sick enough to derive benefit from a transplant, but not so sick so that they are at greater risk for a poor outcome.[13] The LAS makes it more likely that the sickest patients get offered a transplant first and, in addition to blood type, height, and geographic proximity of the donor, is used to determine priority on the transplant waiting list for patients 12 years of age and older (**Box 3**). Prioritization of the transplant list in children less than 12 years of age is based on wait time but also on urgency within a tiered system (**Box 4**).

Surgery

Detailed discussion of the surgical procedure is beyond the scope of this article and is described elsewhere.[14] The most common procedure involves a clamshell incision with bilateral sequential LTx. Of note is that the lymphatics, bronchial circulation, and nervous system are not reanastomosed, which leads to potential limitations in a recipient's ability to clear pulmonary edema or airway secretions.

Living donor LTx lost favor in the United States with the advent of the LAS and the removal of time spent on the list as a criterion. Reasons for the decline in this procedure include the risk to the physical and emotional well-being of the 2 normal donors with no additional benefit in terms of recipient outcomes between living donor and deceased donor transplant.[15]

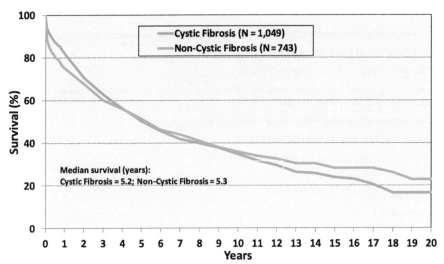

Fig. 1. Pediatric lung transplants. International Society of Heart and Lung Transplantation registry, Kaplan-Meier survival by diagnosis (January 1990 to June 2013). (*Adapted from* Benden C, Goldfarb SB, Edwards LB, et al. The registry of the International Society for Heart and Lung Transplantation: seventeenth official pediatric lung and heart-lung transplantation report–2014; focus theme: retransplantation. J Heart Lung Transplant 2014;33:1025–33.)

Posttransplant Management

Immunosuppression

Immediately posttransplant, most pediatric LTx programs in the United States use induction therapy with lympholytic agents or interleukin (IL)-2 receptor antagonists to decrease the risk of acute rejection. Maintenance immunosuppression consists of a

---

Box 3
The components of the LAS

Blood Type

Diagnosis

Forced vital capacity

Need for supplemental oxygen

Pco_2 and change in Pco_2

Need for mechanical ventilation

Six-minute walk distance

Age

Body mass index

New York Heart Association functional score

Pulmonary arterial pressure

Creatinine

Bilirubin and change in bilirubin

Diabetes

> **Box 4**
> **Prioritization of children less than 12 years of age: criteria for priority 1**
>
> Must have one of the following:
>
> - Be on continuous mechanical ventilation
> - Requiring more than 50% fraction of inspired oxygen to maintain oxyhemoglobin saturations greater than or equal to 90%
> - An arterial or capillary Pco_2 greater than 50 mm Hg
> - A venous Pco_2 greater than 56 mm Hg
> - Pulmonary vein stenosis involving at least 3 vessels
> - A cardiac index less than 2 L/min/m^2
> - Syncope
> - Hemoptysis
> - Suprasystemic pulmonary artery pressure

3-drug regimen that usually comprises a calcineurin inhibitor, a cell cycle toxin, and prednisone or prednisolone (**Table 2**). These agents have many potential side effects and the risk of toxicity can be monitored by following trough concentrations and other laboratory tests (**Box 5**). However, in any individual patient, these concentration levels correlate poorly with the relative degree of immunosuppression.

Unlike other solid organ transplant recipients, pediatric LTx recipients rarely ever wean entirely off any of these medicines. It is essential that patients' home CF centers be aware that there are multiple potential drug interactions and to communicate with the transplant center before initiating any new therapies (**Table 3**).

Antimicrobials

Patients receive antibiotic and antifungal therapy based on their previous native airway cultures and susceptibilities. The donor organ is also cultured before transplant. At our center we perform a bronchoscopy with bronchoalveolar lavage (BAL) within the first 24 hours both to assess the anastomoses and to obtain cultures. Antimicrobial therapies are adjusted based on the results.

Antifungal prophylaxis strategy varies between centers.[16] Candida prophylaxis is routinely administered in the form of oral nystatin or clotrimazole troches. *Pneumocystis jiroveci* prophylaxis is routinely administered shortly after transplant; trimethoprim/sulfamethoxazole is the treatment of choice.

For patients who are cytomegalovirus (CMV) seropositive or for those who receive an organ from a CMV seropositive donor, prophylaxis with ganciclovir is given. The length and mode of therapy vary among different transplant centers.[17] Longer courses of up to 12 months have benefits.[18] Herpes simplex virus (HSV) prophylaxis with acyclovir should be considered when the recipient is not receiving CMV prophylaxis.[19]

Adolescents

Although there are anatomic similarities between adults and adolescents, teenagers present a well-described separate set of challenges for health care teams.[20] Adolescents must cope with their emerging autonomy and need to fit in among their peers. They are more likely to indulge in risk-taking behaviors. Increased incidence of late rejection, graft failure, and death is well described in the adolescent transplant literature.[21,22]

Results from a recent retrospective study of United Network for Organ Sharing (UNOS) data showed improved survival (half-life 4.6 vs 2.5 years) in adolescent LTx

Table 2
Maintenance immunosuppressants and potential adverse effects

Medication	Potential Adverse Effect
Corticosteroids	Hyperglycemia/diabetes Hypertension Osteopenia Glaucoma Infection
Tacrolimus	Renal dysfunction Hypertension Infection (fungal, viral, parasitic) Diabetes/impaired glucose tolerance Dyslipidemia Neurotoxicity (headaches, tremors, seizures, PRES) Malignancy (cutaneous, lymphoid, others)
Cyclosporine	Renal dysfunction Hypertension Infection Neurotoxicity Hirsutism Gingival hyperplasia Malignancy
Mycophenolate mofetil	GI symptoms (nausea, vomiting, diarrhea, abdominal pain) Neutropenia Teratogenicity
Sirolimus	Impaired wound healing Myelosuppression (anemia, neutropenia, thrombocytopenia) Hyperlipidemia Proteinuria Pneumonitis Hepatic artery thrombosis?
Azathioprine and 6-MP	Myelosuppression (especially leukopenia) Malignancy (eg, hepatosplenic T-cell lymphoma [very rare]) Hepatotoxicity (transaminase level increase) Pancreatitis GI symptoms (nausea, vomiting [rare])

Abbreviations: GI, gastrointestinal; 6-MP, 6-mercaptopurine; PRES, posterior reversible encephalopathy syndrome.

Adapted from Busuttil RW, Klintmalm GB, editors. Transplantation of the Liver. 3rd edition. Philadelphia: Elsevier/Saunders; 2015.

recipients transplanted at high-volume pediatric centers compared with those transplanted at adult LTx centers.[23] Multivariable analysis showed that being transplanted at an adult center was an independent risk factor for graft failure in adolescents, with a hazard ratio of 1.5 ($P<.001$). It is the investigators' opinion that any adult center choosing to offer transplants to adolescents must at a minimum have on-site involvement of pediatric care providers such as pediatric pulmonologists, psychologists, child life specialists, coordinators, and social workers to optimize the children's posttransplant outcomes.

Complications

When considering the differential diagnosis in a transplant recipient, it is useful to consider that complications tend to occur along a posttransplant timeline. The immediate posttransplant complications are listed in **Box 6**.

Box 5
Typical surveillance evaluation of a pediatric lung transplant recipient at St Louis Children's Hospital within the first year of transplant.

Bloodwork
- Complete blood count with differential
- Comprehensive metabolic panel, including electrolytes, renal function
- Tacrolimus and mycophenolate concentrations
- Donor-specific antibody assay
- Uric acid, lactate dehydrogenase
- Cholesterol and fasting lipid panel
- Prothrombin time and partial thromboplastin time
- Cytomegalovirus and Epstein-Barr virus polymerase chain reaction (PCR)
- Hemoglobin A1c
- Pregnancy test if appropriate

Pulmonary function testing
- Spirometry
- Lung volumes
- Diffusion capacity

Imaging
- Chest radiograph
- High-resolution chest computed tomography
- Ventilation/perfusion scan

Bronchoscopy
- Evaluation of the anastomoses
- Bronchoalveolar lavage for cultures, stains, or PCR (bacterial, acid fast, fungal, and viral)
- Transbronchial biopsy

Early posttransplant (1–6 months)

Infection Patients with CF come to transplant with chronic airway infection of not only their lower airways but also of their sinuses and trachea. The risk of infection is increased by immunosuppression. Data to support the use of sinus surgery to promote *Pseudomonas* eradication has overall been disappointing.[24] However, in a single center, when combined with daily nasal douching, a reduction in pseudomonal airway colonization was achieved.[25]

Table 3
Drugs and supplements interacting with cytochrome P450 3A4 (CYP3A4) and calcineurin inhibitors (CNI)

CYP3A4 Inhibitors (Increase CNI Blood Levels)	CYP3A4 Inducers (Decrease CNI Blood Levels)
Antimicrobials (fluconazole, ketoconazole, erythromycin, clarithromycin)	Antimicrobials (rifampin, rifabutin)
HIV protease inhibitors (nelfinavir, ritonavir, saquinavir, indinavir)	HIV protease inhibitors (nevirapine, efavirenz)
HCV protease inhibitors (telaprevir, boceprevir)	Antiepileptics (carbamazepine, phenytoin, phenobarbital)
Others: cimetidine, sertraline, grapefruit juice	Others: St John's wort

Abbreviations: HCV, hepatitis C virus; HIV, human immunodeficiency virus.
Adapted from Busuttil RW, Klintmalm GB, editors. Transplantation of the liver. 3rd edition. Philadelphia: Elsevier/Saunders; 2015.

> **Box 6**
> **Immediate posttransplant complications (0–1 month)**
>
> Surgery related
>   Bleeding
>   Vascular anastomotic stenosis
>   Dehiscence of the airway anastomosis
>   Airway anastomotic stenosis
>   Phrenic nerve injury
>   Vocal cord paralysis
>   Atrial arrhythmias
>   Gastrointestinal paresis
>   Distal ileal obstruction syndrome
>
> Primary graft dysfunction
>
> Infection
>   Bacterial
>   Fungal
>   Viral
>
> Immunologic
>   Hyperacute rejection
>   Acute rejection

Fungi are typically considered opportunistic organisms, but, because patients with CF may be chronically colonized before transplant, fungal infection may be seen early.[26,27] Risk factors include acute cellular rejection (ACR), pretransplant colonization, tacrolimus-based immunosuppression, and CMV-positive donor, but not CF.[28] Pulmonary fungal infection is associated with 1-year mortality (hazard ratio, 3.9).[28] Possible therapies include voriconazole, amphotericin (intravenous or inhaled), or echinocandins. Each has its own set of advantages and disadvantages based on mode of delivery, drug interactions, and the specific fungus to be treated.

CMV was a significant pathogen associated with increased mortality within the first year after transplant as well as with the development of chronic lung allograft dysfunction (CLAD).[29,30] However, effective prophylactic regimens have resulted in decreased incidence of infection.[18]

Because this is a time of maximal immunosuppression, even respiratory viral infections (RVIs) may be life threatening.[31,32] RVIs are also associated with the development of CLAD.[33] Therefore, many pediatric LTx centers treat children infected with respiratory syncytial virus (RSV) with ribavirin, although practices are not uniform.[34]

Immunologic At this stage rejection may be cellular or antibody mediated. Both forms are associated with the later development of CLAD. The incidence of ACR is between 18% and 50%.[35,36] ACR may be clinically silent and therefore many transplant centers perform routine surveillance transbronchial biopsies (TBBs) at scheduled intervals within the first 6 to 12 months posttransplant.[37] In experienced hands, TBB can provide important diagnostic information with a good safety profile in even very young children.[38,39]

Patients can present with clinical symptoms, decreased lung function, and/or radiographic infiltrates that are identical to those of a patient with an infection, which highlights the importance of performing appropriate diagnostic testing, including bronchoscopy with BAL and TBB.

When found, ACR is typically treated with 3 days of high-dose methylprednisolone (10–20 mg/kg/d). If ACR is persistent, a second course of methylprednisolone may be given. If ACR is still present, patients then may receive lympholytic therapy with antithymocyte globulin. The primary risk of augmenting immunosuppression is infection. Patients are frequently treated concurrently with antimicrobials.

Antibody-mediated rejection (AMR) may also occur in this phase. AMR in LTx recipients has proved to be both a diagnostic as well as a therapeutic challenge.[40] The evaluation of a patient with clinical allograft dysfunction includes an assessment for the presence of circulating donor-specific antibodies (DSAs), lung biopsy evidence of capillaritis, and capillary endothelial complement (C4d) deposition.[41] The evidence suggests that LTx patients with CF are at higher risk for developing DSA than those without CF.[42] The diagnostic effort is complicated by the potential for autoantibodies, antibodies to self-antigens, to contribute to the development of CLAD.[43] Therefore, the absence of a DSA is not enough to rule out the diagnosis of AMR.

The presence of AMR portends a very poor prognosis and is associated with the development of CLAD.[44] Treatment with a variety of different agents have been described in single case reports, with the most promising perhaps being the addition of bortezomib, a proteasome inhibitor that causes apoptosis of plasma cells.[45] The treatment protocol at our center combines therapy with plasmapheresis, rituximab, intravenous immunoglobulin, and bortezomib; however, the results have been disappointing.

Anastomotic Anastomotic complications can relate to either airway or vascular anastomoses. Vascular anastomotic complications are usually seen in the immediate posttransplant phase. The risk of airway anastomotic stenosis is not associated with the size of the airway, but it is associated with pretransplant BCC, posttransplant fungal pulmonary infection, and days mechanically ventilated.[46] Airway stenosis is treated by balloon dilatation.

Immunosuppression In addition to the increased risk of infection, immunosuppressants commonly used after LTx are associated with a host of potential complications (see **Table 2**). Patients with CF are at increased risk of developing diabetes even without transplant. However, both tacrolimus, a calcineurin inhibitor (CNI), and systemic steroids are known to increase the risk of diabetes.[47] CNIs are also associated with nephrotoxicity,[48] which is more of a problem among patients with CF who, by the time they arrive for transplant, have probably had years of exposure to aminoglycosides and other nephrotoxic antibiotics. CNIs may also cause seizures, headaches, and sleep disturbances.[49,50]

Late postoperative (greater than 6 months)
Infection Although immunosuppression is decreased over time in patients who have not experienced ACR, infection remains a problem throughout the posttransplant course. Pediatric LTx recipients typically stay on triple-drug immunosuppression and therefore are not only at risk for opportunistic infections but also at risk for complications from community-acquired infections.[31–33]

Immunologic Patients continue to be at risk for either ACR or AMR in this phase. Importantly, CLAD begins to emerge as an important complication affecting up to 10% of LTx recipients by the first year and 50% by 3 years from transplant. CLAD is a fairly new term meant to take into consideration that not all patients with allograft dysfunction have obliterative bronchiolitis (OB)/bronchiolitis obliterans syndrome

(BOS).[51] Some may have neutrophil reversible allograft dysfunction (NRAD), whereas others may present with decrease in lung function that is more restrictive, or restrictive allograft syndrome (RAS). CLAD encompasses all of these entities.

Obliterative bronchiolitis/bronchiolitis obliterans syndrome OB is an inflammatory injury to the small airways, which is presumed to result from chronic rejection in LTx. OB is a histopathologic diagnosis. Because the process is initially patchy and inhomogeneous, TBB is often inadequate to make the diagnosis. Open lung biopsy is the gold standard. Therefore, a corresponding clinical syndrome, termed BOS (**Table 4**), was defined that corresponds with OB.[52] However, BOS is not specific to the diagnosis of OB.[53] BOS constitutes most CLAD.[54]

Risk factors for BOS include recurrent acute rejection or a single episode of severe acute rejection. Other risk factors for BOS include lymphocytic bronchiolitis,[55] primary graft dysfunction (PGD),[56] gastroesophageal reflux (GER),[57] RVIs,[33] and the development of anti–human leukocyte antigen (anti-HLA) antibodies.[58]

Chest radiographic findings may be normal or may reveal hyperinflation. High-resolution chest computed tomography scan may show bronchiectasis, decreased vascular markings, and air trapping. Ventilation scan may show retention of xenon. On histology, OB is characterized by a proliferation of fibroblasts into the airway lumen, ultimately forming intraluminal granulation tissue and total obliteration.

The reality is that no intervention in the armamentarium can be expected to do anything more than halt further deterioration in lung function. The exception seems to be in patients with NRAD. They have airway neutrophilia and experience an improvement in lung function when on azithromycin.[59] Therapies that, in some cases, can at least stabilize function for some period of time include antithymocyte globulin, fundoplication for patients with GER, change in immunosuppression from cyclosporine A to tacrolimus, and photopheresis.

Photopheresis is seemingly one of the more promising approaches to treating patients with OB/BOS. A retrospective review of 60 adult LTx recipients showed a slowing in the rate of decline in the FEV_1.[60]

Restrictive allograft syndrome RAS is characterized by a symmetric decline in forced vital capacity and FEV_1 with a decrease in total lung capacity. On histology, inflammation and fibrosis are typically seen.[54]

Posttransplant lymphoproliferative disease The use of immunosuppressive agents places LTx recipients at increased risk for malignancies after their transplants. The most common such malignancy in children is posttransplant lymphoproliferative disease.[61] The spectrum of disease severity varies, with the most severe being true malignancy. Primary infection with Epstein-Barr virus after transplant is the primary risk factor. Pediatric LTx recipients are at high risk.

Table 4 Definition of BOS after acute rejection and infection have been ruled out	
BOS 0	FEV_1 90% of baseline and $FEF_{25\%-75\%}$ 75% of baseline
BOS 0-p	FEV_1 81%–90% of baseline and/or $FEF_{25\%-75\%}$ 75% of baseline
BOS 1	FEV_1 66%–80% of baseline
BOS 2	FEV_1 51%–65% of baseline
BOS 3	FEV_1 50% of baseline

Abbreviation: $FEF_{25\%-75\%}$, average forced expiratory flow during the midportion (25%–75%) of the forced vital capacity.

Potential therapies include reducing immunosuppression, treatment with anti–B-cell antibodies (eg, rituximab), interferon-alpha with or without intravenous immunoglobulin, surgical resection, radiotherapy, and cytotoxic chemotherapy.

Immunosuppression These complications are discussed earlier. In addition, osteopenia may begin to emerge as more of a problem because LTx recipients are rarely able to come off prednisone.

Outcomes

Patients with CF do as well after LTx as any other group (see **Fig. 1**).[10] However, long-term outcomes continue to disappoint. Changes in surgical technique and early postoperative critical care management have resulted in improved early outcomes. However, the inability to adequately prevent or treat CLAD continues to limit long-term success (**Fig. 2**).

Future

Newer techniques and strategies to either address the organ shortage or extend life and optimize clinical state while the patients are waiting on the list are being studied or adopted. These include the following:

Extracorporeal membrane oxygenation (ECMO)
- Ambulatory ECMO is increasingly used as a bridge to LTx. It provides patients in respiratory failure with the potential for ambulation and continued rehabilitation, maximizing the odds for a good transplant outcome.[62]

Donation after cardiocirculatory death (DCD)
- In an attempt to increase the donor pool, some transplant programs accept DCD donors. The outcomes from these donors do not significantly differ from outcomes from donors with brain death.[63]

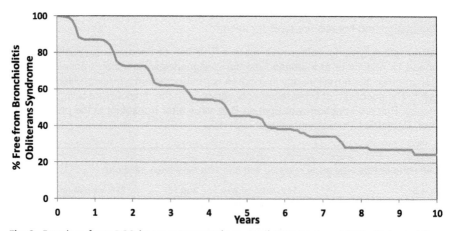

Fig. 2. Freedom from BOS (years posttransplant, April 1994 to June 2014). (*Adapted from* Goldfarb SB, Benden C, Edwards LB, et al. The Registry of the International Society for Heart and Lung Transplantation: eighteenth official pediatric lung and heart-lung transplantation report–2015; focus theme: early graft failure. J Heart Lung Transplant 2015;34:1255–63.)

Ex-vivo lung perfusion (EVLP)

- Donor lungs that do not meet criteria for suitability are never used. EVLP provides an opportunity to assess and improve the function of these lungs. It is essentially a circuit that allows for careful monitoring of oxygenation, compliance, and other parameters. It also allows for the possibility of introducing therapies to the donor lung before transplant. Long-term outcomes of transplanting lungs using EVLP are promising.[64]

Basic science and translational research are focused on improving the understanding of CLAD.

LIVER TRANSPLANTATION
Introduction

Unlike the incidence of end-stage lung disease in CF, which increases with age, the onset of multilobular cirrhosis in CF is usually before 12 years of age. New diagnoses of cirrhosis in teenagers who have been screened previously are rare.[65] The average age of onset of portal hypertension is 11 years.[66] Clinically significant cholestasis and liver synthetic dysfunction generally develop only in very late stages of CF liver disease (CFLD); hepatocellular carcinoma is rare, especially in children.

CFLD is common, but underappreciated because its manifestations are variable and usually not life limiting. Over their lifetimes, most children with CF develop a manifestation of CFLD such as hepatomegaly, hepatic steatosis, increased serum enzyme levels, or focal biliary cirrhosis, but only 5% to 10% develop the most severe form of CFLD, multilobular cirrhosis with portal hypertension. Progression to orthotopic liver transplant (OLT) is rare, with only 39 of 2445 pediatric liver transplant recipients in the Studies of Pediatric Liver Transplantation (SPLIT) database until 2006 having received their graft for CFLD.[67] One review of the UNOS database found 190 isolated OLTs and 15 combined liver-lung transplants (LLTs) over 20 years. Only 26% of the isolated OLT patients were adults, whereas about equal numbers of adults and children received a combined LLT.[68]

Indications

The indications and eligibility criteria for OLT in CF are challenging to define; consideration must be given to comorbidities and risk factors such advanced chronic lung disease, chronic or intercurrent infections (with risk for exacerbation by immunosuppression), and malnutrition; pancreatic insufficiency not only contributes to malnutrition persisting posttransplant but can also interfere with absorption of some immunosuppressive agents.

Children with clinically significant portal hypertension, especially with esophageal varices who either have bled or are at increased risk for bleeding (grade 3), or with ascites or liver synthetic dysfunction, are likely good candidates for OLT. A scoring system attempting to identify those patients likely to benefit from liver transplant and at risk of dying from liver disease was first proposed by Noble-Jamieson and colleagues.[69] Its parameters are related to portal hypertension, hypersplenism, liver synthetic dysfunction, and malnutrition. It was later revised by Milkiewicz and colleagues[70] to include leukocytosis and hyperbilirubinemia.

It should be noted that portal hypertension, generally the main complication of advanced CF liver disease, has been disputed as an indication for OLT. One study of 18 young adults with cirrhosis caused by CFLD and upper gastrointestinal bleeding suggested that long-term transplant-free survival can be achieved with medical and endoscopic therapy alone.[71] Another study in young adults advocated consideration of early OLT before pulmonary deterioration, but then also cautioned that portal hypertension alone as an indication for OLT should be questioned because of the availability of shunt procedures.[72]

Nutritional failure is an additional factor that should suggest consideration of OLT in patients with advanced CFLD. In a small series from Milan, weight, body mass index, lean body mass, bone density, and fat-soluble vitamin levels all improved after liver transplant compared with children who were not transplanted.[73]

If a patient with CFLD cirrhosis is evaluated for OLT and the lung function is satisfactory at baseline, liver transplant alone should be pursued. Lung function can improve in patients with CF after isolated OLT,[74] although this finding has not been consistent across studies.[73] If the pretransplant FEV_1 is repeatedly less than 40% of predicted, consideration should be given to a combined LLT. The outcomes for isolated OLT seem to be better in patients with better baseline lung function. In a study of the European registry, worse outcomes for isolated liver transplant were shown if the pretransplant FEV_1 was less than 50%.[75]

Contraindications

Box 7 lists potential contraindications. Considerations include the absence or presence of infections typical for CF, such as *Aspergillus*, *Pseudomonas*, or *Burkholderia*. Some studies have found a link between posttransplant infectious complications and prior colonization, whereas other groups have found no association with long-term complications or mortality.[70,72,74,76] The decision to use or not use postoperative

---

Box 7
Contraindications to liver transplant

Absolute

- Primary extrahepatic malignancy (unresectable)
- Progressive extrahepatic disease (terminal)
- Severe injury of the nervous system, especially central nervous system (irreversible)
- Sepsis or disseminated viral infection (uncontrolled)

Relative

- Acquired immunodeficiency syndrome (or, in many centers, human immunodeficiency virus infection)
- Advanced or only partially treated systemic infection
- Grade IV hepatic encephalopathy
- Psychosocial factors with potential to severely compromise outcome (eg, substance abuse)
- Primary hepatic malignancy, metastatic and unresponsive to chemotherapy
- Extrahepatic malignancy metastasizing to the liver

Adapted from Suchy F, Sokol R, Balistreri W, editors. Liver disease in children. 4th edition. Cambridge (United Kingdom): Cambridge University Press; 2014.

antibiotics with an isolated OLT should be made on a case-by-case basis based on the preoperative microbiological profile.

As with LTx, excellent, ongoing communication of the liver transplant team with the patients and their families is crucial, beginning at the first encounter. Anticipatory guidance about perioperative and long-term complications, as well as medication side effects, should be provided. Expectations regarding medication adherence and close cooperation with the liver transplant team in all medical decisions need to be clarified. Medical and psychosocial challenges to effective care must be anticipated and acknowledged, and suggestions for solutions offered. Above all, the family must be prepared for the sometimes extraordinary difficulties and sacrifices that a liver transplant may entail, and available resources for advice and support should be explained in advance.

Timing of Transplant

Suitable donor livers are allocated based on a patient's Model for End-stage Liver disease (MELD) or Pediatric End-stage Liver Disease (PELD) score (**Table 5**). Pulmonary status influences the patient's score on the liver transplant waiting list. Exceptions are made in the MELD (for patients 12 years and older) and PELD scoring systems for patients with an FEV_1 less than 40%. These patients receive a predetermined baseline score, with a 10% point increase (mortality equivalent) every 3 months. Separate rules apply to MELD and PELD scores for patients listed for combined LLT.

Table 5 MELD and PELD scores		
Components	MELD (Patients Aged ≥12 y)	PELD (Patients Aged <12 y)
Serum bilirubin	X	X
Serum creatinine	X	—
Serum albumin	—	X
INR	X	X
Dialysis (twice in past 7 d)	X	—
Age (<1 y)	—	X
Growth failure (more than 2 SD < mean)	—	X

Abbreviations: INR, International Normalized Ratio; SD, standard deviations.

Postoperative Management

Postoperatively, the focus of pediatric hepatologists is on prevention of both rejection and infection, and thus requires prudent balancing of the immunosuppressive regimen. The mainstay of immunosuppression is tacrolimus, which is started soon after the allograft is implanted. In the first few months, corticosteroids and mycophenolate are added. At our center, we use induction therapy with high-dose intravenous methylprednisolone for isolated OLT and reserve the addition of thymoglobulin, or an IL-2 receptor antibody such as basiliximab, for cases of combined LLT. **Tables 2** and **6** give overviews of the immunosuppressive drugs used in OLT, with their respective schedules, side effects, and interactions with other medications. **Table 7** lists the schedule for surveillance tests at our center.

Table 6
Schedule for medications after liver transplant at our center

	Prevention of...	Discontinuation After Transplant
Tacrolimus	Allograft rejection	Never (with rare exceptions)
Mycophenolate mofetil		3–6 mo (after corticosteroids)
Prednisone or prednisolone		Around 3 mo (if no rejection)
Famotidine	Gastritis and peptic ulcer	Simultaneous with corticosteroids
Fluconazole	Candidiasis	1 mo
Acyclovir	HSV disease (if CMV negative donor and recipient)	3 mo
Valganciclovir	CMV disease (if CMV positive donor or recipient)	6 mo
Trimethoprim/ sulfamethoxazole	Pneumocystic pneumonia and toxoplasmosis	1 y
Aspirin	Hepatic artery thrombosis	1 y

Complications

Table 8 lists possible short-term and long-term complications after transplant. Many are similar to the complications seen after LTx.

Outcomes

Table 9 discusses outcomes.[68,70,74,75,77–84] Among 2991 children in the SPLIT database transplanted between 1996 and 2006, the 1-year and 5-year survival rates were 89.8% and 84.8%, respectively, and of those who had survived at least 5 years after transplant, 88% had done so with their first allografts.[85] Children undergoing simultaneous LLT may have better outcomes than those who receive LTx only.[78]

Future

Some ongoing questions and controversies surrounding OLT for CF include the following:

- How should clinicians select the patients for whom OLT or LLT is indicated? How is the optimal time point for listing determined?

Table 7
Schedule for surveillance tests after liver transplant at our center

Test	Frequency
CMP, Mg, GGT, fractionated bilirubin, CBC/ diff., PT/INR, tacrolimus trough	Initially twice weekly, then weaned to monthly
Hgb A1c, lipid panel, 25-OH vitamin D	Yearly
Glomerular filtration rate (I-125 iothalamate)	Once after 2 y of age; repeat if abnormal
Bone density (DEXA scan)	Once after 6 y of age; repeat if abnormal
Liver biopsy	Only for cause, no scheduled surveillance Bx

Abbreviations: 25-OH, 25-hydroxy; Bx, biopsy; CBC, complete blood count; CMP, complete metabolic profile; DEXA, dual-energy x-ray absorptiometry; diff, differential; GGT, gamma-glutamyl transferase; Hgb, hemoglobin; PT, prothrombin time.

Table 8
Examples of potential complications after liver transplant

	Early	Middle	Late
Surgical	Wound dehiscence	Diaphragmatic hernia	Biliary stricture
Vascular	Bleeding/hemorrhage, hepatic artery thrombosis, portal vein thrombosis	Portal vein stenosis, hepatic vein stenosis	Portal vein stenosis, hepatic vein stenosis
Infectious	Gram-negative enteric bacteria; *Enterococcus*; *Staphylococcus*; *Candida*; *Clostridium difficile*	HSV, CMV, RSV, influenza, adenovirus, Rotavirus, Pneumocystis, *Toxoplasma*	Any type of infection, largely dependent on comorbidities
Immunologic	ACR, hyperacute (humoral) rejection	ACR, de-novo autoimmune hepatitis	Chronic (ductopenic) rejection, de-novo autoimmune hepatitis
Respiratory	Pleural effusion, pneumonia	Respiratory infections	Respiratory infections
Cardiovascular	Hypotension/shock	Hypertension	Hypertension
Gastrointestinal	Abdominal pain, nausea, vomiting, diarrhea	Eosinophilic GI disease, abdominal adhesions	Eosinophilic GI disease, abdominal adhesions
Metabolic	Hyperlipidemia, hyperglycemia	Hyperlipidemia, hyperglycemia	Hyperlipidemia, hyperglycemia
Neurologic	Hypoxic brain injury, PRES	Seizures, tremors	Neurocognitive delay
Hematologic	Cytopenias	Cytopenias	Cytopenias
Malignant	Recurrent metastases from primary hepatic malignancy	PTLD/lymphoma	PTLD/lymphoma, cutaneous malignancies

Abbreviation: PTLD, posttransplant lymphoproliferative disease.

- What are the indications for a portosystemic shunt and/or splenectomy as a bridge or even an alternative to transplant?
- What is the role of early diagnosis? Can liver transplant be avoided or delayed by early detection and optimal medical management of CFLD? Because there is currently no proven therapy or preventive strategy for CFLD, it is not clear what that means, although it is interesting to speculate what future role new CF transmembrane conductance regulator (CFTR) modulators may play in the prevention or treatment of CFLD. Early diagnosis of CFLD is challenging; no unequivocally useful early biomarkers have been identified to date, although there has recently been a renewed interest in the role of gamma-glutamyl transferase[86]; the roles of various imaging studies such as ultrasonography for prediction of cirrhosis remain to be determined.[87] All these questions await further studies.

Table 9
Outcomes after OLT

	Patient Population	Colonization and Infection	Lung Function	Immunosuppression	Survival	Comments
Milkiewicz et al,[70] 2002	N = 12 M/F = 9:3 Median age 15.1 ± 1.4 y Median FU 38 mo Single-center series	No infectious complications (all had been colonized with *Pseudomonas aeruginosa*, <50% with *Candida* or other organism)	6–9 mo post-OLT mean FVC improved from 61% to 82%	—	100% at last follow-up	—
Fridell et al,[74] 2003	N = 12; median age 10.3 ± 4.5 y Median FU 8.7 y (0.07–15.7) Single-center series	7 out of 12 positive sputum cultures with various organisms One early death (retransplant for primary graft nonfunction, subsequently disseminated candidiasis and aspergillosis). No other infectious complications	No perioperative pulmonary complications; mean FEV$_1$ 73% ≥83% Mean FVC 78% ≥90% from pre-OLT to post-OLT	8 out of 12 tacrolimus 4 out of 12 cyclosporine	1 y 91.6% 5 y 75% 4 retransplants	• All patients had ascites, malnutrition, splenomegaly • 4 patients with variceal GI bleeding • All patients had Roux-en-Y anastomoses, no duct to duct
Barshes et al,[77] 2005	N = 11 M/F = 6:5 Median age 15 y (12–30 y) UNOS review 1987–2004 Combined LLTs	—	Median FEV$_1$, 30% ± 6% Median FVC 44% ± 12%	Variable immunosuppressive regimens with tacrolimus, cyclosporine, mycophenolate, and azathioprine, plus corticosteroids	79% (1 y) 63% (5 y) 3 out of 11 reported deaths: cardiac arrhythmia, viral infection, sepsis	• Median time 282 d on both the liver and the lung waiting lists • Median hospital stay 23.5 d (range 11–64 d)

Study	Demographics	Microbiology	Lung Function	Immunosuppression	Outcomes	Notes
Faro et al,[78] 2007 Kotru et al,[79] 2006	N = 5 Median age 13.6 y Combined LLTs	Pretransplant: all patients with positive sputum cultures, including MRSA, Pseudomonas, or Aspergillus, but no infectious complications	Median FEV_1 21% (14%–36%) Median FVC 29% (25%–50%) Lower lung rejection rates in LLT vs isolated lung transplant (0.2 vs 0.8 per patient year)	Cyclosporine, Azathioprine, and corticosteroids, with or without daclizumab as induction	One patient died POD 11 from liver failure and renal failure; 4 out of 5 alive at median 92 mo (43–112 mo) posttransplant. No cases of bronchiolitis obliterans in the surviving 4 LLT patients	• Median wait time 283 d • Median hospital stay 18 d (11–24 d) • Biliary complications in duct-to-duct anastomoses: 45% in CF vs 12% in non-CF OLT
Melzi et al,[75] 2006	N = 57 Median age 12.2 y (2–27 y) Median follow-up 3.7 y (0–11 y) Questionnaire to European centers Genotype known in 65%; 78% F508del CFRD in 21%	—	FEV_1 was available in 65%: >80% in 22%, 40%–80% in 67% <40% in 11% Half of the patients had post-OLT FEV_1 average increase of 5.9%	—	Alive at last follow-up: 76.7% Mortality higher (P = .02) in patients with FEV_1 <40% 6 mo before transplant	• Pancreatic insufficiency in 98% • Main indications: liver failure, hypersplenism, malnutrition, GI/variceal bleeding • Ascites in 32%
Nightingale et al,[80] 2010	N = 8 M/F = 6:2 Mean age 12.7 y (6.9–16.7 y) Mean FU 9.6 y (4.1–15.5 y) Single-center series	Pretransplant: Pseudomonas (7 out of 8) Aspergillus (3 out of 8) Candida (2 out of 8) Staphylococcus aureus (1 out of 8)	Pretransplant mean FEV_1 80% (59%–116%); generally stable after OLT	Cyclosporin 4 out of 8 Tacrolimus 4 out of 8	2 patients died in first 2 mo: 1 rejection, OKT3, fungemia 2 respiratory and renal failure; fungal infection 6 patients alive and well	• All patients had Roux-en-Y anastomoses, no duct to duct • Weight and BMI z-scores improved in 7 out of 8

(continued on next page)

Table 9
(continued)

	Patient Population	Colonization and Infection	Lung Function	Immunosuppression	Survival	Comments
Arnon et al,[68] 2011	N = 182 (<18 y) Male 63.2% Mean age (SD): 11.3 y (4.7) UNOS database 10/1987–05/2008	Bacterial peritonitis 1.6%	—	—	Graft survival: 1 y 78.6%, 5 y 69.8% Patient survival: 1 y 86.8%, 5 y 78.6%	Mortality: pulmonary, renal failure, hemorrhage, malignancy, graft loss, stroke
Mendizabal et al,[81] 2011	N = 148 (<18 y) Male 62.2% Mean age (SD): 11.1 y (4.7) UNOS database 1987–2008	—	—	—	Patient survival: 30 d 94.6%, 5 y 85.8%	Patient survival lower than for other metabolic or cholestatic liver diseases, but survival benefit by OLT compared with patients on waiting list
Miller et al,[82] 2012	N = 168 OLT and N = 840 no OLT Male 61.3% Mean age (SD): 16.5 y (6.5) 31% adults CF Foundation Patient Registry 1989–2007	P aeruginosa 79.2% B cepacia 5.4% Transplant and nontransplant patients were matched for status	FEV₁ declines after OLT at a rate similar to that of matched, nontransplant control patients with CF	—	3-y mortality after OLT 18.5%; cause of death is more likely liver-related or transplant related than cardiorespiratory	In the transplant group, the FEV₁ 3 y before OLT was lower than in controls but increased in the year before transplant

Study					
Harring et al,[83] 2013	N = 9 M/F 5:4 Age 9–17 y Single-center series One LLT and 1 heart-liver-lung transplant	One patient died from *Aspergillus fumigatus* sepsis 3 wk after transplant	Only baseline FEV_1 reported: 17.8%–92.0%	Induction with methylprednisolone; maintenance with prednisone, tacrolimus, and mycophenolate	1-y and 5-y patient and graft survival 88.9% Mean survival 69.2 mo One death on POD 21	One patient received a double lung transplant 4 y after OLT
Desai et al,[84] 2013	UNOS data October 1987 to August 2009: 294 patients (210 children), 265 of whom received OLT and 29 LLT OLT: 23.7% adults/76.2% children LLT: 72.4% adults/27.5% children	—	—	Comparing 2 eras (before and after tacrolimus), 10/87–12/94 and 01/95–08/09, there were no significant patient survival differences for OLT or LLT in children or adults	Pediatric patient survival (OLT): 1 y 85%, 5 y 75% Pediatric patient survival (LLT): 1 y 83%, 5 y 83% No difference in patient survival or graft survival between OLT and LLT in either age group	Causes of death in children: CF related, sepsis, bleeding, thrombosis, chronic rejection, de-novo autoimmune hepatitis, PTLD

Abbreviations: BMI, body mass index; CFRD, cystic fibrosis–related diabetes; FU, follow-up; FVC, forced vital capacity; MRSA, methicillin-resistant *Staphylococcus aureus*; OKT3, muromonab-CD3; POD, postoperative day.

SUMMARY

Bilateral LTx and OLT offer survival benefits to patients with end-stage CF lung or liver disease if selected appropriately and timed well.[88] It is not an easy path. The medical regimen is complex. The lifelong need to pay close attention to detail is intense and unrelenting. Although quality of life measures are heartening, outcomes as related to morbidity and mortality from complications remain poor and have not changed substantially in the last 20 years for LTx recipients.

It is hoped that, in CF, the emergence of new therapies, such as the genetic modulators, will prevent or so significantly slow the development of end-stage lung and liver disease that, in the near future, articles such as this on transplantation for children with CF will no longer be needed.

REFERENCES

1. Ramsey BW, Davies J, McElvaney NG, et al. A CFTR potentiator in patients with cystic fibrosis and the G551D mutation. N Engl J Med 2011;365(18):1663–72.
2. Wainwright CE, Elborn JS, Ramsey BW, et al. Lumacaftor-ivacaftor in patients with cystic fibrosis homozygous for Phe508del CFTR. N Engl J Med 2015;373(3):220–31.
3. Faro A, Mallory GB, Visner GA, et al. American Society of Transplantation executive summary on pediatric lung transplantation. Am J Transplant 2007;7(2): 285–92.
4. Kerem E, Reisman J, Corey M, et al. Prediction of mortality in patients with cystic fibrosis. N Engl J Med 1992;326(18):1187–91.
5. Liou TG, Adler FR, Cahill BC, et al. Survival effect of lung transplantation among patients with cystic fibrosis. JAMA 2001;286(21):2683–9.
6. Mayer-Hamblett N, Rosenfeld M, Emerson J, et al. Developing cystic fibrosis lung transplant referral criteria using predictors of 2-year mortality. Am J Respir Crit Care Med 2002;166(12 Pt 1):1550–5.
7. Weill D, Benden C, Corris PA, et al. A consensus document for the selection of lung transplant candidates: 2014–an update from the Pulmonary Transplantation Council of the International Society for Heart and Lung Transplantation. J Heart Lung Transplant 2015;34(1):1–15.
8. Alexander BD, Petzold EW, Reller LB, et al. Survival after lung transplantation of cystic fibrosis patients infected with *Burkholderia cepacia* complex. Am J Transplant 2008;8(5):1025–30.
9. Lobo LJ, Noone PG. Respiratory infections in patients with cystic fibrosis undergoing lung transplantation. Lancet Respir Med 2014;2(1):73–82.
10. Benden C, Goldfarb SB, Edwards LB, et al. The registry of the International Society for Heart and Lung Transplantation: seventeenth official pediatric lung and heart-lung transplantation report–2014; focus theme: retransplantation. J Heart Lung Transplant 2014;33(10):1025–33.
11. Liou TG, Adler FR, Cox DR, et al. Lung transplantation and survival in children with cystic fibrosis. N Engl J Med 2007;357(21):2143–52.
12. Sweet SC, Aurora P, Benden C, et al. Lung transplantation and survival in children with cystic fibrosis: solid statistics–flawed interpretation. Pediatr Transplant 2008; 12(2):129–36.
13. Braun AT, Dasenbrook EC, Shah AS, et al. Impact of lung allocation score on survival in cystic fibrosis lung transplant recipients. J Heart Lung Transplant 2015; 34(11):1436–41.
14. Huddleston CB. Pediatric lung transplantation. Semin Pediatr Surg 2006;15(3): 199–207.

15. Date H, Sato M, Aoyama A, et al. Living-donor lobar lung transplantation provides similar survival to cadaveric lung transplantation even for very ill patients. Eur J Cardiothorac Surg 2015;47(6):967–72 [discussion: 972–3].

16. Mead L, Danziger-Isakov LA, Michaels MG, et al. Antifungal prophylaxis in pediatric lung transplantation: an international multicenter survey. Pediatr Transplant 2014;18(4):393–7.

17. Danziger-Isakov LA, Faro A, Sweet S, et al. Variability in standard care for cytomegalovirus prevention and detection in pediatric lung transplantation: survey of eight pediatric lung transplant programs. Pediatr Transplant 2003;7(6):469–73.

18. Finlen Copeland CA, Davis WA, Snyder LD, et al. Long-term efficacy and safety of 12 months of valganciclovir prophylaxis compared with 3 months after lung transplantation: a single-center, long-term follow-up analysis from a randomized, controlled cytomegalovirus prevention trial. J Heart Lung Transplant 2011;30(9):990–6.

19. Miller GG, Dummer JS. Herpes simplex and varicella zoster viruses: forgotten but not gone. Am J Transplant 2007;7(4):741–7.

20. Withers AL. Management issues for adolescents with cystic fibrosis. Pulm Med 2012;2012:134132.

21. Ringewald JM, Gidding SS, Crawford SE, et al. Nonadherence is associated with late rejection in pediatric heart transplant recipients. J Pediatr 2001;139(1):75–8.

22. Bobanga ID, Vogt BA, Woodside KJ, et al. Outcome differences between young children and adolescents undergoing kidney transplantation. J Pediatr Surg 2015;50(6):996–9.

23. Khan MS, Zhang W, Taylor RA, et al. Survival in pediatric lung transplantation: the effect of center volume and expertise. J Heart Lung Transplant 2015;34(8):1073–81.

24. Leung MK, Rachakonda L, Weill D, et al. Effects of sinus surgery on lung transplantation outcomes in cystic fibrosis. Am J Rhinol 2008;22(2):192–6.

25. Vital D, Hofer M, Benden C, et al. Impact of sinus surgery on pseudomonal airway colonization, bronchiolitis obliterans syndrome and survival in cystic fibrosis lung transplant recipients. Respiration 2013;86(1):25–31.

26. Sole A, Salavert M. Fungal infections after lung transplantation. Curr Opin Pulm Med 2009;15(3):243–53.

27. Vadnerkar A, Clancy CJ, Celik U, et al. Impact of mold infections in explanted lungs on outcomes of lung transplantation. Transplantation 2010;89(2):253–60.

28. Danziger-Isakov LA, Worley S, Arrigain S, et al. Increased mortality after pulmonary fungal infection within the first year after pediatric lung transplantation. J Heart Lung Transplant 2008;27(6):655–61.

29. Danziger-Isakov LA, Worley S, Michaels MG, et al. The risk, prevention, and outcome of cytomegalovirus after pediatric lung transplantation. Transplantation 2009;87(10):1541–8.

30. Sharples LD, McNeil K, Stewart S, et al. Risk factors for bronchiolitis obliterans: a systematic review of recent publications. J Heart Lung Transplant 2002;21(2):271–81.

31. McCurdy LH, Milstone A, Dummer S. Clinical features and outcomes of paramyxoviral infection in lung transplant recipients treated with ribavirin. J Heart Lung Transplant 2003;22(7):745–53.

32. Doan ML, Mallory GB, Kaplan SL, et al. Treatment of adenovirus pneumonia with cidofovir in pediatric lung transplant recipients. J Heart Lung Transplant 2007;26(9):883–9.

33. Khalifah AP, Hachem RR, Chakinala MM, et al. Respiratory viral infections are a distinct risk for bronchiolitis obliterans syndrome and death. Am J Respir Crit Care Med 2004;170(2):181–7.

34. Danziger-Isakov LA, Arslan D, Sweet S, et al. RSV prevention and treatment in pediatric lung transplant patients: a survey of current practices among the International Pediatric Lung Transplant Collaborative. Pediatr Transplant 2012;16(6): 638–44.

35. Knoop C, Haverich A, Fischer S. Immunosuppressive therapy after human lung transplantation. Eur Respir J 2004;23(1):159–71.

36. Benden C, Faro A, Worley S, et al. Minimal acute rejection in pediatric lung transplantation–does it matter? Pediatr Transplant 2010;14(4):534–9.

37. Faro A, Visner G. The use of multiple transbronchial biopsies as the standard approach to evaluate lung allograft rejection. Pediatr Transplant 2004;8(4):322–8.

38. Visner GA, Faro A, Zander DS. Role of transbronchial biopsies in pediatric lung diseases. Chest 2004;126(1):273–80.

39. Wong JY, Westall GP, Snell GI. Bronchoscopic procedures and lung biopsies in pediatric lung transplant recipients. Pediatr Pulmonol 2015;50(12):1406–19.

40. Berry G, Burke M, Andersen C, et al. Pathology of pulmonary antibody-mediated rejection: 2012 update from the Pathology Council of the ISHLT. J Heart Lung Transplant 2013;32(1):14–21.

41. Witt CA, Gaut JP, Yusen RD, et al. Acute antibody-mediated rejection after lung transplantation. J Heart Lung Transplant 2013;32(10):1034–40.

42. Lobo LJ, Aris RM, Schmitz J, et al. Donor-specific antibodies are associated with antibody-mediated rejection, acute cellular rejection, bronchiolitis obliterans syndrome, and cystic fibrosis after lung transplantation. J Heart Lung Transplant 2013;32(1):70–7.

43. Hachem RR, Tiriveedhi V, Patterson GA, et al. Antibodies to K-alpha 1 tubulin and collagen V are associated with chronic rejection after lung transplantation. Am J Transplant 2012;12(8):2164–71.

44. Safavi S, Robinson DR, Soresi S, et al. De novo donor HLA-specific antibodies predict development of bronchiolitis obliterans syndrome after lung transplantation. J Heart Lung Transplant 2014;33(12):1273–81.

45. Baum C, Reichenspurner H, Deuse T. Bortezomib rescue therapy in a patient with recurrent antibody-mediated rejection after lung transplantation. J Heart Lung Transplant 2013;32(12):1270–1.

46. Choong CK, Sweet SC, Zoole JB, et al. Bronchial airway anastomotic complications after pediatric lung transplantation: incidence, cause, management, and outcome. J Thorac Cardiovasc Surg 2006;131(1):198–203.

47. Prokai A, Fekete A, Pasti K, et al. The importance of different immunosuppressive regimens in the development of posttransplant diabetes mellitus. Pediatr Diabetes 2012;13(1):81–91.

48. Robinson PD, Shroff RC, Spencer H. Renal complications following lung and heart-lung transplantation. Pediatr Nephrol 2013;28(3):375–86.

49. Wong M, Mallory GB Jr, Goldstein J, et al. Neurologic complications of pediatric lung transplantation. Neurology 1999;53(7):1542–9.

50. Vaughn BV, Ali II, Olivier KN, et al. Seizures in lung transplant recipients. Epilepsia 1996;37(12):1175–9.

51. Sato M. Chronic lung allograft dysfunction after lung transplantation: the moving target. Gen Thorac Cardiovasc Surg 2013;61(2):67–78.

52. Estenne M, Maurer JR, Boehler A, et al. Bronchiolitis obliterans syndrome 2001: an update of the diagnostic criteria. J Heart Lung Transplant 2002;21(3):297–310.

53. Towe C, Chester Ogborn A, Ferkol T, et al. Bronchiolitis obliterans syndrome is not specific for bronchiolitis obliterans in pediatric lung transplant. J Heart Lung Transplant 2015;34(4):516–21.

54. Sato M, Waddell TK, Wagnetz U, et al. Restrictive allograft syndrome (RAS): a novel form of chronic lung allograft dysfunction. J Heart Lung Transplant 2011; 30(7):735–42.

55. Glanville AR, Aboyoun CL, Havryk A, et al. Severity of lymphocytic bronchiolitis predicts long-term outcome after lung transplantation. Am J Respir Crit Care Med 2008;177(9):1033–40.

56. Daud SA, Yusen RD, Meyers BF, et al. Impact of immediate primary lung allograft dysfunction on bronchiolitis obliterans syndrome. Am J Respir Crit Care Med 2007;175(5):507–13.

57. Davis RD Jr, Lau CL, Eubanks S, et al. Improved lung allograft function after fundoplication in patients with gastroesophageal reflux disease undergoing lung transplantation. J Thorac Cardiovasc Surg 2003;125(3):533–42.

58. Girnita AL, Duquesnoy R, Yousem SA, et al. HLA-specific antibodies are risk factors for lymphocytic bronchiolitis and chronic lung allograft dysfunction. Am J Transplant 2005;5(1):131–8.

59. Vanaudenaerde BM, Meyts I, Vos R, et al. A dichotomy in bronchiolitis obliterans syndrome after lung transplantation revealed by azithromycin therapy. Eur Respir J 2008;32(4):832–43.

60. Morrell MR, Despotis GJ, Lublin DM, et al. The efficacy of photopheresis for bronchiolitis obliterans syndrome after lung transplantation. J Heart Lung Transplant 2010;29(4):424–31.

61. Cohen AH, Sweet SC, Mendeloff E, et al. High incidence of posttransplant lymphoproliferative disease in pediatric patients with cystic fibrosis. Am J Respir Crit Care Med 2000;161(4 Pt 1):1252–5.

62. Lehr CJ, Zaas DW, Cheifetz IM, et al. Ambulatory extracorporeal membrane oxygenation as a bridge to lung transplantation: walking while waiting. Chest 2015;147(5):1213–8.

63. Krutsinger D, Reed RM, Blevins A, et al. Lung transplantation from donation after cardiocirculatory death: a systematic review and meta-analysis. J Heart Lung Transplant 2015;34(5):675–84.

64. Tikkanen JM, Cypel M, Machuca TN, et al. Functional outcomes and quality of life after normothermic ex vivo lung perfusion lung transplantation. J Heart Lung Transplant 2015;34(4):547–56.

65. Colombo C, Battezzati PM, Crosignani A, et al. Liver disease in cystic fibrosis: a prospective study on incidence, risk factors, and outcome. Hepatology 2002; 36(6):1374–82.

66. Efrati O, Barak A, Modan-Moses D, et al. Liver cirrhosis and portal hypertension in cystic fibrosis. Eur J Gastroenterol Hepatol 2003;15(10):1073–8.

67. Lin H, Alonso EM, Superina RA, et al. General criteria for transplantation in children. In: Busuttil RW, Klintmalm GB, editors. Transplantation of the liver. Philadelphia: Elsevier/Saunders; 2015. p. 270–87.

68. Arnon R, Annunziato RA, Miloh T, et al. Liver and combined lung and liver transplantation for cystic fibrosis: analysis of the UNOS database. Pediatr Transplant 2011;15(3):254–64.

69. Noble-Jamieson G, Barnes N, Jamieson N, et al. Liver transplantation for hepatic cirrhosis in cystic fibrosis. J R Soc Med 1996;89(Suppl 27):31–7.

70. Milkiewicz P, Skiba G, Kelly D, et al. Transplantation for cystic fibrosis: outcome following early liver transplantation. J Gastroenterol Hepatol 2002;17(2):208–13.

71. Gooding I, Dondos V, Gyi KM, et al. Variceal hemorrhage and cystic fibrosis: outcomes and implications for liver transplantation. Liver Transpl 2005;11(12): 1522–6.

72. Nash KL, Collier JD, French J, et al. Cystic fibrosis liver disease: to transplant or not to transplant? Am J Transplant 2008;8(1):162–9.

73. Colombo C, Costantini D, Rocchi A, et al. Effects of liver transplantation on the nutritional status of patients with cystic fibrosis. Transpl Int 2005;18(2):246–55.

74. Fridell JA, Bond GJ, Mazariegos GV, et al. Liver transplantation in children with cystic fibrosis: a long-term longitudinal review of a single center's experience. J Pediatr Surg 2003;38(8):1152–6.

75. Melzi ML, Kelly DA, Colombo C, et al. Liver transplant in cystic fibrosis: a poll among European centers. A study from the European Liver Transplant Registry. Transpl Int 2006;19(9):726–31.

76. Molmenti EP, Squires RH, Nagata D, et al. Liver transplantation for cholestasis associated with cystic fibrosis in the pediatric population. Pediatr Transplant 2003;7(2):93–7.

77. Barshes NR, DiBardino DJ, McKenzie ED, et al. Combined lung and liver transplantation: The United States Experience. Transplantation 2005;80(9):1161–7.

78. Faro A, Shepherd R, Huddleston CB, et al. Lower incidence of bronchiolitis obliterans in pediatric liver-lung transplant recipients with cystic fibrosis. Transplantation 2007;83(11):1435–9.

79. Kotru A, Sheperd R, Nadler M, et al. Combined lung and liver transplantation: the United States experience. Transplantation 2006;82(1):144–5 [author reply: 145].

80. Nightingale S, O'Loughlin EV, Dorney SF, et al. Isolated liver transplantation in children with cystic fibrosis–an Australian experience. Pediatr Transplant 2010; 14(6):779–85.

81. Mendizabal M, Reddy KR, Cassuto J, et al. Liver transplantation in patients with cystic fibrosis: analysis of United Network for Organ Sharing data. Liver Transpl 2011;17(3):243–50.

82. Miller MR, Sokol RJ, Narkewicz MR, et al. Pulmonary function in individuals who underwent liver transplantation: from the US cystic fibrosis foundation registry. Liver Transpl 2012;18(5):585–93.

83. Harring TR, Nguyen NT, Liu H, et al. Liver transplantation in cystic fibrosis: a report from Baylor College of Medicine and the Texas Children's Hospital. Pediatr Transplant 2013;17(3):271–7.

84. Desai CS, Gruessner A, Habib S, et al. Survival of cystic fibrosis patients undergoing liver and liver-lung transplantations. Transplant Proc 2013;45(1):290–2.

85. Ng VL, Fecteau A, Shepherd R, et al. Outcomes of 5-year survivors of pediatric liver transplantation: report on 461 children from a North American multicenter registry. Pediatrics 2008;122(6):e1128–35.

86. Bodewes FA, van der Doef HP, Houwen RH, et al. Increase of serum gamma-glutamyltransferase associated with development of cirrhotic cystic fibrosis liver disease. J Pediatr Gastroenterol Nutr 2015;61(1):113–8.

87. Leung DH, Ye W, Molleston JP, et al. Baseline ultrasound and clinical correlates in children with cystic fibrosis. J Pediatr 2015;167(4):862–8.e2.

88. Hofer M, Benden C, Inci I, et al. True survival benefit of lung transplantation for cystic fibrosis patients: the Zurich experience. J Heart Lung Transplant 2009; 28(4):334–9.

Psychosocial Challenges/Transition to Adulthood

Carla Frederick, MD

KEYWORDS

• Cystic fibrosis • Transition • Adolescence • Psychosocial

KEY POINTS

• Amazing advancements in the last 20 years afford individuals with CF the opportunity to lead longer, fuller lives.
• The process of transitioning adolescents to adult CF care programs needs to be optimized.
• Adolescent and adult CF care providers need to consider the growing list of psychosocial needs that individuals with CF will encounter.

BACKGROUND

Individuals with cystic fibrosis (CF) are living longer and more active lives. Thanks to medical advances from new drugs, such as inhaled antibiotics, mucus-modifying agents, and the most recent development of CF transmembrane conductance regulator modulator therapies, the median age of survival continues to rise, reaching 39.3 years of age in 2014. Adults now comprise 50.7% of the CF population (**Figs. 1** and **2**).[1,2] There was a time when pediatric CF programs were able to provide care for adults with CF. Adults were not a large portion of their practice, they did not typically have complications outside of the pulmonary or gastrointestinal tract, and they had a long-standing trusting relationship with their pediatric providers. In the 1990s when it became increasingly apparent that transition of adults was needed, adult CF care centers were few and far between. This prompted the Cystic Fibrosis Foundation (CFF), which accredits CF care centers around the United States, to mandate that all centers with more than 40 adults establish an adult program by the year 2000. This mandate was met with some resistance but today with more than half of individuals with CF being older than the age of 18, there is a well-established network of adult programs to care for this population.

Disclosure Statement: The author has nothing to disclose.
Department of Medicine, WCHOB Lung & Cystic Fibrosis Center, State University of New York at Buffalo, 219 Bryant Street, Buffalo, NY 14222, USA
E-mail address: cfrederick@upa.chob.edu

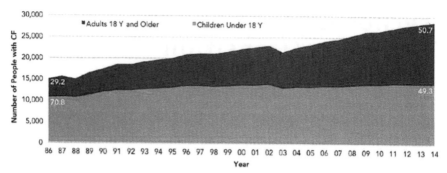

Fig. 1. Number of children and adults with CF: 1986 to 2014. (*From* Cystic Fibrosis Foundation Patient Registry. 2014 Annual Data Report. Bethesda, Maryland; ©2015 Cystic Fibrosis Foundation.)

Pediatric and adult programs are developing expertise and more enthusiastic attitudes in the area of transition.[3] The existence of adult programs and the aging of adults bring a variety of additional clinical questions and concerns to surface. When should an individual be transitioned from a pediatric to an adult program? What skills do teenagers need to care for themselves as young adults? What kind of infrastructure is necessary within a CF care center to make transition successfully happen? How will individuals with CF feel about this change? How will parents and caretakers adjust to transition? The answers to these questions are not black and white. Each CF care center has a unique population and structural set-up that demands customization of transition to best suit their needs. CF care centers across the country differ dramatically in size, geography, and socioeconomic composition. However, common components of transition include early introduction of the topic of transition; fostering skills of independence and self-management; education about CF and adult-focused issues, such as employment and fertility; introduction to adult care team members and making adult care facility tours available; and recognition of the emotional component of transition. A timeline (**Fig. 3**) may be helpful to conceptualize the process.

TRANSITION TO ADULTHOOD

The American Academy of Pediatrics defines transition as "the planned movement of adolescents with chronic medical conditions to adult health care with the goal to

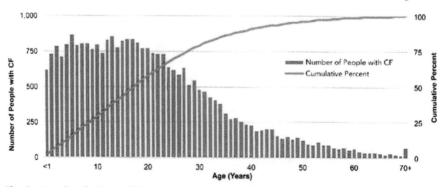

Fig. 2. Age distribution of CF population in 2014. (*From* Cystic Fibrosis Foundation Patient Registry. 2014 Annual Data Report. Bethesda, Maryland; ©2015 Cystic Fibrosis Foundation.)

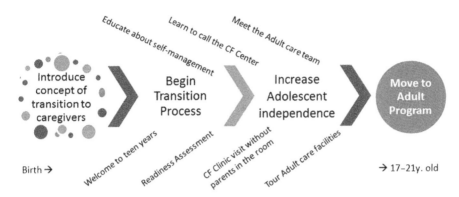

Fig. 3. Transition timeline.

maximize lifelong functioning and potential through the provision of high-quality, developmentally-appropriate health care services that continue uninterrupted as the individual moves from adolescence to adulthood."[4] Note that "transition" is a dynamic process over time as opposed to "transfer," which is a single point in time entailing the hand-off of care from one provider to another. Successful transition is broken down into two main categories: preparation of the individual with CF and family, and preparation of the adult CF care center.

Preparation of Individuals with Cystic Fibrosis and Their Families

Individuals with CF and their families need to be aware that transition to an adult care program takes place as a normal part of growing up just like graduating from one school to another. Before a child sets foot in high school or college, he or she goes through years of education to develop a base of knowledge and often a specific orientation to help him or her become familiar with the new environment. Learning about transition well before it happens can help prepare an individual. Transfer to an adult care center cannot be abruptly announced when someone turns 18 without creating confusion, reluctance, and a variety of other untoward emotions. Early discussion of transition, even in the first years of life, can be framed as a picture of optimism and expectation of an independent adult future.

Preparing individuals with CF and their caregivers for transition involves providing clear expectations, ongoing education, introducing them to adult care team members and facilities, and recognizing commonly encountered emotions. Expectations delivered are two-fold. First, individuals with CF should expect to live well into adulthood and should hear that message early and often from their pediatric care team. The communication of this expectation affords individuals and their families the opportunity to plan for the future instead of having tunnel vision for the present time. Adolescence is a hazardous time for individuals with chronic medical conditions. Several challenges to be expected are listed in **Table 1**.[5] Normal adult development involves maturing into a mindset that extends past the adolescent attitude of immediate self-gratification. Taking this into account, if hope for the future is nonexistent, an adolescent may engage in higher risk, pleasure-driven behaviors rather than more responsible health-sustaining actions. Thus, the introduction of transition to adult care should be rooted in the expectation that people with CF need to develop self-care skills to support them in their later years.

Table 1
Adolescent challenges and the potential impact of CF

Adolescent Challenges	Potential Impact of/on CF
Rapid physical growth	Delayed growth (height and weight gain) Decreased body fat (especially women) Prevalence of eating disorders may exceed that of the general population
Pubertal changes	Delay in genital development (male) Delay in menarche (female)
Sexual development	Delay in dating and sexual relationships Sexual dysfunction Misunderstanding of fertility Issues with reproduction
Development of personal identity	Poor body image Low self-esteem and self-concept
Autonomy and independence	Dependency Parental overprotection
Development of interpersonal relationships	Social isolation Difficulty forming intimate relationships Fear of rejection leading to secrecy about illness
Planning for the future	Increased uncertainty of future Decreased expectations for self Delay in planning for future Need for realistic planning Use of denial as coping strategy
Risk-taking behavior	Sexual and substance abuse may be less than in general population, but still present Poor adherence to medications and therapy

The second layer of expectations to be delivered in the process of transition are the specifics of when transfer of care will take place and what is required for successful navigation of the adult care program. Setting a goal age or time of transfer, commonly at age 18 or after high school, is akin to establishing another milestone that occurs with age, such as driving, voting, or graduation. A concrete timeframe can help normalize the change that will take place and highlight its importance and improve patient satisfaction.[6] Along with establishing a set time for transfer, communication of basic skills that are expected for independence in an adult care program is helpful. These expectations and self-identified competencies have been presented and measured in several ways. Questionnaires and checklists have been implemented by some CF centers (**Fig. 4**). Initiation of readiness assessments early in the process of transition can allow for targeted education and intervention in areas that need improvement while providing a framework of what is expected in an adult care program. Care teams may find that the more difficult parties to transition are the parents of an individual with CF because of the intense investment of time, energy, and emotion to maintain their child's health. For that reason, assessment of parent readiness may be beneficial given a specific center's needs (**Fig. 5**). These checklists in themselves are intended to be tools for organizing the many facets of transition that need to be addressed before moving from one care program to the next. Sawicki[7] developed and studied a Transition Readiness Assessment Questionnaire. In analysis it was found that 70% of youth and 67% of parents believed that they/their child could manage their care but less than half of them reported thinking about health care transition to

Use the following scale to rank your answers to the statements below

1 = No way	2 = Once in a while	3 = Maybe	4 = Most of the time	5 = Yes, for sure

	1	2	3	4	5	Comments
I can describe my CF to others						
If I don't understand something about CF I know where to get information						
I know how my health may change in the future						
I speak up for myself and tell others what I need						
I prepare and take my own breathing/respiratory treatments						
I prepare and take my own medications (pills, enzymes...)						
When I get sick I know how to get the help that I need						
I make my own phone calls to the CF Center if...						
... I am sick						
...I need an appointment						
... I need medication refills						
I take part in health care discussions about me						
I understand how my CF will affect the way I develop through puberty						
I have thought about a career and am working towards it						
I am aware of the risks if I use alcohol, drugs or cigarettes						

Do you have any questions or thoughts about transition? Please write them below.

_____

_____

_____

_____

Name:_____   Date Completed: _____

Fig. 4. Patient readiness checklist.

adulthood and less than one-third had a plan to transition. These findings illustrate the sparse understanding of the process of transition and support the fact that more work needs to be done to prepare individuals with CF and their families for this major life change.

Self-management is the set of behaviors that help individuals to choose, monitor, and sustain daily treatment and to manage the effects of illness on their lives. Education about CF and self-management skills can build the foundation for successful transition. A variety of resources are available from the CF Patient Resource Center that can be used spanning all age ranges.[8] Ensuring that individuals know how different medications and therapies work can help them understand their treatment regimen. Education alone, however, does not guarantee adherence to a treatment regimen,[9]

Use the following scale to rank your answers to the statements below						
1 = No way	2 = Once in a while		3 = Maybe		4 = Most of the time	5 = Yes, for sure

	1	2	3	4	5	Comments
My child understands what CF is and can describe it to others						
I understand CF and can describe it to others						
My child knows how CF may affect his/her health in the future						
My child speaks up *to tell me* what he/she needs						
My child speaks up *to tell members of the CF team (doctors, nurses, respiratory therapist, nutritionist, social work)* what he/she needs						
I feel comfortable leaving the room during a CF clinic visit						
My child prepares and takes his/her own breathing treatments						
My child prepares and takes his/her own medications (pills, enzymes)						
I feel comfortable with my child preparing his/her own breathing treatments and medications						
When my child gets sick, he/she knows how to get the help that he/she needs						
My child makes his/her own phone calls to the CF Center when he/she...						
...is sick						
...needs an appointment						
...needs medication refills						
I feel comfortable with my child making his/her own phone calls to the CF Center when he/she...						
...is sick						
...needs an appointment						
...needs medication refills						
My child takes part in health care discussions						
I have talked to my child about the risks of alcohol, drugs, and cigarettes						

Name:_____   Date Completed: _____

Fig. 5. Parent readiness checklist.

which is a challenge that spans all ages. Assessment of barriers to adherence is a major upcoming goal of the Success with Therapies Research Consortium of the CFF.[10,11] Although not strong, a recent Cochrane Review found some evidence to suggest that self-management education may result in positively changing a small number of behaviors in patients and caregivers.[12]

It is important for teenagers to meet the adult CF care team. An ideal concept that some larger centers may be able to use is that of a dedicated transition clinic. A transition clinic is one where both pediatric and adult providers see patients in the same visit along with the multidisciplinary team of therapists and ancillary staff to allow for maximum overlap of care. For most centers, logistics do not allow for this to be a practical consideration. It has been shown that some overlap in involvement of pediatric and adult providers that is achieved by a transition clinic or other means results in improved satisfaction among young adults with CF.[13–15] Adult providers can often make a point to meet individuals and their families in the pediatric clinic setting before the first official adult clinic appointment. Hospital and clinic tours guided by either pediatric or adult care team members can help transitioning individuals gain familiarity in their new health care environment.[16] Regular meetings with pediatric and adult care providers focused on discussing individuals in the process of transition can help foster a collaborative effort to attend to the most active issues in an adolescent's health care.[17,18]

Emotions surrounding transition vary from pride and excitement to anxiety and reluctance to leave a long and trusted relationship. Parents and patients may have divergent feelings about transition. Validation of these emotions and appreciation of the sensitivity of the time should be considered. At the same time, pediatric and adult providers should aim to foster self-efficacy and independence and convey confidence in the necessity and importance of transitioning. In other chronic disease populations, overprotection has been associated with decreased quality of life, whereas self-efficacy is associated with a sense of well-being.[19] In general, when effort is made to create a formal transition process to a well-established program, patients and parents report satisfaction.[6,20] Further discussion of mental health in this age population and depression and anxiety screening is found later in this article.

Preparation of the Adult Cystic Fibrosis Care Center

All CF centers with more than 40 adults are required to have an adult CF program. The requirements of an adult program as established by the CFF Care Center Accreditation Committee are as follows:

- Physician leadership: appropriately trained physicians with CF care experience
- A multidisciplinary team: ideally as many of the following ancillary care providers as possible: respiratory therapist, dietician, social worker, pharmacist, physical therapist, psychologist, case manager, patient advocate, chaplain
- Participation in the CFF National Patient Registry (CFF-NPR)
- Compliance with clinical and research requirements

Adult care providers face many challenges and this is one reason why transition can be difficult. Support received from adult institutions for care of individuals with CF and other chronic illnesses is often less than that of their pediatric counterparts in the outpatient and inpatient realms. As the adult population grows, it is essential to have access to resources necessary to maintain excellence in care for this increasingly complex and aging population.

Although there has been much center-based research on transition perceptions and practices, there is a paucity of data regarding the relationship of transition processes and health care outcomes. One small study did demonstrate that formal transition process avoided negative health outcomes during this time of change[21] but larger scale studies are needed to identify which if any of these interventions lead to improved patient outcomes. There is no one-size-fits-all approach to achieving success in transition; however, the CF care team needs to be thoughtful in planning out how the process of transition will take place over time and ensure their population has an appropriately resourced center.

PSYCHOLOGICAL EFFECTS OF LIVING WITH CYSTIC FIBROSIS

In addition to the task of successful transition to adult care centers, there are a variety of psychosocial issues encountered in caring for adolescents and adults with CF.

Depression and anxiety, the complexity of navigating the health care system and insurance, employment considerations, living independently, and starting a family are among many challenges that individuals now commonly encounter with longer lives. Many people with CF are resilient, courageous, and even seemingly motivated by their existential dilemma. That being said, children and adults with chronic medical conditions have been shown to be at increased risk for depression and anxiety.[22,23] Several studies have examined the specific prevalence of these conditions in individuals with CF. Many of these studies conducted with small sample sizes found increased rates of depression and anxiety in the CF population. To gather more robust data the most complete study to date, The International Depression Epidemiologic Study (TIDES), was completed in 2014.[24] This massive collaborative effort screened 1286 adolescents and 4739 adults with CF and 4102 parent caregivers for symptoms of depression and anxiety. Two well-validated tools, the Center for Epidemiologic Studies Depression Scale and Hospital Anxiety and Depression Scale, were used to screen for depression and anxiety, respectively. Results of this study showed screens positive for depression in 10% of adolescents, 19% of adults, and more than 30% of parent caregivers (**Fig. 6**). Screens positive for anxiety were found in 22% of adolescents, 32% of adults, 36% of fathers, and 48% of mothers (**Fig. 7**).

Depression and anxiety are associated with negative clinical consequences. Psychological distress in CF is associated with decreased health-related quality of life,[25,26] decreased adherence to prescribed therapies,[27,28] decreased pulmonary function,[2,29] increased hospitalization, and increased health care costs.[30] Several risk factors for depression and anxiety were identified with these data including older age; female gender; lower pulmonary function; lower body mass index; and recent changes in health status, such as receiving intravenous antibiotics, hemoptysis, or pneumothorax. Given the important clinical implications and the high yield of identifying treatable diagnoses, the International Committee on Mental Health in Cystic Fibrosis, a multidisciplinary committee formed in 2013, created the CFF and European Cystic Fibrosis Society consensus statements for screening and treating depression and anxiety.[31] Recommendation statements, all of which received 100% consensus, are seen in **Box 1**. After implementation of these guidelines and prescribing appropriate treatment, the next step is to assess improvement in specific health outcomes and identify areas that are still in need of more targeted intervention. Limited data

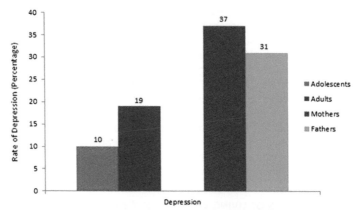

Fig. 6. Depression in patients with CF. (*Data from* Quittner A. Prevalence of depression and anxiety in patients with cystic fibrosis and parent caregivers: results of The International Depression Epidemiological Study across nine countries. Thorax 2014;69:1090–7.)

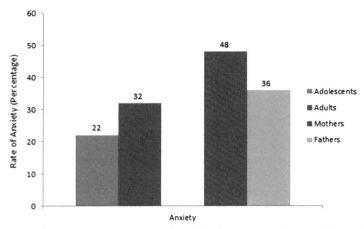

Fig. 7. Anxiety in patients with CF. (*Data from* Quittner A. Prevalence of depression and anxiety in patients with cystic fibrosis and parent caregivers: results of The International Depression Epidemiological Study across nine countries. Thorax 2014;69:1090–7.)

suggest that this process of screening, monitoring, and treatment does in fact reduce rates of depression.[32] In addition, the process of screening for depression has been demonstrated to be successfully disseminated and implemented across care centers and achieved excellent patient and parent satisfaction.[33]

Chronic illness can lead to feelings of "otherness" and a recent recommendation from the CFF concerning infection prevention and control may add to this. Guidelines for infection prevention and control were published by the CFF in 2013.[34] To avoid cross-contamination and exchanging potentially harmful pathogens, individuals with CF are recommended to be physically isolated from one another. The psychological implications of isolation include feelings of being ostracized and the inability to seek physical contact with others who share similar disease-related challenges. Social media, blogs, telemedicine, and video conferencing are potential ways to obviate these restrictions but optimization and acceptance of these methods is still a work in process.[35]

SOCIAL AND ECONOMIC EFFECTS OF LIVING WITH CHRONIC ILLNESS

Living with CF has several unique social and economic consequences. The treatment burden for individuals with CF and their families often increases over time. Morbidity and mortality have been demonstrated to be related to socioeconomic status even after adjusting for prescription practices and other potential confounders.[36] Disparities in allocation of lung transplantation have also been shown to be related to poverty.[37] This problem is not unique to CF but is one to be mentioned and in need of attention. Access to care and prescribed medication are barriers that can affect each individual with CF. The CFF has a variety of resources to assist families.[38] Social workers are part of each care team and can assist in overcoming these obstacles that can adversely affect patient outcomes.

PLANNING A LIFE WITH CYSTIC FIBROSIS
Education and Career Choices

Education and career choices involve a unique set of considerations for an individual with CF. Individuals with CF attain a variety of educational achievements as is

Box 1
Recommendation statement

1. For all individuals with CF and caregivers, the CFF/European Cystic Fibrosis Society International Committee on Mental Health (ICMH) recommends that ongoing education and preventative, supportive interventions, such as training in stress management and the development of coping skills, aligned with appropriate developmental stage and disease events be offered.

2. For all individuals with CF undergoing medical procedures, the ICMH recommends that behavioral approaches be used to reduce the risk of distress.

3. The ICMH recommends that children with CF ages 7 to 11 be clinically evaluated for depression and anxiety when caregiver depression or anxiety scores are elevated, or when significant symptoms of depression or anxiety in the child are reported or observed by patients, caregivers, or members of the CF multidisciplinary teams.

4. The ICMH recommends annual screening for depression and anxiety with the Patient Health Questionnaire (PHQ)-9 and Generalized Anxiety Disorder (GAD)-7 for adolescents and adults with CF (ages 12 to adulthood).

5. The ICMH recommends offering annual screening for depression and anxiety to *at least* one primary caregiver of children and adolescents with CF (ages 0–17) using one of the following approaches, depending on staffing and resources:
   a. Screening with the PHQ-9 and GAD-2
   b. Screening with the PHQ-8 and GAD-7
   c. Screening with the PHQ-2 and GAD-2

6. The ICMH recommends that any treatment of depression and anxiety in individuals with CF and caregivers be based on clinical diagnosis.
   a. A health care provider with appropriate training and expertise should evaluate the clinical significance of elevated screening scores and presenting symptoms to perform a differential diagnosis before initiating treatment.

7. For caregivers of individuals with CF who have clinically significant symptoms of depression/anxiety, the ICMH recommends referral for treatment to primary care or mental health services after initial assessment with the CF team.

8. For all individuals with CF and symptoms of depression/anxiety, the ICMH recommends a flexible, stepped care model of clinical intervention developed and implemented in close collaboration with patients and caregivers, the multidisciplinary CF team, and other treatment providers or consultants, such as primary care or mental health specialist.
   a. CF teams must identify who will be responsible to initiate and coordinate care and monitor treatment effects.

9. The ICMH recommends that in children with CF ages 7 to 11, who have clinically significant depression or anxiety, evidence-based psychological interventions are recommended as the first-line treatment.

10. For individuals with CF ages 12 to adulthood and mild depression or anxiety symptoms, the ICMH recommends education about depression/anxiety, preventative or supportive interventions, and rescreening at the next clinic visit.

11. For individuals with CF ages 12 to adulthood and moderate depression or anxiety, the ICMH recommends offering or providing a referral of evidence-based psychological interventions, including cognitive behavior therapy or interpersonal therapy.
   a. When psychological intervention is unavailable, declined, or not fully effective, antidepressant treatment should be considered.

12. For individuals with CF ages 12 to adulthood and severe depression, the ICMH recommends use of combined evidence-based psychological intervention and antidepressant pharmacotherapy.

13. For individuals with CF ages 12 to adulthood and severe anxiety, the ICMH recommends offering exposure-based CBT.
   a. When exposure-based CBT is unavailable, declined, or not fully effective, antidepressant medications can be considered.

14. The ICMH recommends that the selective serotonin reuptake inhibitors citalopram, escitalopram, sertraline, and fluoxetine are appropriate first-line antidepressants for most individuals with CF, ages 12 to adulthood, requiring pharmacotherapy.
    a. In selecting an antidepressant and adjusting its dosage, close monitoring of therapeutic effects, adverse effects, drug-drug interactions, and medical comorbidities is recommended.
15. The ICMH recommends that lorazepam be considered for short-term use in individuals with CF with moderate-to-severe anxiety symptoms, associated with medical procedures, who have not responded to behavioral approaches.

demonstrated by annual CFF-NPR data.[1] Results of 2014 CFF-NPR data showed that 24.2% of adults obtained a high school diploma, 33% completed some college, 28.8% received a college degree, and 7% earned a masters or doctoral level degree. This range of accomplishment demonstrates the great potential of adults with this chronic disease. Completion of high school and pursuit of postsecondary education is a benefit in itself regardless of the subsequent vocational implications.[39] Those that are able to balance physical and emotional health should be encouraged to seek formal education if desired. Disease severity may make this goal challenging; however, disease severity in itself should not be a reason to avoid higher education efforts. CF center social workers can often provide information regarding available educational financial assistance. In addition to seeking financial counsel, young adults with CF pursuing postsecondary education should consider the college or university location. Remote and online classes are available through many institutions that may be convenient. If an individual is considering an out of town location for postsecondary education, identification of an accredited CF care center so that health information can be shared and investigating insurance coverage of health care services in the area should be done before enrollment. Colleges are obligated to follow Section 504 of the Rehabilitation Act of 1973, which states that no entity that receives federal funds can discriminate against a person based on disability. This protects students at colleges from discrimination based on their disease and requires that appropriate accommodations are made. Individuals with CF can receive helpful assistance from an Office of Disabled Students at many universities and colleges, such as a private air-conditioned room, a reduction in minimum hours required each semester if necessary, parking privileges on campus, and the foreknowledge that alternative methods of obtaining assignments or taking examinations may be necessary based on health-related absences. A CF center social worker may need to provide documentation of the student's disability to acquire the specific accommodations that help achieve success.

Vocational Planning

According to the 2014 CFF-NPR, 35.3% of adults with CF were working full time, 11.6% were working part time; 25.3% were students, and 4.4% were homemakers.[1] Early in life, optimally as the concept of transition is introduced, parents should be informed that career planning will be necessary as their child grows older. The CF care center team should be proactive about discussing the implications of CF on career planning. Pursuit of a given career should be based on an individual's interests and aptitude. Physical abilities and environmental risks should be considered; however, there are few careers that are strictly not recommended for people with CF. Government-funded vocational rehabilitation programs are available in all states at no cost and provide job training, placement, and assistance with school tuition.

Logistical features of career opportunities for individuals with CF that are helpful to consider include the benefits package offered by the employer, disability insurance coverage, life insurance, flexibility in work hours, flexible use of vacation and sick leave, additional paid or unpaid sick time, and the option of working from home. Other factors to take into account include consideration of exposures that may adversely affect health in a particular career setting. Work environments that have pulmonary irritants, exposure to viruses, such as working with young children, or employment with high stress can adversely impact physical well-being. A balance of these considerations with the life-goals of the individual with CF is necessary on an individualized basis to arrive at the best solution.

Family Planning and Pregnancy

Another challenge somewhat different than their peers that young adults with CF face is that of family planning and pregnancy. Anticipatory counseling of teenagers concerning sexuality and reproduction needs to include these issues. Men with CF have normal sexual pleasure and function; however, they are usually infertile secondary to absence of the vas deferens. Traditional fertility is found in 1% to 2% of men, many of whom are diagnosed in adulthood.[40–42] For those men who are not able to conceive naturally, artificial insemination with donor sperm, or microsurgical epididymal aspiration of spermatozoa with intracytoplasmic sperm injection into the oocyte are ways to achieve the goal of becoming a biologic father. Adoption is another option for those who are not interested in or able to pursue these options.

Women with CF have slightly lower rates of fertility than women without CF; however, many can become pregnant.[43,44] Reproductive anatomy is not altered in women with CF but rather thicker cervical mucus with decreased water content and rheologic properties are the proposed mechanisms for a relative challenge in achieving conception. Nonetheless, more than 200 women per year with CF have successful pregnancies (**Fig. 8**).[1] All children are obligate carriers; the risk of children having CF depends on the father's carrier status. Women seeking pregnancy should be referred to a high-risk obstetrician; however, given the low number of women with CF seen in their practice, most require partnership in management with the CF center for optimal care. Awareness of physiologic hemodynamic changes during pregnancy, careful assessment of CF maintenance medications, attention to the increased complexity

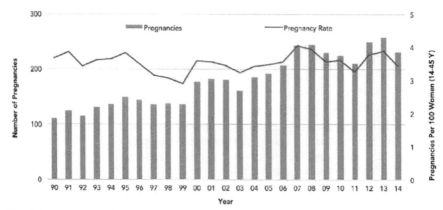

Fig. 8. Pregnancies and pregnancy rates in women ages 14 to 45 years with CF 1990 to 2014. (*From* Cystic Fibrosis Foundation Patient Registry. 2014 Annual Data Report. Bethesda, Maryland; ©2015 Cystic Fibrosis Foundation.)

of CF-related diabetes, and the need for prompt and aggressive treatment of increased pulmonary symptomatology is necessary for maintenance of health during pregnancy.

Education regarding contraception and fertility is a responsibility of the primary care and CF provider. Men with CF should not assume they are infertile but rather have semen analysis to assess for natural reproductive potential. Methods of contraception for women with CF are largely similar to those for women without CF. However, it is important to consider the decrease in efficacy of hormonal methods of contraception with concurrent use of antibiotics and CF transmembrane conductance regulator modulators. All individuals with or without CF should use barrier contraception to prevent the transmission of sexually transmitted diseases.

The issue of counseling or family planning extends beyond the physical process of conception. Genetic counseling and CF carrier screening for the partner of the individual with CF should be offered to allow for informed risk of becoming pregnant with a child with CF. A sensitive topic but an important one to be addressed is that although the lifespan of individuals with CF is increasing, many face the possibility of early death and the inability to participate in the long-term responsibility of raising a child. Also important to note is that women with severe lung disease should be informed that pregnancy often increases panel-reactive antibodies, which complicate the process of matching for lung transplantation depending on the proximity of the pregnancy to the need for lung transplantation. No parent is guaranteed freedom from disabling illness that impairs child-rearing; however, the known reality of the progressive nature of CF warrants an honest, nonjudgmental discussion and disclosure of medical information so that an individual with CF and his or her partner can make an informed decision that best aligns with their values.

SUMMARY

From the time of diagnosis, pediatric providers should convey the expectation that with new therapies, all patients with CF will live to adulthood and even to old age. Individuals with CF, caretakers, specialists, and primary care providers alike should embrace this attitude. Discussion and education about transitioning to adult care should being early in life to integrate with other normal parts of development and maturity. A young person with CF can look forward to this transition as one among many accomplishments they will achieve in their lifetime. That being said, individuals with CF still have tremendous physical and psychological burden of disease. As psychosocial challenges arise in the lives of individuals with CF, providers should develop diagnostic and management expertise similar to that of other physical manifestations of CF to support optimal health for their patients. The future for individuals with CF has never looked more promising. New therapies and a focus on planning for a full life should bring a sense of optimism to individuals with CF, their families, and care providers.

REFERENCES

1. Cystic Fibrosis Foundation Patient Registry 2014 Annual Data Report. Bethesda (MD): Cystic Fibrosis Foundation; 2015. Available at: http://www.cff.org/2014-Annual-Data-Report/.
2. Yohannes A. Relationship between anxiety, depression, and quality of life in adult patients with cystic fibrosis. Respir Care 2012;57:550–6.
3. Schidlow D. Transition in cystic fibrosis: much ado about nothing? A pediatrician's view. Pediatr Pulmonol 2002;33(5):325–6.

4. Transition of care provided for adolescents with special health care needs. American Academy of Pediatrics Committee on Children with Disabilities and Committee on Adolescence. Pediatrics 1996;98:1203–6.

5. Yankaskas J. Cystic fibrosis adult care: consensus conference report. Chest 2004;125:1S–39S.

6. Chaudry S. Evaluation of a cystic fibrosis transition program from pediatric to adult care. Pediatr Pulmonol 2013;48(7):658–65.

7. Sawicki G. Ready, set, stop: mismatch between self-care beliefs, transition readiness skills and transition planning among adolescents, young adults, and parents. Clin Pediatr 2014;53(11):1062–8.

8. www.cff.org. Living with CF. 2015. Available at: https://www.cff.org/Living-with-CF/. Accessed May 18, 2016.

9. Parcel GS. Self-management of cystic fibrosis: a structural model for educational and behavioral variables. Soc Sci Med 1994;38(9):1307–15.

10. Mclean K. Barriers to adherence in adolescents with CF and their parents: qualitative coding of contextual factors. Pediatr Pulmonol 2015;50(12):441–2.

11. Modi A. Barriers to treatment adherence for children with cystic fibrosis and asthma: what gets in the way? J Pediatr Psychol 2006;31(8):846–58.

12. Savage E. Self-management education for cystic fibrosis. Cochrane Database Syst Rev 2014;(9):CD007641.

13. Townshend J. Patient's perceptions of the transition from pediatric to adult care. Pediatr Pulmonol 1998;17:393–4.

14. Nasr S. Transition program from pediatric to adult care for cystic fibrosis patients. J Adolesc Health 1992;13:682–5.

15. Abdale B. Evaluation of patient satisfaction with the transition from a pediatric hospital to an adult centre [abstract]. Pediatr Pulmonol 1994;10:291–2.

16. Pownceby J. The coming of age project: a study of the transition from paediatric to adult care and treatment adherence amongst young people with cystic fibrosis; summary report, 1996, Cystic Fibrosis Trust.

17. Schidlow D. Life beyond pediatrics: transition of chronically ill adolescents from pediatric to adult health care systems. Med Clin North Am 1990;74:1113–20.

18. Nobili R. Pediatric-to-adult care transition program: the Milan experience [abstract]. Pediatr Pulmonol 1996;13:338.

19. Joekes K. Self-efficacy and overprotection are related to quality of life, psychological well being and self-management in cardiac patients. J Health Psychol 2007;12:4–16.

20. Fernandes S. Transition and transfer of adolescents and young adults with pediatric onset chronic disease: the patient and parent perspective. J Pediatr Rehabil Med 2014;7(1):43–51.

21. Tuchman L. Health outcomes associated with transition from pediatric to adult cystic fibrosis care. Pediatrics 2013;132(5):847–53.

22. Moussavi S. Depression, chronic diseases, and decrements in health: results from the World Health Surveys. Lancet 2007;370:851–8.

23. Pinquart M, Shen Y. Depressive symptoms in children and adolescents with chronic physical illness: an updated meta analysis. J Pediatr Psychol 2011;36:375–84.

24. Quittner A. Prevalence of depression and anxiety in patients with cystic fibrosis and parent caregivers: results of The International Depression Epidemiological Study across nine countries. Thorax 2014;69:1090–7.

25. Riekert K. The association between depression, lung function, and health-related quality of life among adults with cystic fibrosis. Chest 2007;132:231–7.

26. Havermans T. Quality of life in patients with cystic fibrosis: association with anxiety and depression. J Cyst Fibros 2008;7:581–4.

27. Grenard J. Depression and medication adherence in the treatment of chronic diseases in the United States: a meta-analysis. J Gen Intern Med 2011;26:1175–82.
28. Smith B. Depressive symptoms in children with cystic fibrosis and parents and its effects on adherence to airway clearance. Pediatr Pulmonol 2010;45:756–63.
29. Goldbeck L. Prevalence of symptoms of anxiety and depression in German patients with cystic fibrosis. Chest 2010;138:929–36.
30. Snell C. Depression, illness severity, and healthcare utilization in cystic fibrosis. Pediatr Pulmonol 2014;49(12):1177–81.
31. Quittner A. International Committee on Mental Health in Cystic Fibrosis: Cystic Fibrosis Foundation and European Cystic Fibrosis Society consensus statements for screening and treating depression and anxiety. Thorax 2016;71(1):26–34.
32. Goetz D. The relationship between depression screening and patient outcomes in children and adults with CF. Pediatr Pulmonol 2015;50(12):441.
33. Roach C. Routine depression screening: patient perceptions and satisfaction. Pediatr Pulmonol 2015;50(12):421.
34. Saiman L. Infection prevention and control guideline for cystic fibrosis: 2013 update. Infect Control Hosp Epidemiol 2014;35:S1–67.
35. Singh S. Using video conferencing for parent patient advisory group in era of infection control. Pediatr Pulmonol 2015;50(12):451.
36. OConnor G. Median household income and mortality rate in cystic fibrosis. Pediatrics 2003;111:333–9.
37. Quon B. Disparities in access to lung transplantation for patients with cystic fibrosis by socioeconomic status. Am J Respir Crit Care Med 2012;186(10): 1008–13.
38. 2016. Available at: https://www.cff.org/Help-Affording-Your-Care/. Accessed May 18, 2016.
39. Burker E. Psychological and educational factors: better predictors of work status than FEV1 in adults with cystic fibrosis. Pediatr Pulmonol 2004;38(5):413–8.
40. Kaplan E. Reproductive failure in males with cystic fibrosis. N Engl J Med 1968; 279:65–9.
41. Kotloff R. Fertility and pregnancy in patients with cystic fibrosis. Clin Chest Med 1992;13:623–35.
42. Seale T. Reproductive defects in patients of both sexes with cystic fibrosis: a review. Ann Clin Lab Sci 1985;15:152–8.
43. Geddes D. Cystic fibrosis and pregnancy. J R Soc Med 1992;85:36–7.
44. Oppenheimer E. Cervical mucus in cystic fibrosis: a possible cause of infertility. Am J Obstet Gynecol 1970;108:673–4.

New Therapeutic Approaches to Modulate and Correct Cystic Fibrosis Transmembrane Conductance Regulator

 CrossMark

Thida Ong, MD[a], Bonnie W. Ramsey, MD[b],*

KEYWORDS

- CFTR modulator • Personalized medicine • Therapeutics • Potentiator • Corrector

KEY POINTS

- Cystic fibrosis transmembrane conductance regulator (CFTR) mutations can be classified into defects that lead to reduced quantity or reduced function of CFTR protein, impairing critical salt and fluid homeostasis in multiple organs.
- Classification of mutations is a framework for therapeutic approaches to identify compounds that improve CFTR presence at the cell surface (corrector therapy) or augment channel function of the nascent protein (potentiator therapy).
- Ivacaftor (Kalydeco), the first approved CFTR potentiator for individuals with class III (gating) mutations, and Arg117H have demonstrated significant and sustained multi-system improvement.
- The combination of ivacaftor and lumacaftor (Orkambi) was approved in 2015 for individuals homozygous for the Phe508del mutation. Its long-term clinical impact is not yet known.
- Novel systems and disease markers that address and monitor individualized response to therapies are being developed and will serve as important tools to explore current and future CFTR modulators.

T. Ong has nothing to disclose. B.W. Ramsey reports grants from 12th Man Technologies, Catabasis, Corbus Pharmaceuticals, Cornerstone Therapeutics, Flatley Discovery Lab LLV, Gilead Sciences, Inc, GlycoMimetics, Inc, Insmed, Inc, La Jolla Pharmaceutical, Mpex Pharmaceuticals, Inc, Nibalis Therapeutics, Inc, Nordmark, Novartis Pharmaceuticals Corp., Pharmaxis Ltd., Respira Therapeutics, Inc, Sanofi, Savara Pharmaceuticals, Synedgen, Inc, the Cystic Fibrosis Foundation, Vertex Pharmaceuticals, outside the submitted work; and NIH funding: P30DK089507 and ULITR000423.

[a] Division of Pulmonary and Sleep Medicine, Department of Pediatrics, Seattle Children's Hospital, University of Washington, 4800 Sand Point Way Northeast, M/S OC.7.720, Seattle, WA 98105, USA; [b] Department of Pediatrics, Seattle Children's Research Institute, Center for Clinical and Translational Research, University of Washington, 2001 8th Avenue, Suite 400, M/S CW8-5B, Seattle, WA 98121, USA
* Corresponding author.
E-mail address: Bonnie.Ramsey@seattlechildrens.org

Pediatr Clin N Am 63 (2016) 751–764
http://dx.doi.org/10.1016/j.pcl.2016.04.006
0031-3955/16/$ – see front matter © 2016 Elsevier Inc. All rights reserved.

pediatric.theclinics.com

INTRODUCTION

The science of personalized medicine is taking shape in the cystic fibrosis (CF) community with genotype-directed therapies available for more than half of the CF population. Personalized or precision medicines approach the treatment of disease by accounting for an individual's variability in genes, environment, and lifestyle.[1]

This momentum in precision medicine launched with the basic understanding of CF as a result of mutations in the cystic fibrosis transmembrane conductance regulator (CFTR) gene.[2–4] In the decades since CFTR gene identification, knowledge of CFTR mutations and their pathophysiologic consequences has rapidly expanded, leading to the development of small-molecule therapies that target specific CFTR variants that have some level of CFTR protein produced.[5] These small-molecule therapies are defined as CFTR modulators, a novel class of precision medicines directed to improve CFTR function and/or presence at the cell surface level.

In this review, we focus on therapeutic approaches, known as "potentiators" and "correctors" that explore our understanding of specific CFTR variants and aim to augment or repair function of the CFTR protein.

APPROACHING CYSTIC FIBROSIS TRANSMEMBRANE CONDUCTANCE REGULATOR: REVIEW OF STRUCTURE AND FUNCTION

CFTR, located in the apical membranes of epithelial cells in multiple exocrine organs, is a chloride and bicarbonate ion channel that regulates salt and fluid homeostasis.[6] The CFTR glycoprotein has multiple membrane-integrated subunits that form 2 membrane-spanning domains (MSDs), 2 intracellular nucleotide-binding domains (NBDs), and a regulatory (R) domain, which acts as a phosphorylation site.[7,8] MSD1 and MSD2 form the channel pore walls. Opening and closing of the pore is through ATP interactions with cytoplasmic NBD domains, leading to conformational changes of MSD1 and MSD2.[9] Gating and conductance is regulated through R domain phosphorylation with protein kinase A (PKA).[7]

The intricate regions of CFTR require processing and maturation to allow precise folding. CFTR structure must satisfy rigorous quality standards to be exported from the endoplasmic reticulum and subsequently transported to the cell surface. CFTR that fails to meet these standards is destined to endoplasmic reticulum–associated protein degradation (ERAD).[7] Such a complex quality-control system operates at the detriment of efficiency, decreasing export production of even wild-type CFTR to 33% of similar family cell transporters.[10]

CF is a result of mutations that alter CFTR in these domains or the way these domains interact with each other. Ultimately, these defects affect the function or quantity of the channel at the cell surface.[5] With nearly 2000 disease-causing mutations identified in CFTR, variants have historically been categorized in 5 or 6 functional classifications (**Fig. 1**).[8,11] Class I mutations lead to a lack of protein synthesis, such as those with a premature termination codon present. Class II mutations are unable to mature, leading to early degradation through the mechanism of ERAD and resulting in CFTR rarely reaching the cell surface. Class III mutations are considered gating defects with abnormal regulation that make the pore nonfunctioning. Class IV defects have inefficient CFTR function with defective chloride conductance. Class V and VI mutations are those that lead to decreased quantity of CFTR at the cell surface as a result of promoter or splicing defects (V) or increased turnover from the cell surface (VI).

These categories of molecular mechanisms provide a useful framework to consider personalized therapeutic approaches (**Table 1**), but present an oversimplification in that a single variant can disrupt multiple functional classes. Phe508del, the most

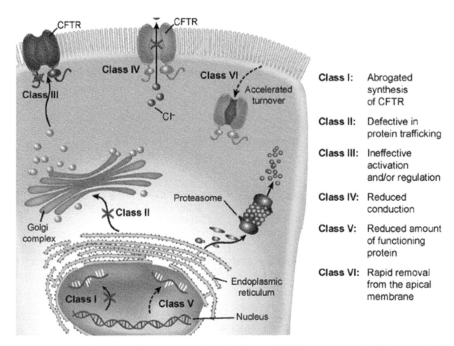

Fig. 1. Functional classes of CFTR mutations. Defects of CFTR are categorized into a lack of protein synthesis (class I), incomplete maturation and early degradation (class II), abnormal gating and regulation (class III), inefficient chloride conductance (class IV), decreased number of CFTR transcripts (class V), and increased turnover of CFTR from the cell surface (class VI). (*From* Banjar H, Angyalosi G. The road for survival improvement of cystic fibrosis patients in Arab countries. International Journal of Pediatrics and Adolescent Medicine 2015;2:49.)

common CFTR allele, is a prime example of this complexity. Deletion of phenylalanine leads to instability and abnormal folding of the NBD1 region and increased ERAD, categorizing it classically as a class II mutation.[12,13] A small portion of synthesized protein, however, is able to traffic to the cell membrane, but has increased degradation like a class VI mutation. Additionally, Phe508del alters protein stability of NBD1 and MSD2, 2 important structural domains needed to open the channel, leading to defective gating as in a class III mutation.[5] Personalized therapeutic approaches need to consider the potential diversity of effects a single mutation may determine.

HIGH-THROUGHPUT SCREENING TO IDENTIFY CYSTIC FIBROSIS TRANSMEMBRANE CONDUCTANCE REGULATOR MODULATORS

Identifying modulators has been bolstered by the advent of high-throughput screening (HTS). HTS uses robotic drug screening of more than a million molecules in cell-based fluorescence assays of membrane potential or halide efflux to identify candidate compounds that restore CFTR activity in vitro.[14–16] HTS defined 2 approaches to identify modulators, termed potentiators and correctors. Potentiators are candidate agents that demonstrate improved CFTR chloride conductance in the absence of preincubation time for synthesis of new protein. It is presumed that potentiators augment ATP activation of the pore of nascent CFTR transcripts that have successfully trafficked to the cell surface. Candidate agents, termed correctors, focus on improved processing and chaperoning of CFTR. The corrector therapies rescue CFTR activity only after

Table 1
CFTR mutation classes and summary of approved or potential therapies

Class	Impact on CFTR Protein	Common Mutation (Legacy Name)	Approved Therapy (Dose)	Therapies in Development
I	Lack of protein synthesis (reduced quantity)	Trp1282X (W1282X)	—	Ataluren (Phase 3)
II	Abnormal processing with misfolding keeping it from reaching cell surface (reduced quantity)	Phe508del (deltaF508)	Lumacaftor/Ivacaftor (400 mg every 12 h/250 mg every 12 h)	VX-661/Ivacaftor (Phase 3)
III	Reaches cell surface, but gating defect impairs function (reduced function)	Gly551Asp (G551D)	Ivacaftor (6 y+: 150 mg every 12 h; 2–5 y <14 kg: 50 mg every 12 h; 2–5 y ≥14 kg: 75 mg every 12 h)	VX-661/Ivacaftor (Phase 3)
IV	Reaches cell surface, but conductance defect leads to faulty opening (reduced function)	Arg117His (R117H)	Ivacaftor (6 y+: 150 mg every 12 h; 2–5 y <14 kg: 50 mg every 12 h; 2–5 y ≥14 kg: 75 mg every 12 h)	VX-661/Ivacaftor (Phase 3)
V	Created in insufficient quantities (reduced quantity)	3849 + 10 kb C→G	—	—
VI	Rapid turnover (reduced quantity)	Cys1400X (4326delTC)	—	—

incubation time with the agent to promote stability and cell-surface trafficking of CFTR protein.

HTS is an automated process that screens blindly to identify hundreds of chemical compounds with the outcome of CFTR-mediated chloride secretion (**Fig. 2**). These compounds are deemed "hits" but require multiple cycles of medicinal chemistry, including validation in a second assay, such as human bronchial epithelial cells. Among these "validated hits," lead compounds are identified with a chemical scaffold that optimizes potency and selectivity. Ultimately, development candidates are refined in animal studies to develop drugs that are tested for safety and efficacy in clinical trials.[17]

AUGMENTING CYSTIC FIBROSIS TRANSMEMBRANE CONDUCTANCE REGULATOR ACTIVITY: THE POTENTIATOR APPROACH

CFTR variants that benefit from the potentiator approach have absent or limited pore function, characteristic of functional class III or IV mutations. Potentiators can function through enhancing the open configuration or improving the gating of the CFTR channel. Gly551Asp-CFTR is the most prevalent gating mutation, present in 4% to 5% of individuals with CF.[18] This variant is thought to interfere with the NBD1 and its ability to interface with NBD2, a function crucial for pore opening.[19]

Production of ivacaftor (Kalydeco) is proof-of-concept of CFTR modulation. Hundreds of thousands of chemical compounds were screened through HTS to identify CFTR potentiator candidates and of these, ivacaftor (formerly known as VX-770) was selected for further development because of its favorable pharmacokinetic profile

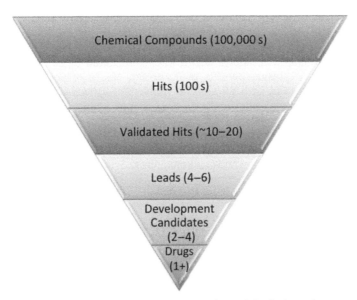

Fig. 2. Summary of CFTR modulator drug discovery through high-throughput screening.

and its ability to augment various CFTR mutants.[17] Ivacaftor was rigorously tested in cell models and demonstrated an increase in chloride secretion for Gly551Asp/Phe508del-CFTR by approximately 10-fold, nearly 50% of activity seen with wild-type CFTR. This improvement was also reflected in improved mucociliary beating and increased apical fluid level. With these encouraging in vitro data, initial human trials with ivacaftor were started.

The safety profile of ivacaftor was evaluated in a phase 2 randomized placebo-controlled trial of 39 adults with at least 1 copy of Gly551Asp-CFTR.[20] In addition to a reassuring safety profile with similar adverse event rates in placebo and treated groups, subjects demonstrated a significant improvement in lung function, the most responsive at a dose of 150 mg/d. Additionally, markers of CFTR activity, including nasal potential difference and sweat chloride concentration, were shown to have significant improvements. With this evidence, ivacaftor was evaluated in a phase 3 trial, known as STRIVE, that enrolled 161 subjects, 12 years and older, with at least 1 copy of the Gly551Asp mutation.[21] Individuals were randomized in a double-blind trial to receive 150 mg ivacaftor or placebo twice daily for 48 weeks. Within 2 weeks of therapy, the ivacaftor group demonstrated a 10.6% improvement in the primary end point: change from baseline of percent of predicted forced expiratory volume in 1 second (FEV_1). This effect was sustained through the 48 weeks of the study. Important secondary outcomes included a 55% reduction in pulmonary exacerbations through week 48, an increase in 2.7 kg of weight through week 48, and improved quality of life in respiratory domains, as determined by validated questionnaire. Biomarkers as in the phase 2 trial also demonstrated improvement in sweat chloride with ivacaftor, and the adverse event rates were similar in both groups. In fact, the serious adverse event rate was lower in the treated group compared with placebo (24% vs 42%) primarily driven by a decreased number of pulmonary exacerbations in the treated group. Similar magnitude of outcomes were confirmed and validated in a second phase 3 trial, known as ENVISION, which enrolled children ages 6 to 11 years with Gly551Asp-CFTR.[22]

The Food and Drug Administration (FDA) approved ivacaftor in 2012 for those 6 years and older with 1 copy of Gly551Asp-CFTR. Commonly reported side effects and monitoring recommendations on the prescribing label are summarized in **Box 1**. An open-label trial, known as PERSIST, monitored those on STRIVE and ENVISION, noting sustained benefits of 9.4% and 10.3% of absolute change in FEV_1 and weight gain at both 96 and 144 weeks.[23] Pulmonary exacerbation rate decreased in adolescents and adults, but not in the younger cohort, who had a much lower baseline frequency of pulmonary exacerbations.

In a phase 4 observational study, known as GOAL, Rowe and colleagues[24] monitored 151 individuals with Gly551Asp-CFTR over a 6-month period after they initiated ivacaftor. Their report extended and confirmed phase 3 data with consistent and rapid improvement in FEV_1% predicted and weight gain. Sweat chloride, as a marker of

---

Box 1
Warnings and precautions of approved cystic fibrosis transmembrane conductance regulator modulator therapy and suggested monitoring

Ivacaftor

Absorption	Take tablet with fat-containing food.
Elevated liver transaminases	Monitor alanine and aspartate transaminases before initiation, every 3 mo in the first year, and annually thereafter.
Cataracts	Eye examination before initiation and follow-up for patients younger than 18 y.
Drug interactions (St John wort, rifampin)	Decreases exposure to ivacaftor and coadministration is not recommended.
Drug interactions (ketoconazole, fluconazole)	Increases exposure to ivacaftor. Dose adjustment of is needed.
Drug interactions (Seville oranges, grapefruit)	Increases exposure to ivacaftor. Avoid food containing grapefruit or Seville oranges.

Lumacaftor-Ivacaftor

Absorption	Take tablet with fat-containing food.
Elevated liver transaminases	Monitor alanine and aspartate transaminases before initiation, every 3 mo in the first year, and annually thereafter.
Liver disease	Childs-Pugh score classification and dose adjustment may be necessary. Caution in patients with advanced liver disease.
Cataracts	Eye examination before initiation and follow-up for patients younger than 18 y.
Chest discomfort, dyspnea, breathing difficulties	Additional monitoring recommended for patients with forced expiratory volume in 1 s % predicted <40 during therapy initiation.
Drug interactions (hormonal contraceptives)	Decreased efficacy of hormonal contraception. Alternative methods of contraception and anticipation of menstrual-related adverse reactions.
Drug interactions (benzodiazepines, immunosuppressants, digoxin, corticosteroids, antidepressants, proton pump inhibitors)	Decreases efficacy of these medications. Dose adjustment, level monitoring if applicable, or alternative agent recommended. Coadministration not recommended.
Drug interactions (St John wort, rifampin, phenytoin)	Decreases exposure to lumacaftor-ivacaftor and coadministration is not recommended.
Drug interactions (ketoconazole, itraconazole, voriconazole, clarithromycin)	Increases exposure to lumacaftor-ivacaftor. Dose adjustment may be needed when initiating therapy.

CFTR function, demonstrated reduction to near-normal values. Important subsets within the GOAL study provided preliminary information with mechanistic implications for these clinical outcomes, noting improvement in mucociliary clearance by gamma-scintigraphy and early neutralization of gastrointestinal pH. In addition, there were more initial indications that CFTR modulation may impact the microbiologic milieu in the CF airway. The number of patients with *Pseudomonas aeruginosa* colonization decreased[25] and colonization with the anaerobe, *Prevotella*, increased. The relative abundance of *Prevotella* has been associated with higher lung function in patients with CF.[26]

Beyond Gly551Asp-CFTR, ivacaftor has been studied in additional gating mutations. The KONNECTION trial enrolled 39 patients 6 years and older with at least 1 copy of a non-Gly551Asp gating mutation, including G178R, S549N, S549R, G551S, G970R, G1244E, S1251N, S1255P, and G1349D.[27] In an adjusted model, the treatment group had a similar magnitude of clinical outcomes with absolute change in FEV_1% predicted, body mass index, and validated respiratory domain score to the patients with Gly551Asp-CFTR in the STRIVE study.[21]

The potentiator approach also would augment function in typical class IV mutations with limited conductance, in which chloride and bicarbonate ion flow is only partially present. In a randomized, double-blind, placebo-controlled trial, the KONDUCT study enrolled 69 patients 6 years and older with 1 copy of Arg117His-CFTR, a known class IV mutation.[28] The primary end point was absolute change in FEV_1% predicted. The KONDUCT trial demonstrated an approximately 2% absolute FEV_1% predicted change for all patients who did not achieve statistical significance. The response to ivacaftor was age related. Patients 6 to 11 years of age in the treated group had a near-normal baseline FEV_1 of 97.5% predicted and showed no treatment response with an absolute FEV_1 change of −2.8%. Patients 18 years and older with more established lung disease with mean FEV_1 of approximately 60% had a 5% absolute improvement in lung function. Based on this evidence in the older patients, the FDA has approved ivacaftor for additional gating mutations, and Arg117His-CFTR for ages 6 years and older.

Ivacaftor pharmacokinetic and safety data were recently evaluated in children with specific gating mutations as young as 2 years, which has ultimately led to FDA approval for children as young as 2 years with specific gating mutations G551D, G1244E, G1349D, G178R, G551S, S1251N, S1255P, S549N, S549R, and R117H.[29,30] With FDA approval of ivacaftor monotherapy for individuals 2 years and older with CF who carry at least 1 copy of a class III mutation or Arg117His, this drug is available to treat almost 10% of the CF population in the United States and many countries worldwide.

Yet, the most common mutation associated with CF is Phe508del, with nearly half of patients in the United States homozygous for this mutation. Although Phe508del is categorized as a class II mutation (see the preceding section: Approaching cystic fibrosis transmembrane conductance regulator: review of structure and function), a limited amount of Phe508del-CFTR does make it to the cell surface, making it a feasible target for the potentiator approach.[31] Thus, there was significant interest in testing ivacaftor monotherapy in the homozygous and heterozygous Phe508del population. In addition, ivacaftor improved channel open probability and chloride ion conductance in cultured human bronchial epithelial (HBE) cells from patients homozygous for Phe508del, which was an encouraging in vitro finding.[17] The DISCOVER study, a phase 2 trial, enrolled 140 patients with 2 copies Phe508del and randomized to placebo or ivacaftor at 150-mg dose twice daily.[32] The study was not powered to measure efficacy, and demonstrated safety of ivacaftor in Phe508del homozygous patients with similar adverse events reported in placebo and ivacaftor groups (89.3% vs 87.5%). In the 16-week trial duration, followed by a 96-week open-label extension, the ivacaftor-treated group had no significant improvement in lung function, rate of pulmonary exacerbation, or improvement in validated respiratory symptoms score. Thus, ivacaftor has not been approved as monotherapy for patients homozygous for Phe508del.

IMPROVED CYSTIC FIBROSIS TRANSMEMBRANE CONDUCTANCE REGULATOR PROCESSING: THE CORRECTOR APPROACH

CFTR modulators, termed "correctors," focus on improved cellular processing to increase its presence at the cell surface.[33] This approach can function through stabilizing CFTR and facilitating folding, minimizing ERAD, or encouraging stability at the cell membrane.

Given the prevalence of Phe508del-CFTR in the CF population, the corrector or rescue approach has targeted individuals with at least 1 copy of this mutation. Lumacaftor is a corrector compound, identified by HTS. The molecular mechanisms of lumacaftor monotherapy are not well understood; however, studies suggest lumacaftor stabilizes domain interactions between NBD1 and MSD2 to improve Phe508del-CFTR cellular processing.[13,33] In vitro models with cultured HBE cells demonstrated increased chloride secretion by 14% compared with non-CF HBE cells.[15,34] Phase 2 testing of lumacaftor monotherapy in patients homozygous for Phe508del was powered to detect differences in CFTR function by sweat chloride.[35] The study detected small, but significant improvement in sweat chloride in a dose-dependent effect, particularly with the maximum dose of 200 mg twice daily. This dose did not translate to significant changes in clinical outcomes, including lung function, rates of pulmonary exacerbation, or validated patient-reported outcome scores. These data combined with in vitro work made clear that neither lumacaftor nor ivacaftor monotherapy is an effective treatment for the homozygous Phe508del-CFTR population in contrast to ivacaftor monotherapy on class III (Gly551Asp-CFTR) or class IV (Arg117His) mutations.[15,21,34,35]

COMBINING POTENTIATOR AND CORRECTOR APPROACHES

As described previously, the Phe508del mutation spans multiple functional classes and thus a combined corrector and potentiator approach may be necessary to reach a threshold therapeutic effect. HBE cell work identified augmented effect of ivacaftor on CFTR function after lumacaftor exposure on homozygous Phe508del-CFTR HBE cells in support of this concept.[34] Lumacaftor, however, induces cytochrome P450 metabolism of ivacaftor, reducing its effects and requires higher dosing.[35] Higher-dose ivacaftor (250 mg twice daily) in combination with lumacaftor (600 mg daily or 400 mg twice daily) was studied in a dose-escalation phase 2 trial in patients with 1 or 2 copies of Phe508del-CFTR.[36] Patients received an initial 28 days of lumacaftor monotherapy before addition of the ivacaftor. The lumacaftor monotherapy period was associated with a decline in FEV_1% predicted and increased sensation of chest tightness and dyspnea in a subgroup of patients. In contrast, combined therapy (lumacaftor plus ivacaftor) over the subsequent 28 days demonstrated a 6% increase in FEV_1% predicted in Phe508del homozygous, resulting in a net increase of 3% in FEV_1% predicted over the total 56-day treatment period. A cohort of patients heterozygous for Phe508del was studied and did not demonstrate improvement in FEV_1 or other clinical markers of disease. Thus, the 2 phase 3 trials described as follows were limited only to patients homozygous for Phe508del.

Combination lumacaftor-ivacaftor (Orkambi) underwent 2 phase 3 trials, known as TRAFFIC and TRANSPORT, over a 24-week study period.[37] Each study was powered to detect an absolute change in FEV_1 in a randomized, double-blind, multicenter trial for patients 12 years and older with 2 copies of Phe508del allele. Just more than 1100 people were enrolled in the 2 studies and were randomized to 2 dosing arms of lumacaftor (600 mg once daily or 400 mg twice daily) and the same dose of ivacaftor (250 mg twice daily). Absolute change in FEV_1 significantly improved in each dosing arm with a range of 2.6% to 4.0% compared with placebo. Secondary outcome analysis pooled for patients treated in the lumacaftor 400 mg twice daily dosing arm demonstrated a 39% lower rate of pulmonary exacerbations compared with placebo and a 0.24-increase in body mass index. Adverse events, pooled across the studies were 17.3% to 22.8% in the lumacaftor-ivacaftor–treated groups and 28.6% in placebo, with the most common serious adverse event of pulmonary exacerbations. Common adverse events reported more frequently with treatment groups were primarily respiratory, including dyspnea and chest tightness (see **Box 1**). Elevation of liver function tests led to discontinuation or interruption of lumacaftor-ivacaftor treatment in 7 patients. Based on the overall efficacy and safety data, lumacaftor (400 mg twice daily)–ivacaftor (250 mg twice daily) was approved by the FDA for individuals 12 years and older with 2 Phe508del alleles, estimated to impact 8500 individuals in the United States.[18,38]

ADDITIONAL MODULATOR THERAPIES

VX-661 is another first-generation corrector targeted to Phe508del-CFTR. Early phase 2 results demonstrated safety with well-tolerated doses of 100 mg once daily and 50 mg twice daily of VX-661 in combination with 150 mg twice daily of ivacaftor.[39] The study was performed in 39 people 18 years and older with 2 copies of Phe508del over a 12-week interval. In the small subset of patients with 100-mg dosing of VX-661 in combination with ivacaftor, FEV_1% predicted improved 4.4% at 4 weeks and 3.0% at 12 weeks compared with placebo. The study was of similar magnitude in FEV_1% predicted for individuals with Phe508del and Gly551Asp already on ivacaftor. VX-661 at 100 mg and 150 mg once daily in addition to ivacaftor 150 mg twice daily had an approximately 4% improvement in FEV_1% predicted at 4 weeks. VX-661 in combination with ivacaftor is currently in a phase 3 study evaluating for absolute change in FEV_1% predicted.[40] The combination therapy is being tested in patients homozygous and heterozygous for Phe508del. Patients will be classified into 4 cohorts based on genotype and presumed amount of CFTR function in the second mutation: (1) Phe508del/Phe508del homozygous, (2) Phe508del/gating defect allele (eg, class III), (3) Phe508del/residual function CFTR allele (eg, class IV), (4) Phe508del/minimal CFTR function allele (eg, class I, II).

Additional modulators are entering or are currently in phase 2 trials in the CF Foundation drug-development pipeline. Riociguat (BAY 63-2521) is a soluble guanylate cyclase stimulator that increases nitric oxide, a pathway related to improved maturation and function of CFTR.[41] QBW251 is a potentiator currently being tested in people with 1 or 2 copies of Phe508del-CFTR as well as healthy patients.[42] Miglustat is an enzyme inhibitor presumed to improve impaired trafficking of Phe508del-CFTR protein and is being tested in patients homozygous for Phe508del-CFTR.[43,44] New molecules are being developed to target inhibition of S-nitrosoglutathione reductase (GSNOR) that also may improve cellular trafficking of Phe508del-CFTR. N91115 is an oral GSNOR inhibitor in phase 2 trials with adults homozygous for Phe508del-CFTR on lumacaftor/ivacaftor therapy.[45]

ALTERNATE THERAPEUTIC APPROACHES: BEYOND CORRECTORS AND POTENTIATORS

CFTR modulators require some production of the protein transcript to improve or repair its function. Important therapeutic approaches, such as genetic modulation or gene-editing, target altered translation of the CFTR gene, but are not traditionally classified as CFTR modulators. Read-through agents or premature termination codon (PTC) suppressor therapies target approximately 10% of the CF population.[18] Ataluren, a PTC suppressor therapy reached a phase 3 trial, but did not demonstrate a significant relative change in baseline $FEV_1\%$ predicted (−2.5% ataluren vs −5.5% placebo, $P = .12$).[46] A 5.7% relative change in $FEV_1\%$ predicted was seen in non-tobramycin users compared with 1.4% in those treated with inhaled tobramycin in post hoc subgroup analysis, suggesting that aminoglycoside therapy may interfere with ataluren effect. A second phase 3 trial in patients not receiving inhaled aminoglycosides is currently in progress.[47] New in vitro work with the most common PTC mutations, W1282X and G542X, suggests constructs that respond to PTC suppression may have partial CFTR function that could be augmented with CFTR modulator use, lumacaftor and ivacaftor.[48]

APPROACHES TO MAXIMIZE THE BENEFIT OF CYSTIC FIBROSIS TRANSMEMBRANE CONDUCTANCE REGULATOR MODULATORS

Tremendous progress has been made in the development of CFTR modulators. The goal remains to expand personalized therapy, targeted at the basic defect in CFTR to every person with CF. More CFTR modulators are in the pipeline, and additional approaches continue to be developed and refined. As this novel class of medications expand, methods to predict and monitor treatment response become crucial. These methods must take into account the rarity of CFTR mutations and how to determine an individual's personalized response to therapy.

New systems, such as organoids to use as personal human model systems, are being assessed to predict response over a wide range of mutations.[49–51] Dekkers and colleagues[49] established primitive organoids from rectal punch biopsy cultures with intestinal stem cells. These cultures contain an internal lumen and serve as a functional assay of CFTR by swelling in response to forskolin. This assay allows an ex vivo approach to detect organoid-based fluid transport and can serve as an efficient strategy to test variability in drug response in rare CFTR mutants.[50]

Individual phenotypic responses are also being considered through N-of-1 clinical trial design. Single subjects are monitored in a multi-crossover design of a randomized schedule to receive treatment or placebo with frequent outcome measurements to assess efficacy and profile adverse events.[52,53] This study design may be a useful strategy to estimate individual treatment effects, but requires significant investment to design and monitor for outcomes. Additionally, outcome measures must be carefully chosen to distinguish baseline chronic disease variability over time from treatment effect. An N-of-1 study was recently completed for ivacaftor in patients with residual function CFTR mutations.[54]

LESSONS FROM IVACAFTOR

Ivacaftor provides additional important lessons going forward, including the potential role of biomarkers more sensitive to early physiologic changes in young patients, such as lung clearance index.[55] A phase 4 study of lumacaftor/ivacaftor, known as the PROSPECT study, is in progress to attempt to identify biomarkers of CFTR and CF disease progression in response to treatment.[56] Post approval studies can be augmented with data from the CF Foundation National Patient Registry (CFFNPR) for assessment of hospitalization risk and P aeruginosa infection as in the GOAL study or to estimate the long-term impact of modulators with comparative rates of lung function decline.[24,57] CFFNPR was also a useful adjunct to identify clinical and sociodemographic variables of baseline lung function, geography, and race as factors that may influence ivacaftor prescription.[58] Nongenetic determinants that play an important role in uptake and adherence of modulator therapy deserve ongoing attention to maximize clinical benefit of modulator therapies as they integrate into daily care.

SUMMARY

CFTR modulators are proof-of-concept that personalized therapies can be integrated into clinical practice. These new therapies provide hope that the course of disease will be forever changed in people with CF. Evidence from the CFFPNR fuels this hope with a recent study demonstrating ivacaftor-treated Gly551Asp-CFTR patients have a nearly 50% reduction in the rate of decline of lung function compared with F508del control patients matched by propensity score.[57] Moving forward, future generations of modulators and adjunct systems to test and monitor these medications will continue to develop. The CF community remains steadfast to identify personalized therapies for all people with CF.

REFERENCES

1. Collins FS, Varmus H. A new initiative on precision medicine. N Engl J Med 2015; 372(9):793–5.
2. Kerem B, Rommens JM, Buchanan JA, et al. Identification of the cystic fibrosis gene: genetic analysis. Science 1989;245(4922):1073–80.
3. Riordan JR, Rommens JM, Kerem B, et al. Identification of the cystic fibrosis gene: cloning and characterization of complementary DNA. Science 1989; 245(4922):1066–73.
4. Rommens JM, Iannuzzi MC, Kerem B, et al. Identification of the cystic fibrosis gene: chromosome walking and jumping. Science 1989;245(4922):1059–65.
5. Cutting GR. Cystic fibrosis genetics: from molecular understanding to clinical application. Nat Rev Genet 2015;16(1):45–56.
6. Lindsell P. Functional architecture of the CFTR chloride channel. Mol Membr Biol 2014;31(1):1–16.
7. Riordan JR. CFTR function and prospects for therapy. Annu Rev Biochem 2008; 77:701–26.
8. Rowe SM, Miller S, Sorscher EJ. Cystic fibrosis. N Engl J Med 2005;352(19): 1992–2001.
9. Muallem D, Vergani P. Review. ATP hydrolysis-driven gating in cystic fibrosis transmembrane conductance regulator. Philos Trans R Soc Lond B Biol Sci 2009;364(1514):247–55.
10. Loo MA, Jensen TJ, Cui L, et al. Perturbation of Hsp90 interaction with nascent CFTR prevents its maturation and accelerates its degradation by the proteasome. EMBO J 1998;17(23):6879–87.
11. Welsh MJ, Smith AE. Molecular mechanisms of CFTR chloride channel dysfunction in cystic fibrosis. Cell 1993;73(7):1251–4.
12. Rabeh WM, Bossard F, Xu H, et al. Correction of both NBD1 energetics and domain interface is required to restore DeltaF508 CFTR folding and function. Cell 2012;148(1–2):150–63.

13. Solomon GM, Marshall SG, Ramsey BW, et al. Breakthrough therapies: cystic fibrosis (CF) potentiators and correctors. Pediatr Pulmonol 2015;50(Suppl 40): S3–13.

14. Pedemonte N, Lukacs GL, Du K, et al. Small-molecule correctors of defective DeltaF508-CFTR cellular processing identified by high-throughput screening. J Clin Invest 2005;115(9):2564–71.

15. Van Goor F, Straley KS, Cao D, et al. Rescue of DeltaF508-CFTR trafficking and gating in human cystic fibrosis airway primary cultures by small molecules. Am J Physiol Lung Cell Mol Physiol 2006;290(6):L1117–30.

16. Verkman AS. Drug discovery in academia. Am J Physiol Cell Physiol 2004;286(3): C465–74.

17. Van Goor F, Hadida S, Grootenhuis PD, et al. Rescue of CF airway epithelial cell function in vitro by a CFTR potentiator, VX-770. Proc Natl Acad Sci U S A 2009; 106(44):18825–30.

18. Cystic Fibrosis Foundation Foundation Patient Registry Annual Data Report 2013. Available at: https://www.cff.org/mwg-internal/de5fs23hu73ds/ progress?id=Qoy1lnAqzZMDOZ5gLAFJIGGa_5b8l5Wz9q2z32CJslU,&dl. Accessed October 30, 2015.

19. Bompadre SG, Sohma Y, Li M, et al. G551D and G1349D, two CF-associated mutations in the signature sequences of CFTR, exhibit distinct gating defects. J Gen Physiol 2007;129(4):285–98.

20. Accurso FJ, Rowe SM, Clancy JP, et al. Effect of VX-770 in persons with cystic fibrosis and the G551D-CFTR mutation. N Engl J Med 2010;363(21):1991–2003.

21. Ramsey BW, Davies J, McElvaney NG, et al. A CFTR potentiator in patients with cystic fibrosis and the G551D mutation. N Engl J Med 2011;365(18):1663–72.

22. Davies JC, Wainwright CE, Canny GJ, et al. Efficacy and safety of ivacaftor in patients aged 6 to 11 years with cystic fibrosis with a G551D mutation. Am J Respir Crit Care Med 2013;187(11):1219–25.

23. McKone EF, Borowitz D, Drevinek P, et al. Long-term safety and efficacy of ivacaftor in patients with cystic fibrosis who have the Gly551Asp-CFTR mutation: a phase 3, open-label extension study (PERSIST). Lancet Respir Med 2014; 2(11):902–10.

24. Rowe SM, Heltshe SL, Gonska T, et al. Clinical mechanism of the cystic fibrosis transmembrane conductance regulator potentiator ivacaftor in G551D-mediated cystic fibrosis. Am J Respir Crit Care Med 2014;190(2):175–84.

25. Heltshe SL, Mayer-Hamblett N, Burns JL, et al. Pseudomonas aeruginosa in cystic fibrosis patients with G551D-CFTR treated with ivacaftor. Clin Infect Dis 2015;60(5):703–12.

26. Zemanick ET, Harris JK, Wagner BD, et al. Inflammation and airway microbiota during cystic fibrosis pulmonary exacerbations. PLoS One 2013;8(4):e62917.

27. De Boeck K, Munck A, Walker S, et al. Efficacy and safety of ivacaftor in patients with cystic fibrosis and a non-G551D gating mutation. J Cyst Fibros 2014;13(6): 674–80.

28. Moss RB, Flume PA, Elborn JS, et al. Efficacy and safety of ivacaftor in patients with cystic fibrosis who have an Arg117His-CFTR mutation: a double-blind, randomised controlled trial. Lancet Respir Med 2015;3(7):524–33.

29. Vertex Pharmaceuticals: Vertex receives U.S. Food and Drug Administration approval of Kalydeco (ivacaftor) for children with cystic fibrosis ages 2 to 5 who have specific mutations in the CFTR gene. 2015. Available at: http:// investors.vrtx.com/releasedetail.cfm?ReleaseID=902211. Accessed November 25, 2015.

30. U.S. National Institutes of Health in ClinicalTrials.gov: Study of ivacaftor in cystic fibrosis subjects 2 through 5 years of age with a CFTR gating mutation. 2012. Available at: https://clinicaltrials.gov/ct2/show/study/NCT01705145. Accessed November 25, 2015.

31. Sermet-Gaudelus I, de Blic J, LeBourgeois M, et al. Potentiating and correcting mutant CFTR in patients with cystic fibrosis. In: Mall MA, Elborn JS, editors. Cystic fibrosis. 64. Sheffield (United Kingdom): European Respiratory Society; 2014. p. 129–49.

32. Flume PA, Liou TG, Borowitz DS, et al. Ivacaftor in subjects with cystic fibrosis who are homozygous for the F508del-CFTR mutation. Chest 2012;142(3):718–24.

33. Rowe SM, Verkman AS. Cystic fibrosis transmembrane regulator correctors and potentiators. Cold Spring Harb Perspect Med 2013;3(7) [pii:a009761].

34. Van Goor F, Hadida S, Grootenhuis PD, et al. Correction of the F508del-CFTR protein processing defect in vitro by the investigational drug VX-809. Proc Natl Acad Sci U S A 2011;108(46):18843–8.

35. Clancy JP, Rowe SM, Accurso FJ, et al. Results of a phase IIa study of VX-809, an investigational CFTR corrector compound, in subjects with cystic fibrosis homozygous for the F508del-CFTR mutation. Thorax 2012;67(1):12–8.

36. Boyle MP, Bell SC, Konstan MW, et al. A CFTR corrector (lumacaftor) and a CFTR potentiator (ivacaftor) for treatment of patients with cystic fibrosis who have a phe508del CFTR mutation: a phase 2 randomised controlled trial. Lancet Respir Med 2014;2(7):527–38.

37. Wainwright CE, Elborn JS, Ramsey BW. Lumacaftor-ivacaftor in patients with cystic fibrosis homozygous for Phe508del CFTR. N Engl J Med 2015;373(18): 1783–4.

38. Business Wire: FDA approves Orkambi (lumacaftor/ivacaftor)–the first medicine to treat the underlying cause of cystic fibrosis for people ages 12 and older with two copies of the F508del mutation. 2015. Available at: www.businesswire.com/news/home/20150702005760/en/. Accessed July 5, 2015.

39. Vertex Pharmaceuticals: Vertex announces data from 12-week phase 2 safety study of VX-661 in combination with ivacaftor in people with cystic fibrosis who have two copies of the F508del mutation. 2015. Available at: http://investors.vrtx.com/releasedetail.cfm?ReleaseID=902790. Accessed October 30, 2015.

40. Vertex Pharmaceuticals, Inc. Vertex reviews recent progress and announces upcoming milestones in the development of multiple combinations of medicines that target the underlying cause of cystic fibrosis. 2014. Available at: http://investors.vrtx.com/releasedetail.cfm?ReleaseID=875448. Accessed October 15, 2015.

41. Zaman K, Carraro S, Doherty J, et al. S-nitrosylating agents: a novel class of compounds that increase cystic fibrosis transmembrane conductance regulator expression and maturation in epithelial cells. Mol Pharmacol 2006;70(4):1435–42.

42. Cystic Fibrosis Foundation: Drug development pipeline. 2015. Available at: https://tools.cff.org/research/drugdevelopmentpipeline/. Accessed November 25, 2015.

43. U.S. National Institutes of Health in ClinicalTrials.gov. Effect of Miglustat on the nasal potential difference in patients with cystic fibrosis homozygous for the F508del mutation (MIGLUSTAT-CF). 2014. Available at: https://clinicaltrials.gov/ct2/show/NCT02325362. Accessed November 25, 2015.

44. Leonard A, Lebecque P, Dingemanse J, et al. A randomized placebo-controlled trial of miglustat in cystic fibrosis based on nasal potential difference. J Cyst Fibros 2012;11(3):231–6.

45. U.S. National Institutes of Health in ClinicalTrials.gov. Study of N91115 in patients with CF homozygous for the F508del-CFTR mutation (SNO-6). 2015. Available at: https://clinicaltrials.gov/ct2/show/NCT02589236. Accessed November 25, 2015.

46. Kerem E, Konstan MW, De Boeck K, et al. Ataluren for the treatment of nonsense-mutation cystic fibrosis: a randomised, double-blind, placebo-controlled phase 3 trial. Lancet Respir Med 2014;2(7):539–47.

47. U.S. National Institutes of Health in ClinicalTrials.gov. Study of ataluren (PTC124) in cystic fibrosis. 2014. Available at: https://clinicaltrials.gov/ct2/show/NCT02107859. Accessed November 25, 2015.

48. Xue X, Mutyam V, Mobley J, et al. Identification and functional analysis of the alternate amino acids inserted as CFTR premature STOP codons during nonsense suppression. Pediatr Pulmonol Suppl 2015;41:280.

49. Dekkers JF, Wiegerinck CL, de Jonge HR, et al. A functional CFTR assay using primary cystic fibrosis intestinal organoids. Nat Med 2013;19(7):939–45.

50. Dekkers R, Vijftigschild LA, Vonk AM, et al. A bioassay using intestinal organoids to measure CFTR modulators in human plasma. J Cyst Fibros 2015;14(2):178–81.

51. Mou H, Brazauskas K, Rajagopal J. Personalized medicine for cystic fibrosis: establishing human model systems. Pediatr Pulmonol 2015;50(Suppl 40):S14–23.

52. Duan N, Kravitz RL, Schmid CH. Single-patient (n-of-1) trials: a pragmatic clinical decision methodology for patient-centered comparative effectiveness research. J Clin Epidemiol 2013;66(Suppl 8):S21–8.

53. Lillie EO, Patay B, Diamant J, et al. The n-of-1 clinical trial: the ultimate strategy for individualizing medicine? Per Med 2011;8(2):161–73.

54. U.S. National Institutes of Health in ClinicalTrials.gov. Pilot study testing the effect of ivacaftor on lung function in subjects with cystic fibrosis and residual CFTR function. 2012. Available at: https://clinicaltrials.gov/ct2/show/results/NCT01685801. Accessed November 25, 2015.

55. Davies JC. Cystic fibrosis: bridging the treatment gap in early childhood. Lancet Respir Med 2013;1(6):433–4.

56. U.S. National Institutes of Health in ClinicalTrials.gov. A two-part multicenter prospective longitudinal study of CFTR-dependent disease profiling in cystic fibrosis (PROSPECT). 2015. Available at: https://clinicaltrials.gov/ct2/show/NCT02477319. Accessed October 29, 2015.

57. Sawicki GS, McKone EF, Pasta DJ, et al. Sustained benefit from ivacaftor demonstrated by combining clinical trial and cystic fibrosis patient registry data. Am J Respir Crit Care Med 2015;192(7):836–42.

58. Sawicki GS, Dasenbrook E, Fink AK, et al. Rate of uptake of ivacaftor use after U.S. Food and Drug Administration approval among patients enrolled in the U.S. Cystic Fibrosis Foundation patient registry. Ann Am Thorac Soc 2015; 12(8):1146–52.

Index

Note: Page numbers of article titles are in **boldface** type.

Pediatr Clin N Am 63 (2016) 765–774
http://dx.doi.org/10.1016/S0031-3955(16)41046-1
0031-3955/16/$ – see front matter

Moving?

Make sure your subscription moves with you!

To notify us of your new address, find your **Clinics Account Number** (located on your mailing label above your name), and contact customer service at:

Email: journalscustomerservice-usa@elsevier.com

800-654-2452 (subscribers in the U.S. & Canada)
314-447-8871 (subscribers outside of the U.S. & Canada)

Fax number: 314-447-8029

Elsevier Health Sciences Division
Subscription Customer Service
3251 Riverport Lane
Maryland Heights, MO 63043

*To ensure uninterrupted delivery of your subscription, please notify us at least 4 weeks in advance of move.

Printed and bound by CPI Group (UK) Ltd, Croydon, CR0 4YY

03/10/2024

01040394-0001